PUBLISHER'S NOTE

One of the stunning photographic achievements of the 1980 television year was a documentary film, "The Invisible World," that explored the realms of our interior and exterior universe. The film was the winner of many awards, including the Emmy and the Christopher.

The publishers are grateful to the many people responsible for the television documentary, which was the inspiration for this book, in particular to Alex Pomasanoff, the show's writer, producer, and director, and to Edward Garrick, the associate producer — and to the photographers whose genius uncovered this invisible world.

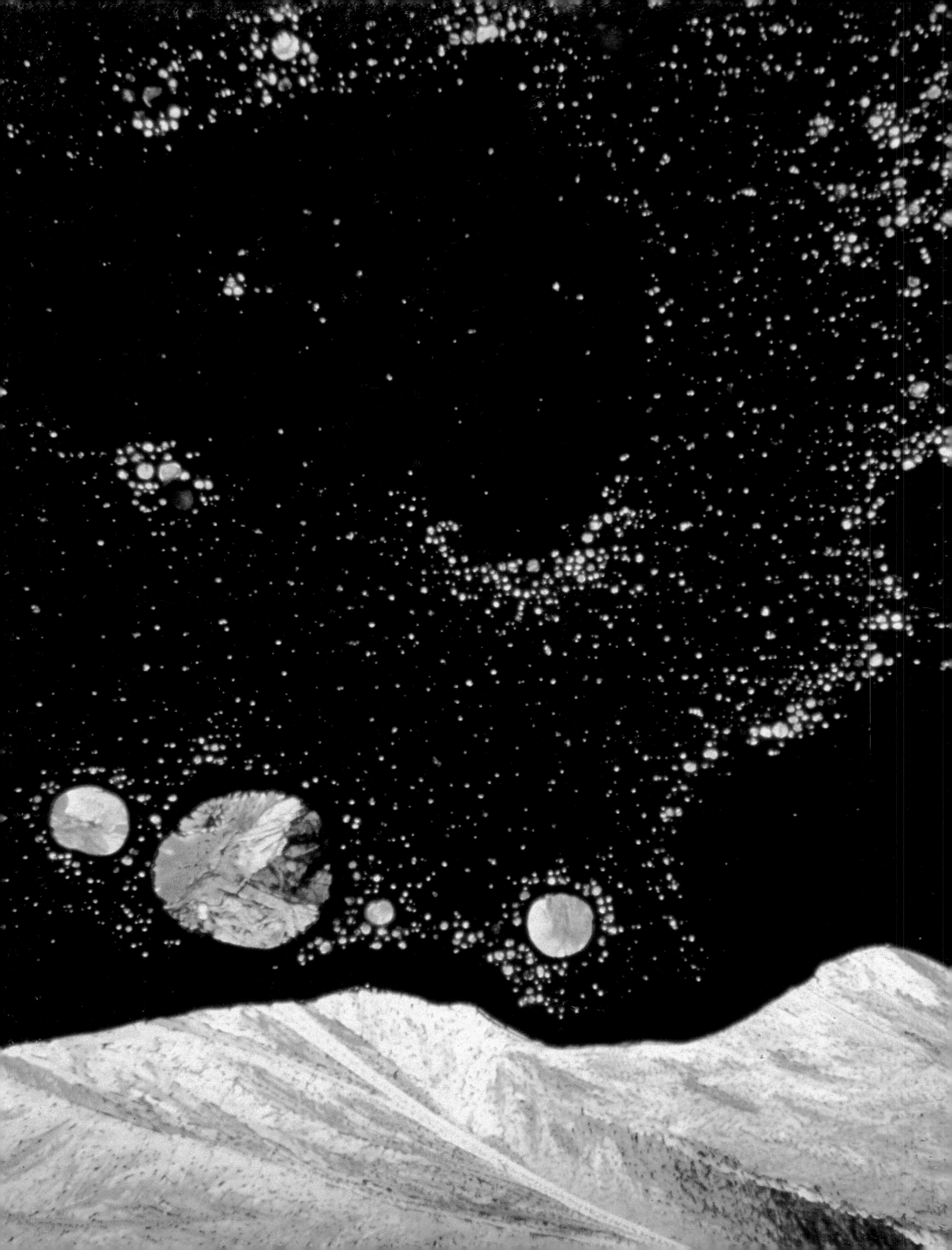

THE INVISIBLE WORLD

Sights Too Fast, Too Slow, Too Far, Too Small
for the Naked Eye to See

HOUGHTON MIFFLIN COMPANY BOSTON 1981

Frontis: **WINTER WONDERLAND**

This magical snow-covered vista is actually trans-stilbene, a crystal often used in chemical analysis. Magnification: × 150.

Library of Congress Cataloging in Publication Data

Pomasanoff, Alex.
The invisible world.

1. Photography—Scientific applications. 2. Photomicrography. I. Title.
TR721.P65 778.3'1 81-2105
ISBN 0-395-31326-0 AACR2

Printed in the United States of America

H 10 9 8 7 6 5 4 3 2 1

To the photographers, scientists, and technicians whose photographs made this book possible: Dr. Guenther Albrecht-Buehle, Dr. Luis J. Alvarez, Dr. J. D. H. Andrews, Dr. Halton Arp, John V. Atkinson, H. S. Baird, Robert C. Beebe, James M. Bell, George Brangan, Dr. Garry T. Cole, Dr. Albert Crewe, John Gustav Delly, David Donofrio, I. F. Dumitrescu, Dr. Harold E. Edgerton, Dr. Wolf H. Fahrenback, Dr. Donald Fawcett, Dr. Edward Fomalont, David Gnizak, Joseph Goren, Dr. David Gorham, Andre Gorzynski, Dr. D. A. Griffiths, Dr. A. J. Gwinnett, Michael Hadland, Art Hansen, Jan Hinsch, Dr. Alfred Hulstrunk, Dr. Ian Hutchings, Dr. Michael Isaacson, Dr. Susumo Ito, Kendall Johnson, Dr. William Jordan, Dr. E. Lazarides, DoSuk Duke Lee, Dr. Roderick MacLeod, G. Marshall, Dan McCoy, Joseph D. McKenzie, Charles Miller, Dr. Thelma Moss, Dr. Erwin W. Mueller, Dr. William Nutting, Dr. David M. Phillips, Louis Raboni, Dr. Jean-Paul Revel, Dorothy Rutherford, David Scharf, Dr. Gary S. Settles, Ralph L. Shook, Dr. Lee D. Simon, Stephen Skirius, Dr. Robert F. Smith, Howard Sochurek, William A. Sokol, Theodore Thomas, Dr. J. Kim Vandiver, John C. Walsh, Dr. Robley C. Williams,

. . . and to: AGA Corporation, AURA, Inc., Battelle Memorial Institute, Cerro Tololo Observatory, Daedalus Enterprises, Inc., H. S. Dakin Co., Earth Satellite Corporation, Eastman Kodak Company, Fermi Lab, Field Museum of Natural History, Chicago, George Eastman House, John Hadland, Ltd., Hale Observatories, Hawker-Siddeley Dynamics, Ltd., Holosonics, Inc., Kitt Peak National Observatory, E. Leitz, Inc., NASA, Nikon, Inc., Oxford Scientific Films, Parker Pen Company, Stanford Research Institute, Carl Zeiss, Inc.,

. . . and special thanks to: Dennis Kane, National Geographic Society, Washington, D.C., and Tom Skinner, WQED-TV, Metropolitan Pittsburgh Public Broadcasting, Inc.

CONTENTS

THE INVISIBLE WORLD

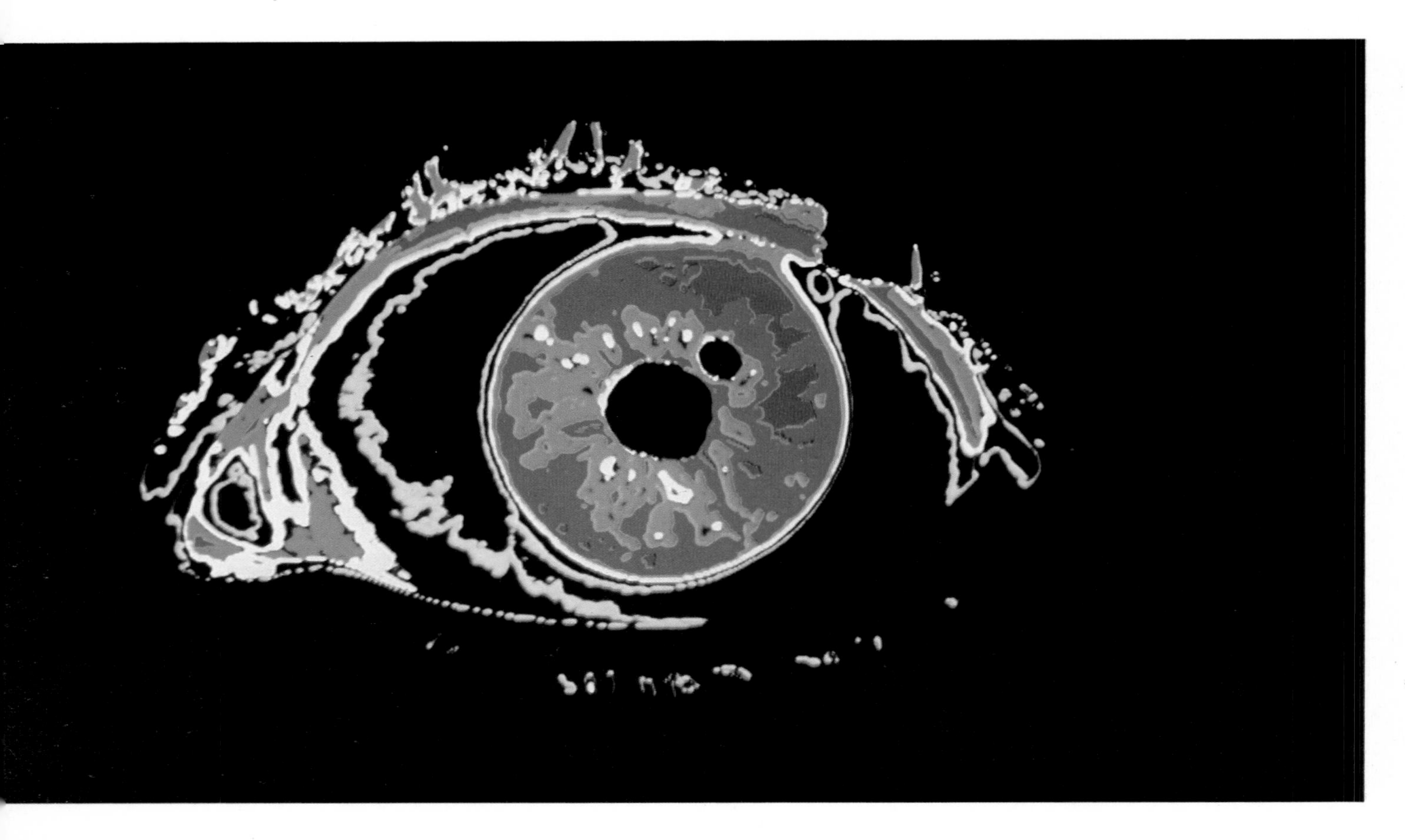

HUMAN EYE
The human eye, color-enhanced by a computer for a bold new view of its outward appearance.

INTRODUCTION

We are visual creatures, dependent on our sense of sight as our most vital link with the world around us. Most of what we know comes to us through our eyes, organs so marvelously developed that they can focus on a tiny particle of dust or a planet 400 million miles away, adapt instantly from light to dark, trace motion, and differentiate between thousands of shadings of colors.

Yet despite our eyes' amazing powers and remarkable sensitivity, there are countless sights around us to which we are totally blind. Our normal vision is but a narrow window on a vast and awesome universe, a universe of sights and happenings that are too fast or too slow, too faint or too minute for the human eye to record. And when we get beyond the spectrum of visible light, we find even more foreign realms—dimensions of energy, such as x rays and heat, that elude our sense of sight.

In the time it takes to blink an eye, a host of exotic cameras and other imaging tools can transport us into these invisible worlds. In conjunction with microscopes, telescopes, strobe lights, radiation detectors, and even computers, cameras can now reveal once-hidden sights. Possessed of powers to explore and reveal in ways that our unaided eyes cannot, cameras are extending enormously the once limited reach of our vision and knowledge, altering forever our image of the world.

In this book, we will take a visual journey into the invisible world—a journey inspired by the National Geographic Society television special "The Invisible World" and made possible by the many people whose pictures make up this book.

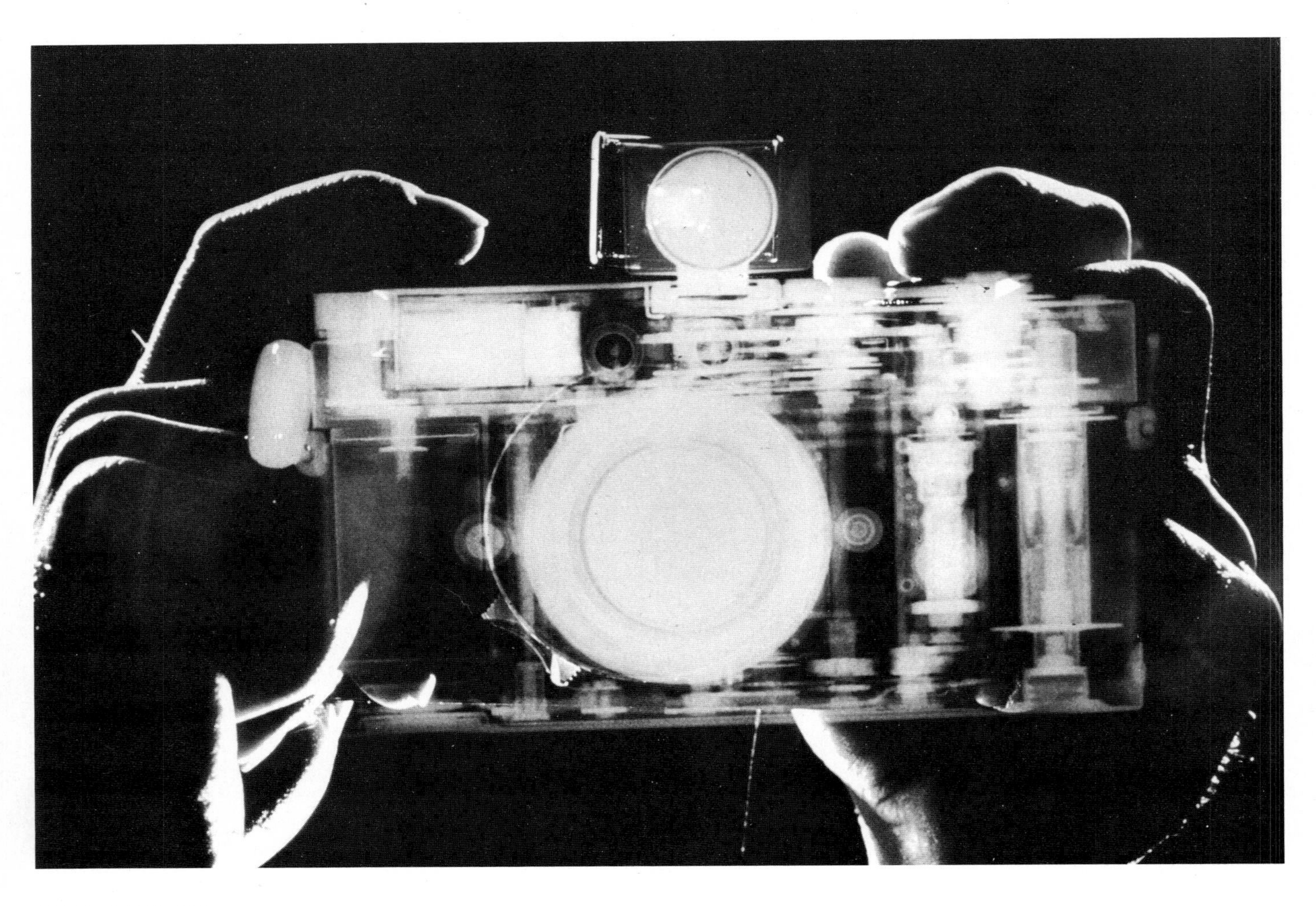

MECHANICAL EYE
The camera's eye has the power to reveal an otherwise invisible world. This composite photo combines both conventional and x-ray photography.

VISIONS OF VISION

As sense organs our eyes are magnificent examples of evolutionary development. When they are considered as optical instruments, however, their powers of perception are rather limited. And when we look at our eyes under high magnification, they take on unexpected appearances, no longer resembling the familiar objects we know.

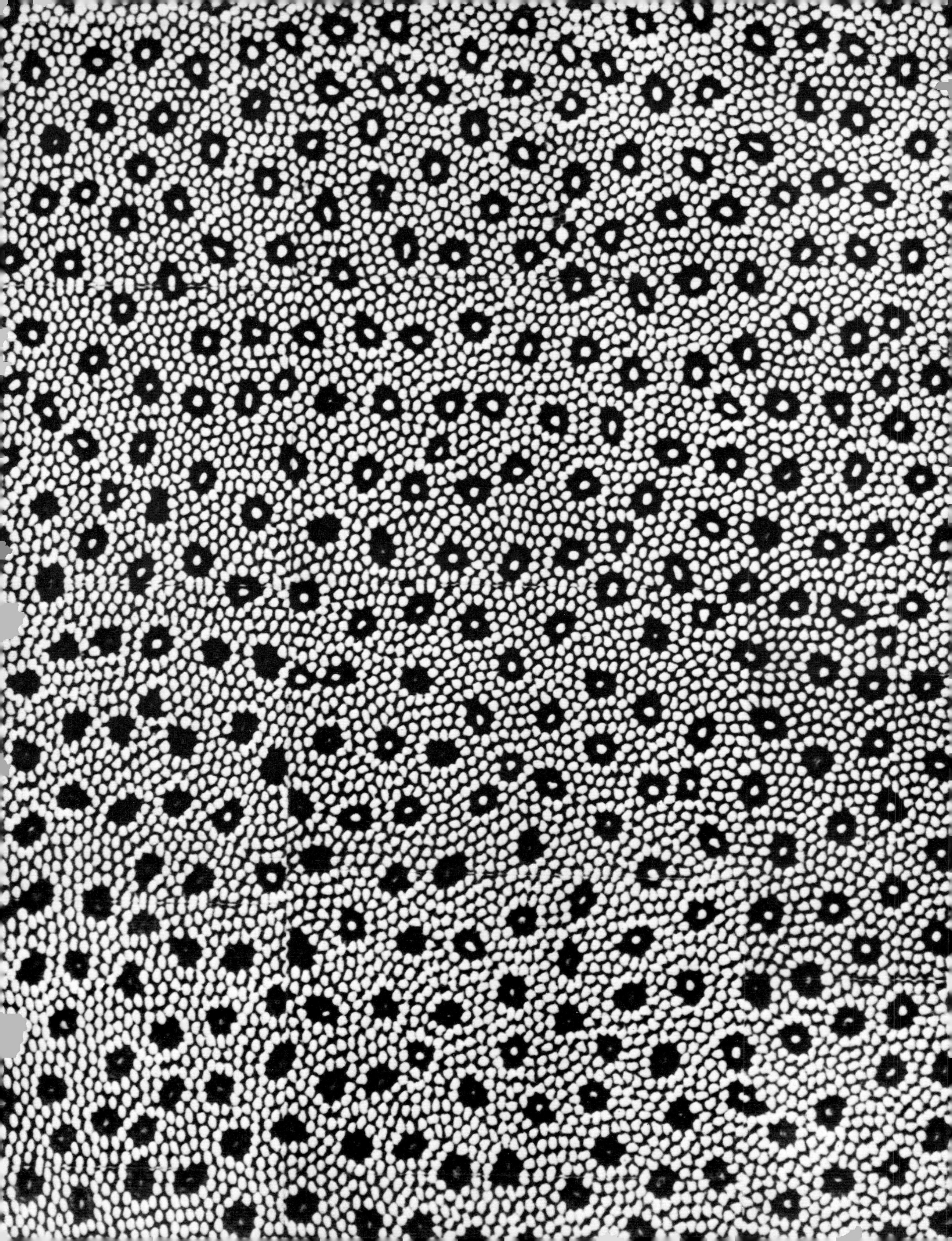

◁ **PRIVATE EYE**

The rods and cones of a human eye magnified 10,000 times by an electron microscope. Located at the back of the retina, they are the sensitive light-receptor cells that provide us with our first sensations of sight. Cones function in daylight and give us color vision. Rods function in low illumination and give vision only in shades of gray.

IN SIGHT ▷

Blood vessels in the iris of the human eye, magnified 125 times. The vessels have been injected with latex, giving them their three-dimensional appearance.

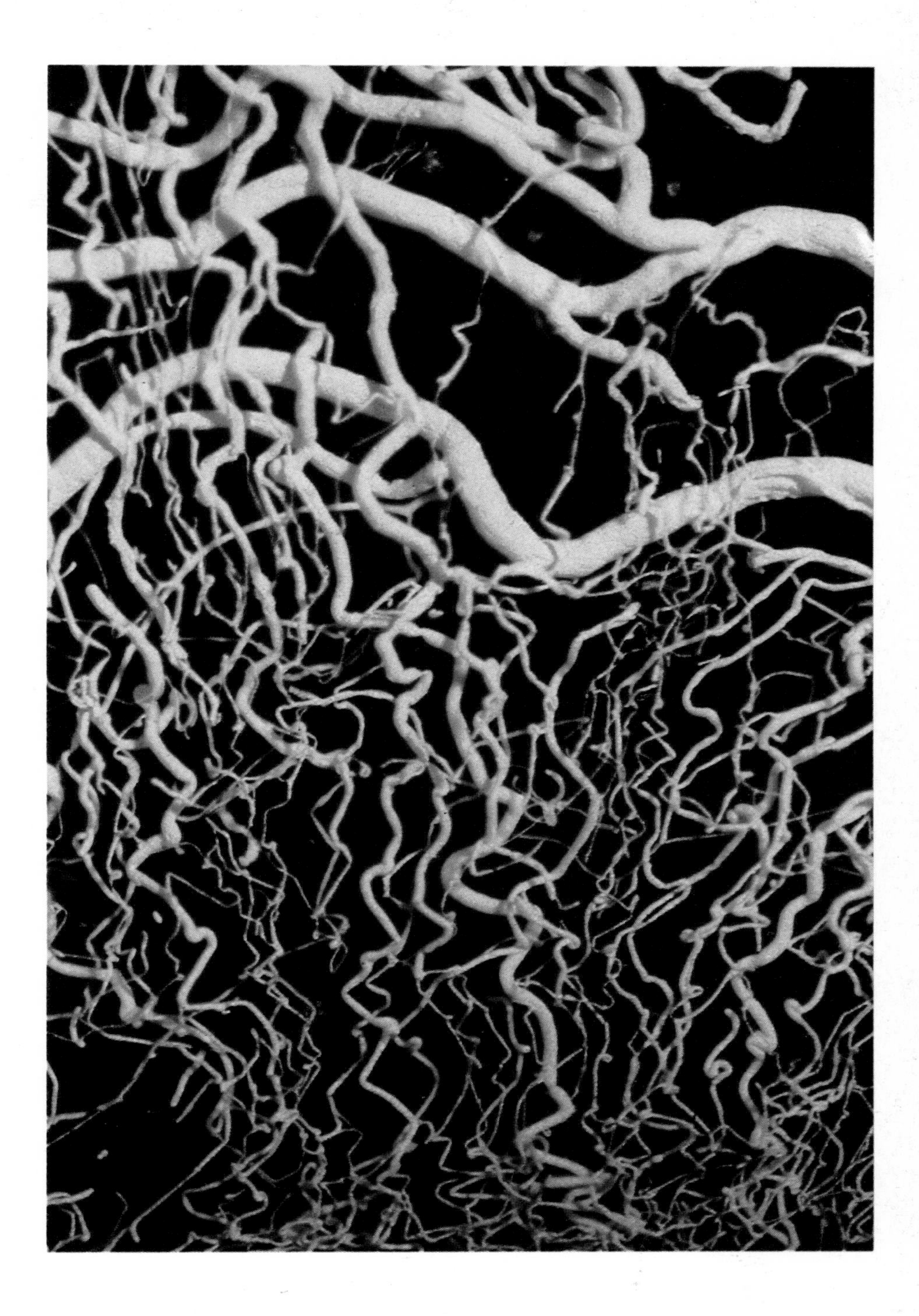

MICROWORLDS

Even up close our eyes can barely see objects that are one three hundredth of an inch in diameter—a fraction the size of a tiny grain of sand. Though this may seem quite small in human scale, it is but the threshold of a microcosm beyond the limits of our eyes.

Until the invention of the microscope some four hundred years ago, the world consisted totally of what the naked eye could see. When man first glimpsed a magnified drop of pond water, it provoked unparalleled wonder. It was filled with countless unknown creatures, and it seemed at first inconceivable that living things could be so small—that a single drop of water could contain a miniature world.

The microscope quickly became an indispensable tool of exploration and discovery. Bacteria were seen for the first time in 1674. Blood was revealed to be composed of millions of free-floating corpuscles. The sight of a cell dividing seemed a miracle of nature—another astonishing discovery that would quickly revolutionize biology and medicine.

Over the years the microscope has improved enormously. It has revealed ever-smaller sights, but it too is limited. Even today the best optical lenses can magnify objects little more than 2000 times.

A powerful new instrument called the scanning electron microscope (SEM) has recently overcome this boundary and penetrated a whole new uncharted level of detail and size. Seeing with a beam of focused electrons rather than with light, it can magnify objects in apparent three dimension hundreds of thousands of times. The transmission electron microscope (TEM)—an even more powerful instrument—transmits a shower of electrons through an object to form an image. It can magnify tens of millions of times.

Today we are seeing ever deeper into the still mysterious microworld. At each new level of magnification unexpected structure and complexity are revealed . . . and as happened when man peered at a miniature world he had never seen before, nearly every new sight offers a new discovery.

LIFE IN A WATER DROP

A single drop of water abounds with a variety of delicate microlife. These tiny invisible creatures help form the vital basis of the world's entire food chain. Magnification: × 250.

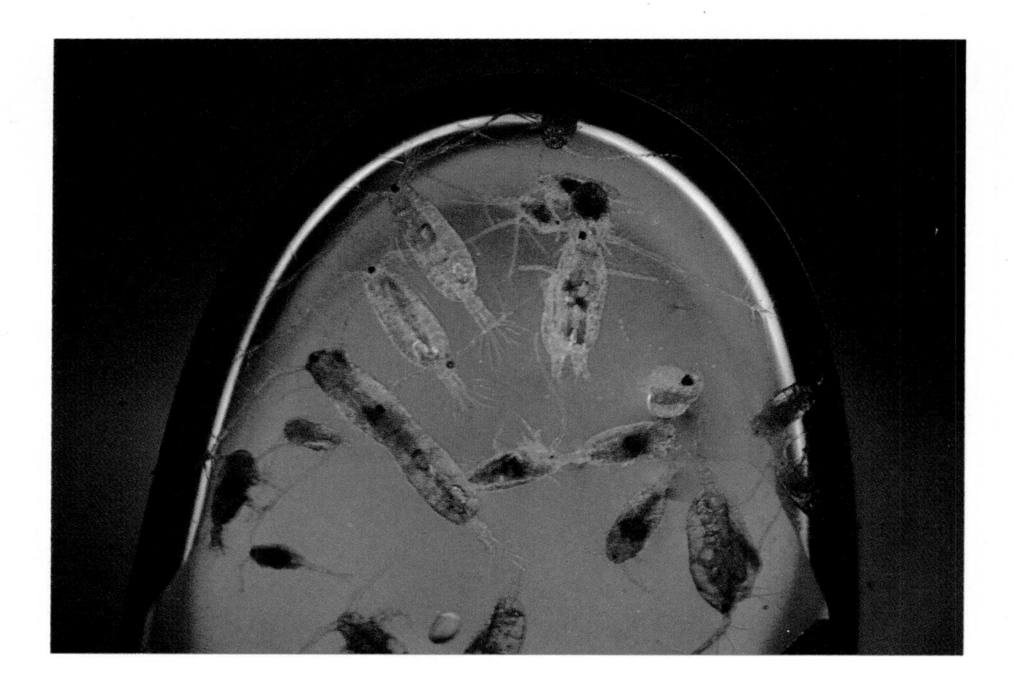

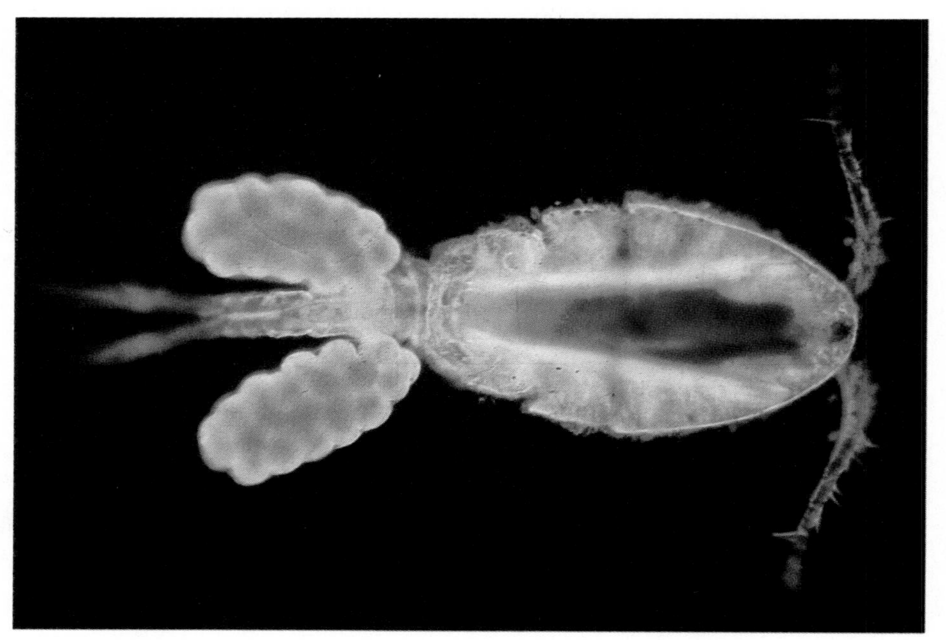

CYCLOPS

Although it looks like a spaceship from some alien world, this creature is a type of water flea known as *Cyclops*. The flea is common in fresh water. The apparent tail fins are actually egg sacs. Magnification: × 350.

WATER FLEA

A young female water flea known as *Daphnia,* magnified 63 times. A small egg is growing inside the transparent body. The offspring will be born as fully developed miniature versions of the mother.

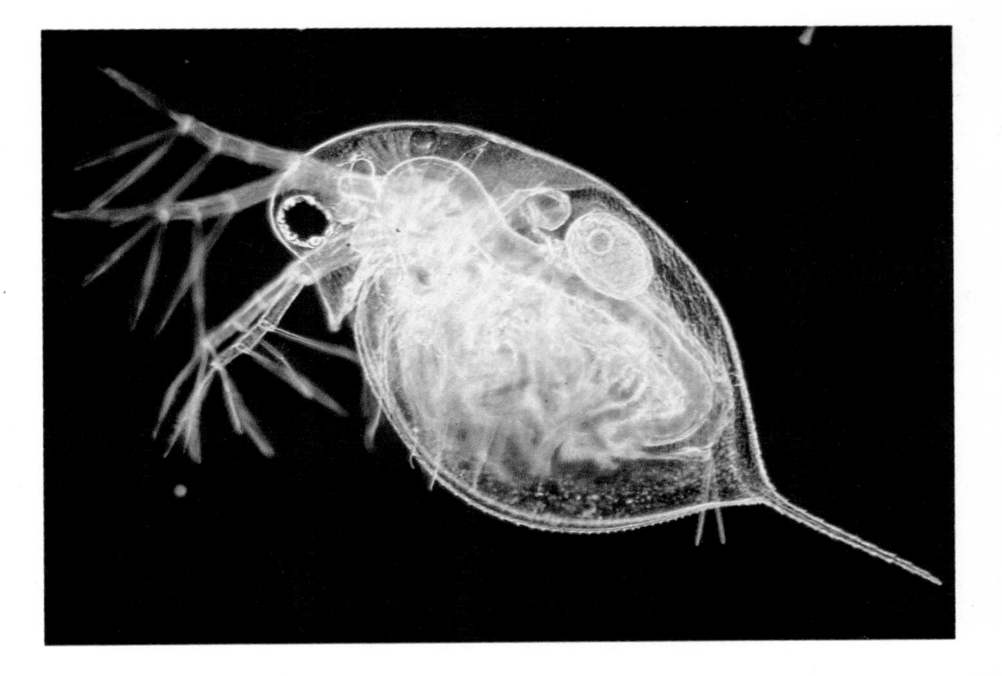

BABY JELLYFISH

What looks like a sea monster is actually a microscopic baby jellyfish, named Anthomedusa. Magnification: × 250.

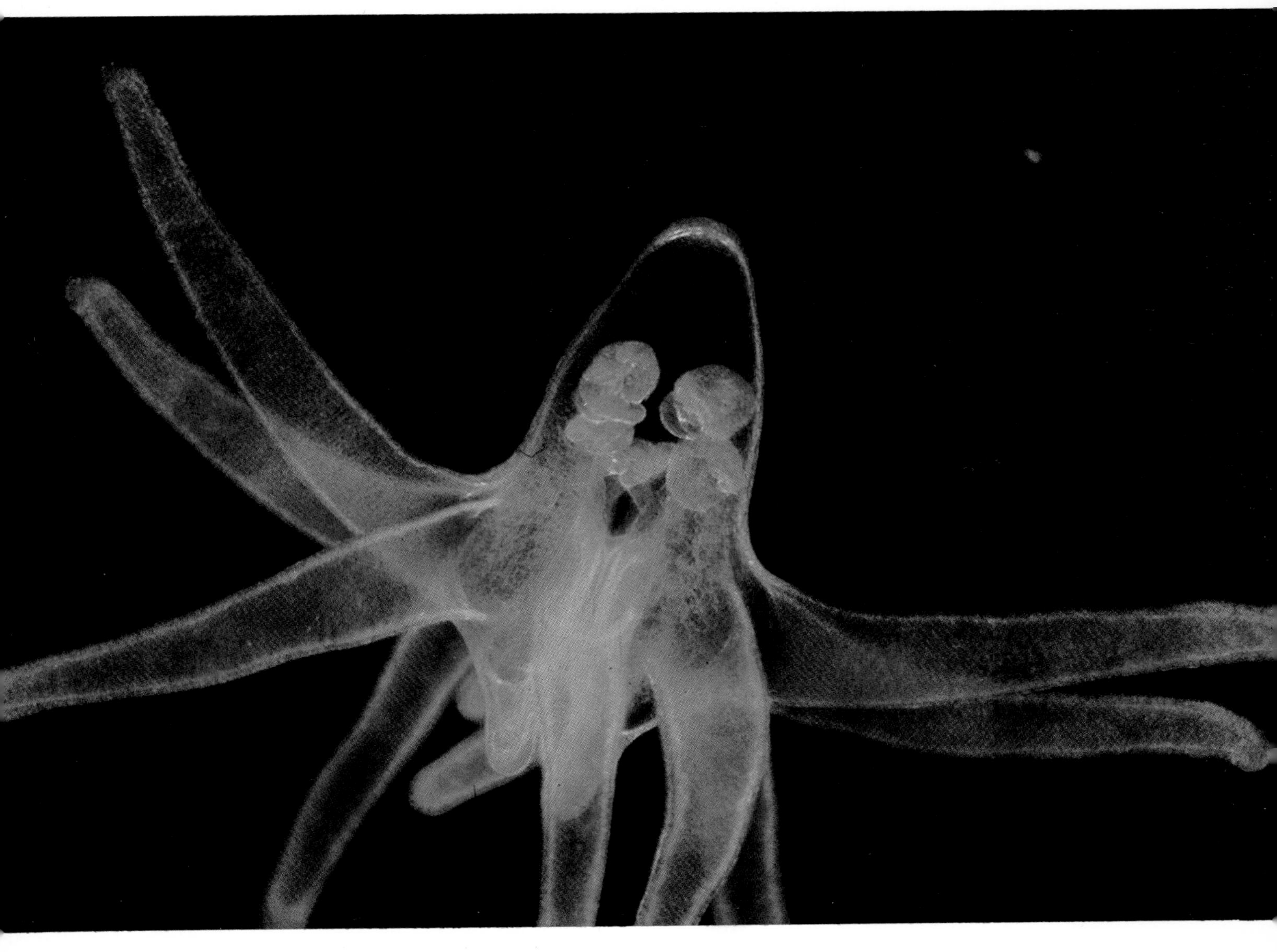

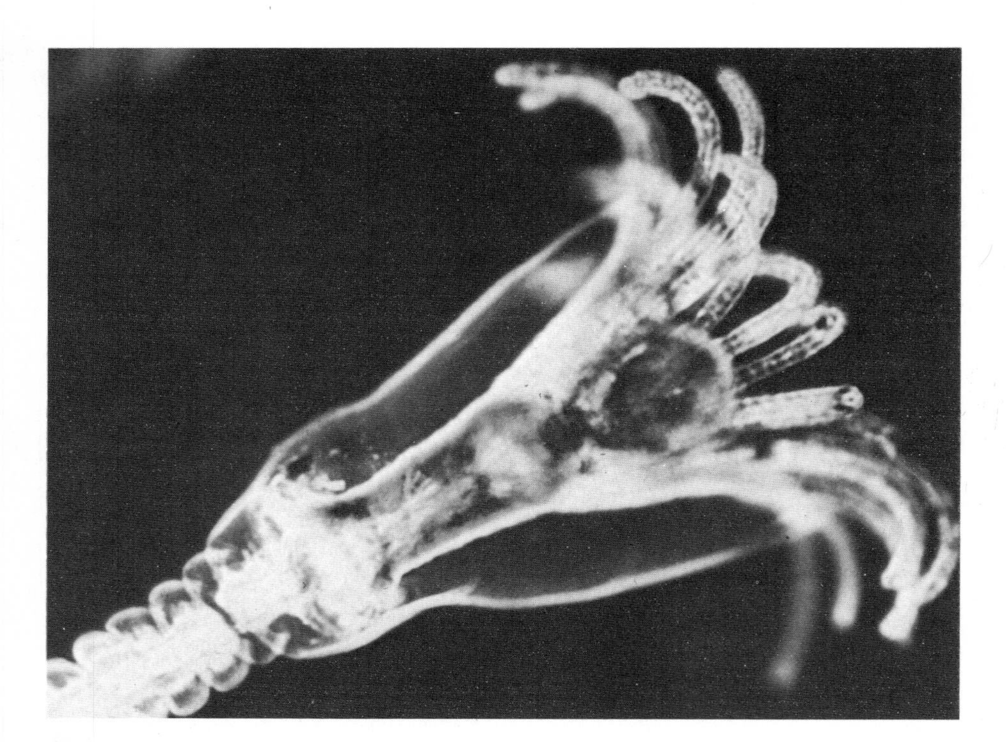

OBELIA HYDROID

Obelia, a microscopic marine protozoan, thrives in shallow ocean tide pools. During its life cycle, it takes on several forms. Obelia hydroid is not a single creature, but a colony made up of thousands of individual organisms. Hydroid colonies often cling to submerged rocks, and sometimes grow large enough to be seen as very tiny specks.

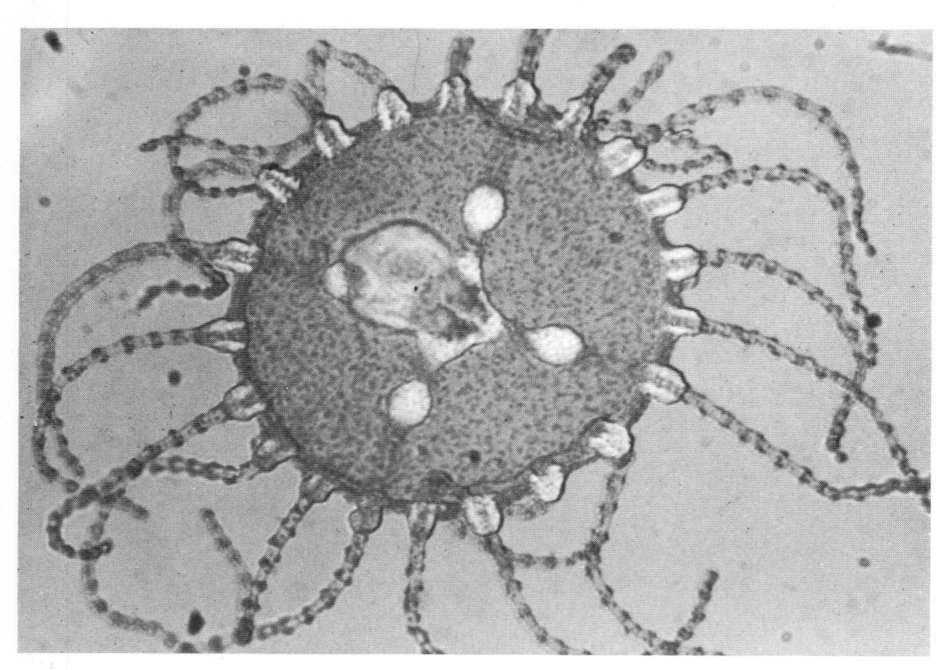

OBELIA MEDUSA

The medusa is a singular form of obelia, many times smaller than the hydroid colony. It swims freely in the water, feeding on even smaller creatures, and searching for a mate. When new obelias are created, they form hydroid colonies . . . and the life cycle continues.

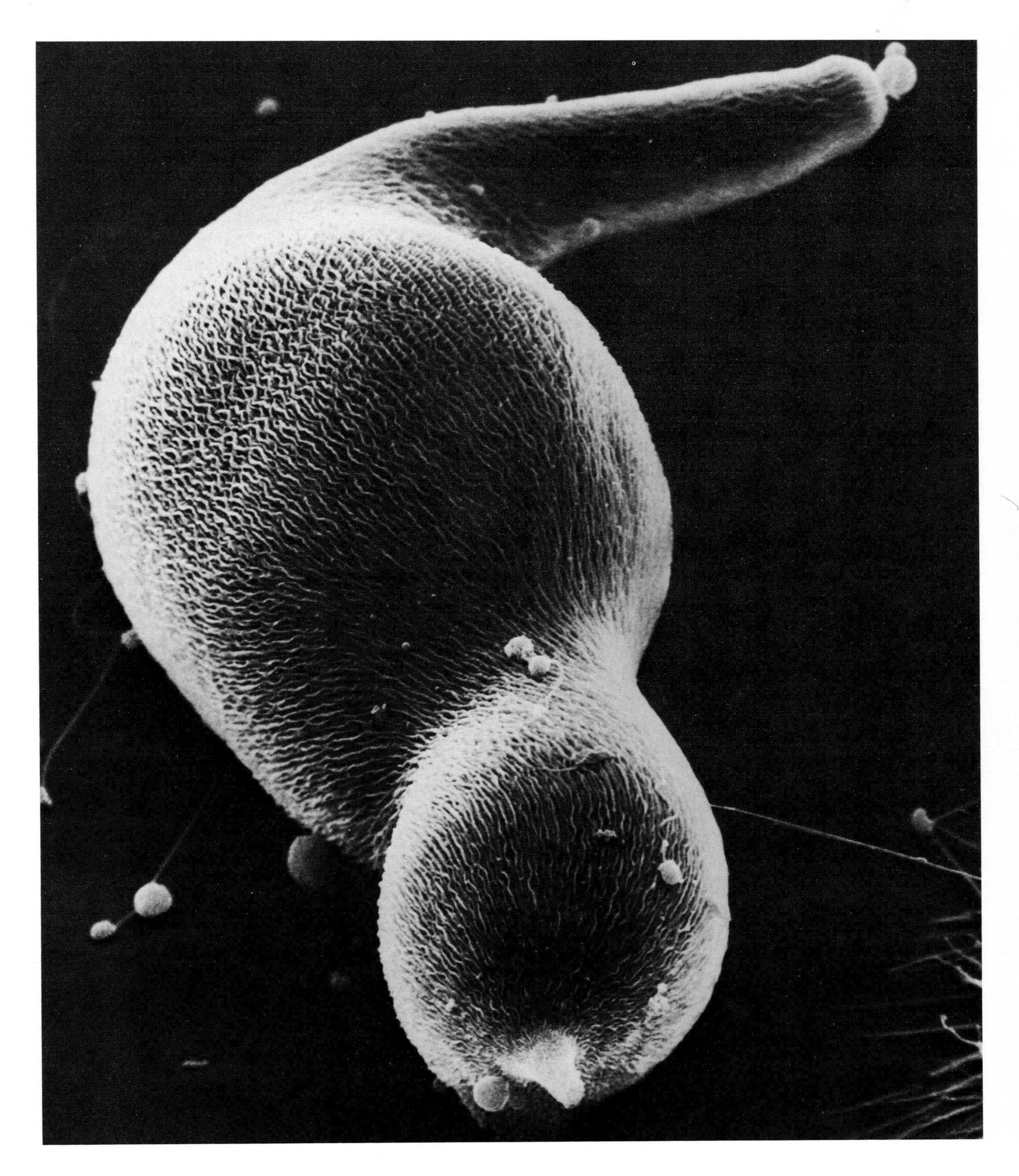

PROTOZOAN
This miniature parasite known as Scyzogregori is found inside clams. No one knows exactly why it is there or how it survives. It moves about by contracting and stretching its supple body. Magnification: × 1000.

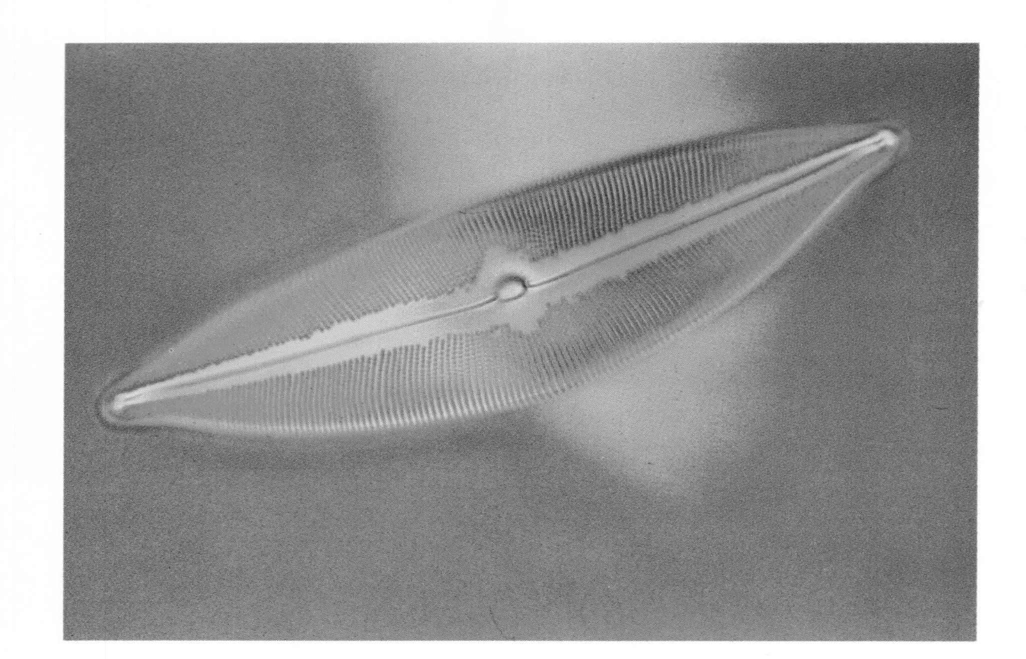

DIATOM

Microscopic jewels of the sea, diatoms remained undiscovered until the end of the eighteenth century. Microscopes had to become powerful enough to resolve an object one thousandth of an inch long—about the average size of a diatom. Diatoms are single-celled plants, and they thrive in the world's oceans in almost infinite numbers. Magnification: × 500.

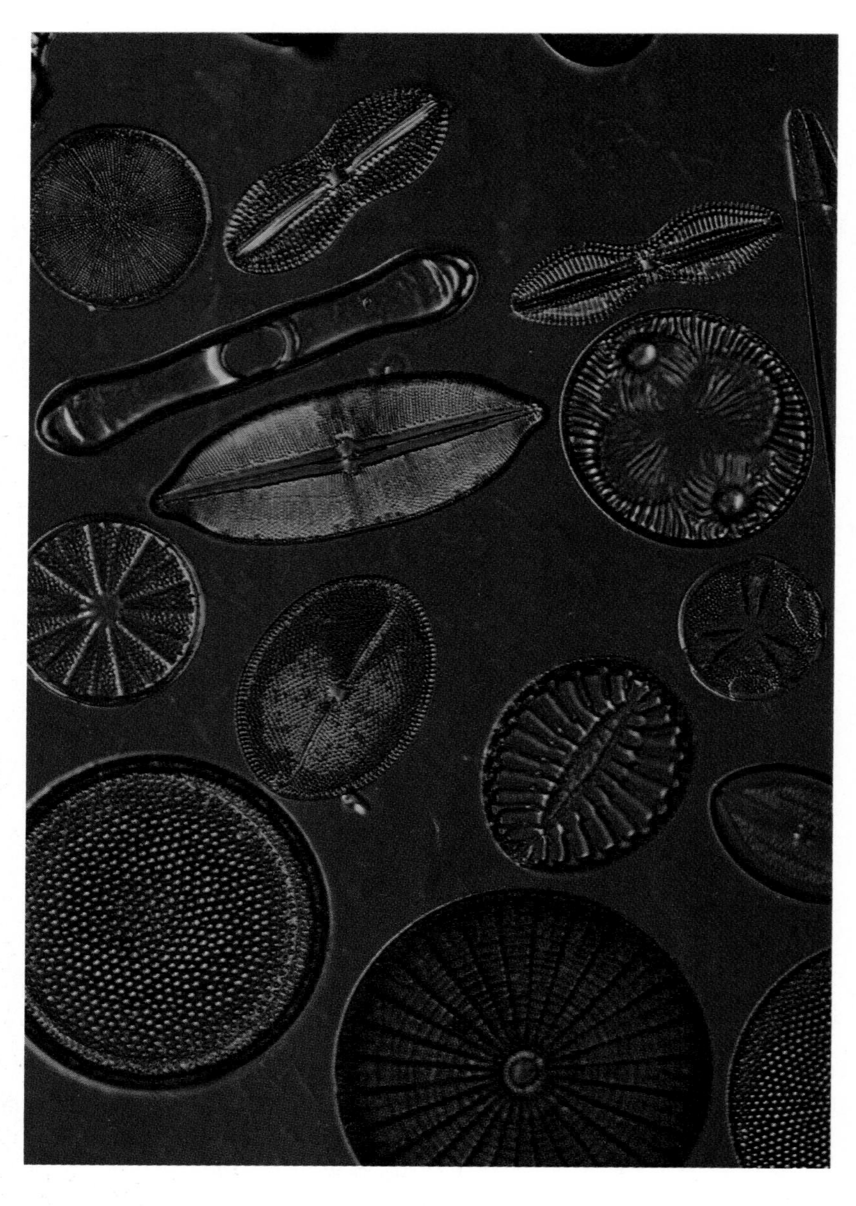

COLLECTION OF DIATOMS

Diatoms are so small that it would take ten million to cover the surface of a half dollar. They reproduce by dividing . . . and they do it often. The division of a single diatom will result in one billion diatoms in less than a month. Magnification: × 200.

AMOEBA

An amoeba is crawling over the tightly woven threads of a piece of nylon. It will constantly change its wrinkled, clothlike appearance in order to move. The much tinier rod-shaped organisms nearby are bacteria. Magnification: × 2500.

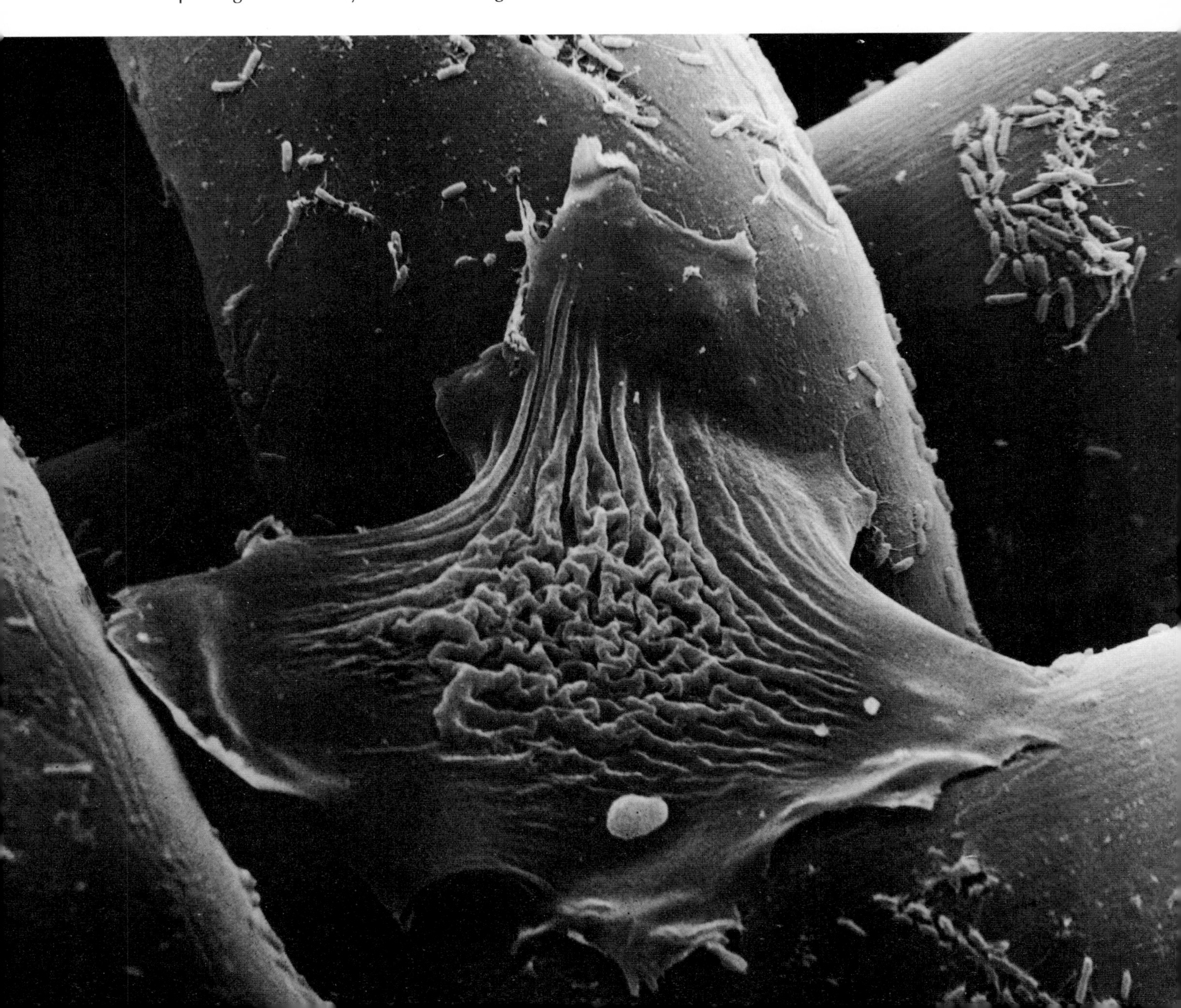

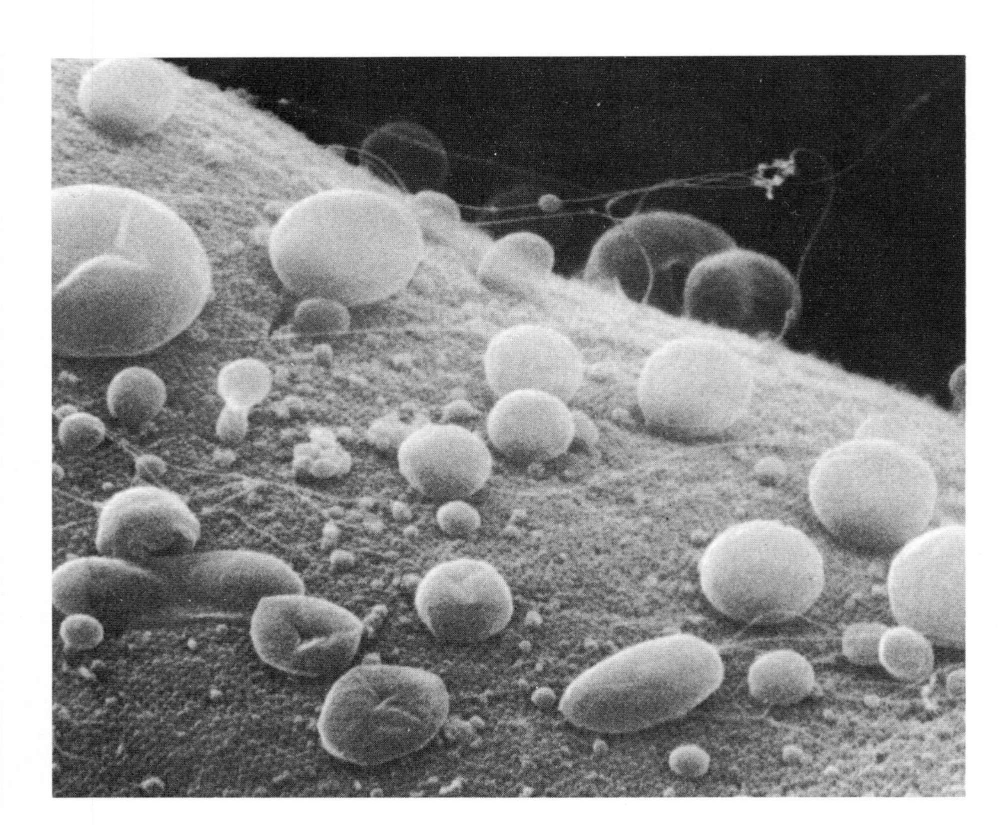

MICROMOUSE

Millions of spherical bacteria find a happy home on the intestinal lining of a mouse. They are ever-present and perform a vital role in normal digestion. Scientists call them bacterial flora. Magnification: × 8000.

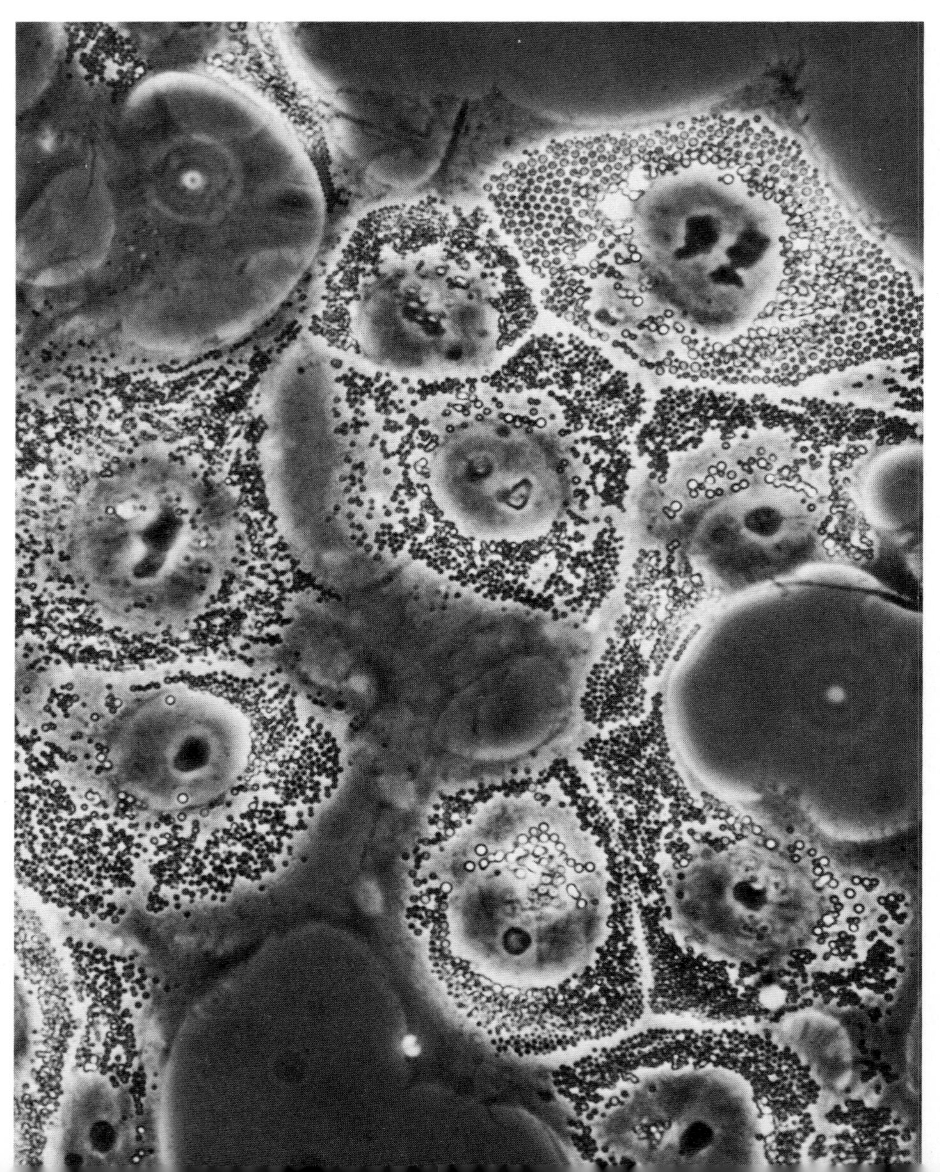

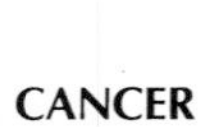

CANCER

Living cancer cells, magnified 250,000 times. When grown in a laboratory culture, cancer cells will go on multiplying forever. This characteristic makes them ideal subjects for numerous biological experiments totally unrelated to cancer research.

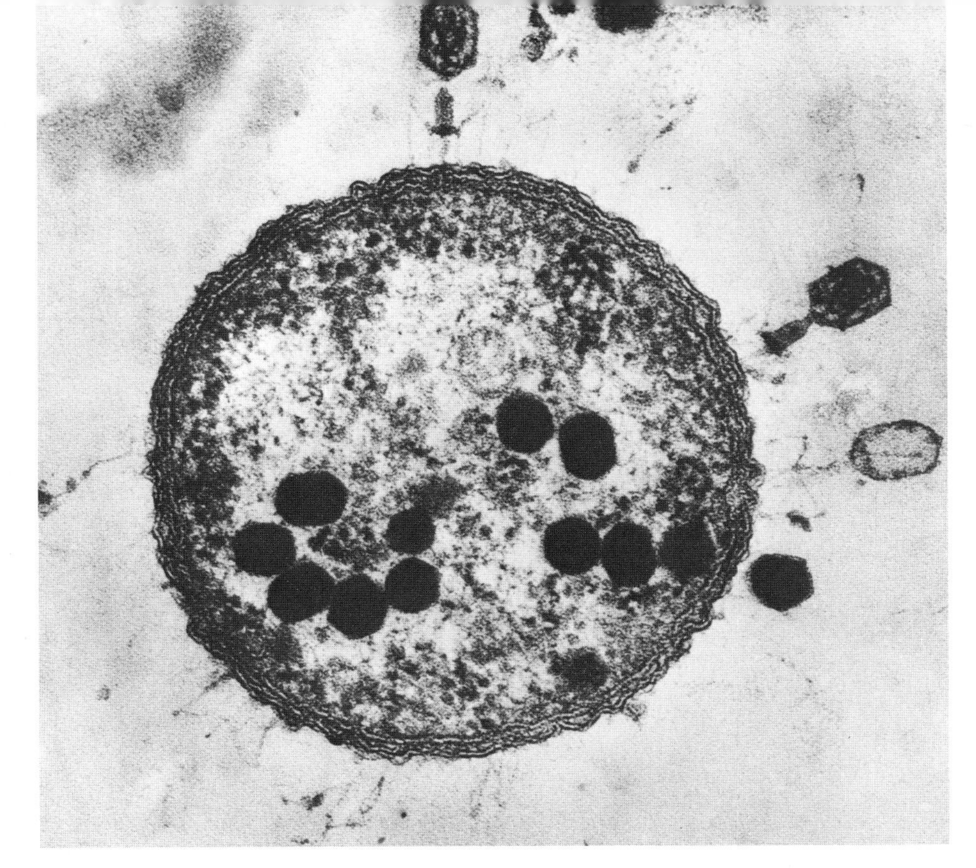

VIRUS ATTACK

Like lunar landing modules, two T2 viruses sit on the surface of an *Escherichia coli* bacterium. Viruses are really more like biological hypodermic needles. The hexagonal crystalline bodies are filled with the genetic chemical DNA, which the viruses inject into their victims. The bacterium's own DNA is then reprogrammed to produce more viruses. The dark spots inside the bacterium are newly made viruses. Magnification: × 10,000,000.

VIRUSES

This is not a picture of health. Each tiny dot is a polio virus. Magnification: × 65,000.

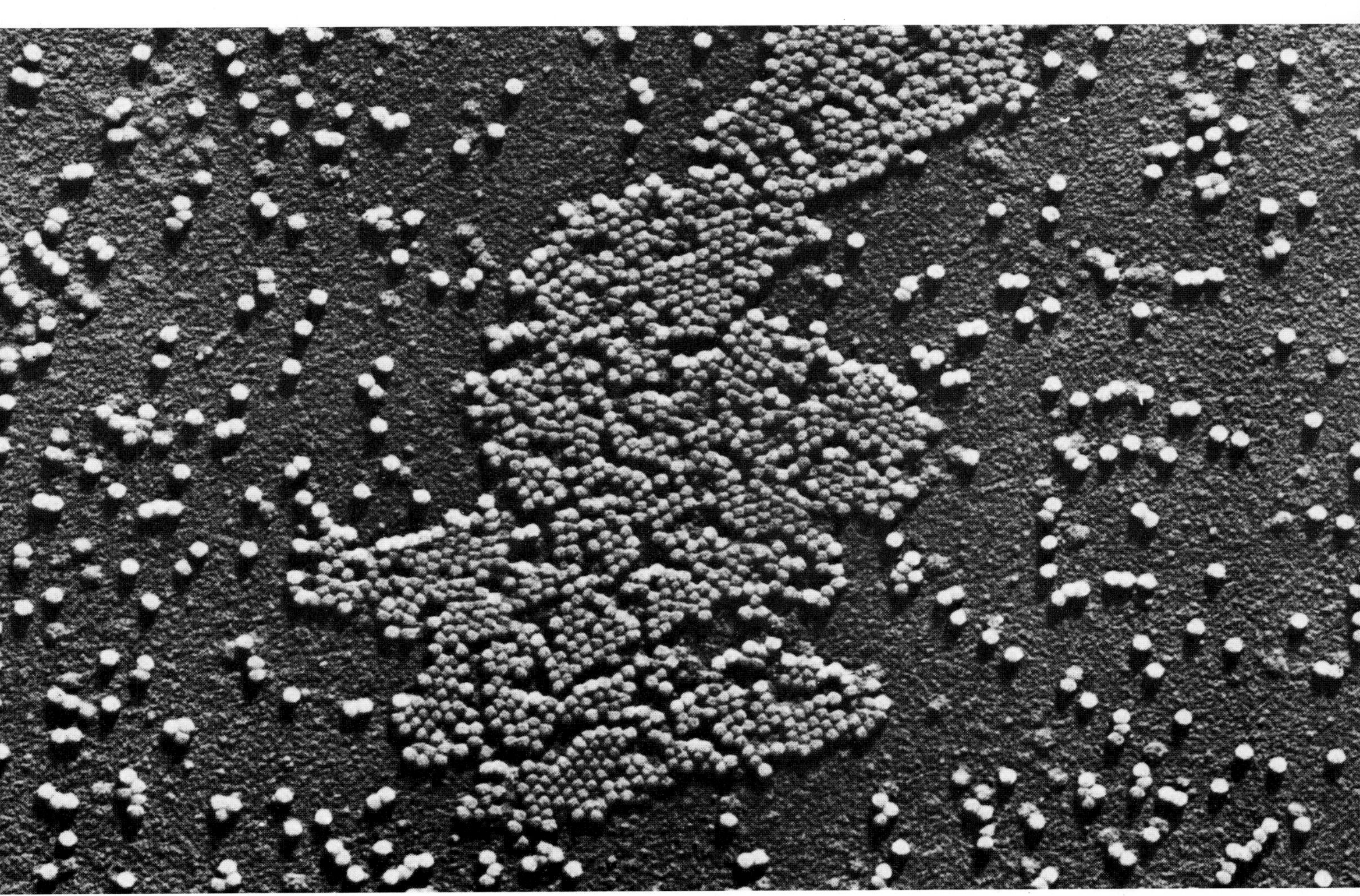

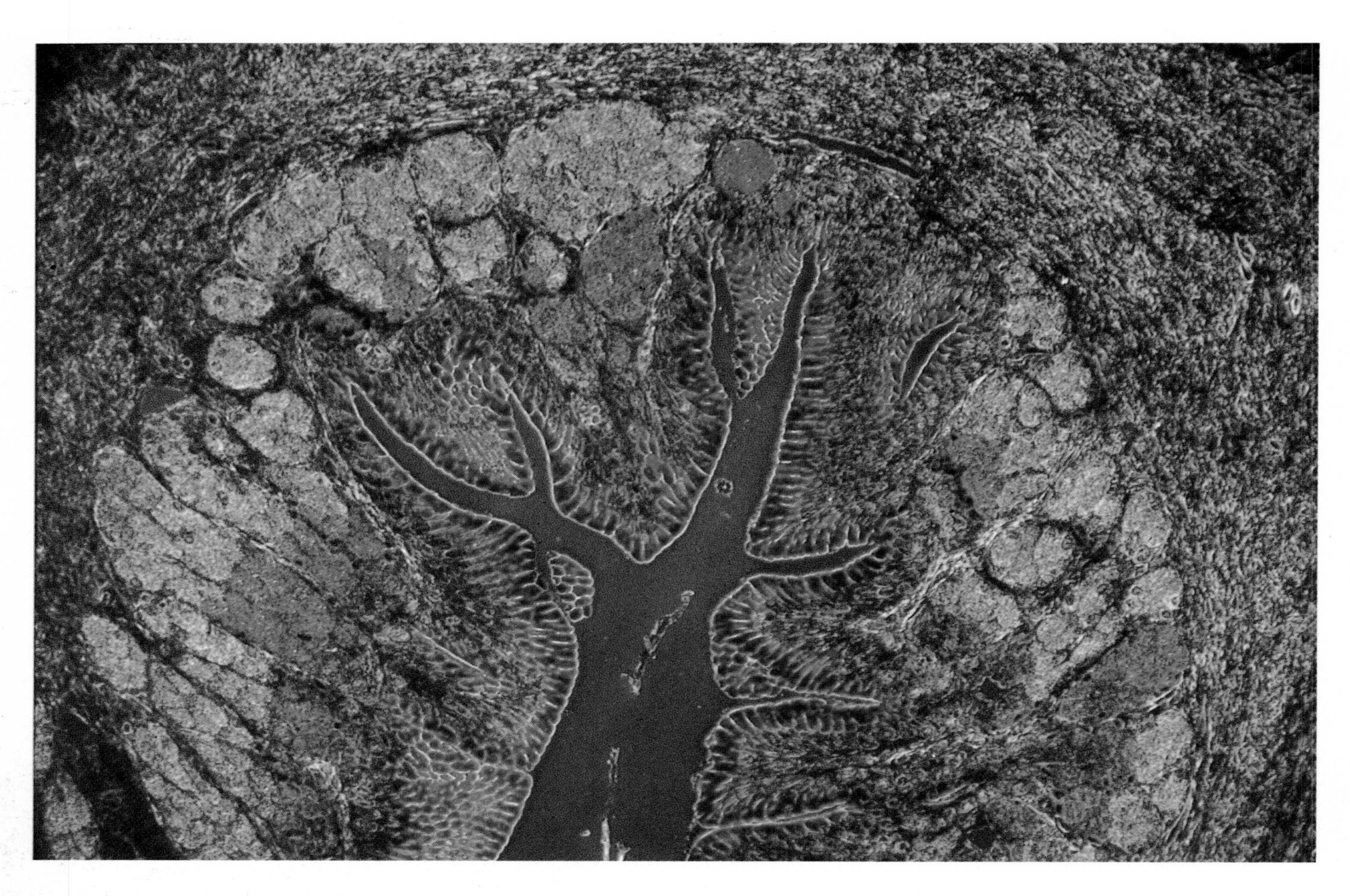

NEWT GUT
A tiny section of a newt's stomach magnified 30 times.

CRYSTALSCAPES

Most of the solid physical world—everything that isn't a gas or a liquid—has an underlying crystalline structure. Crystals are the natural shapes that molecules form when they group together. When viewed through a microscope, crystals vividly show us the invisible shapes and symmetries that form the world we see.

HEXANITRODIPHENYLAMINE
High-explosive crystals, magnified 35 times.

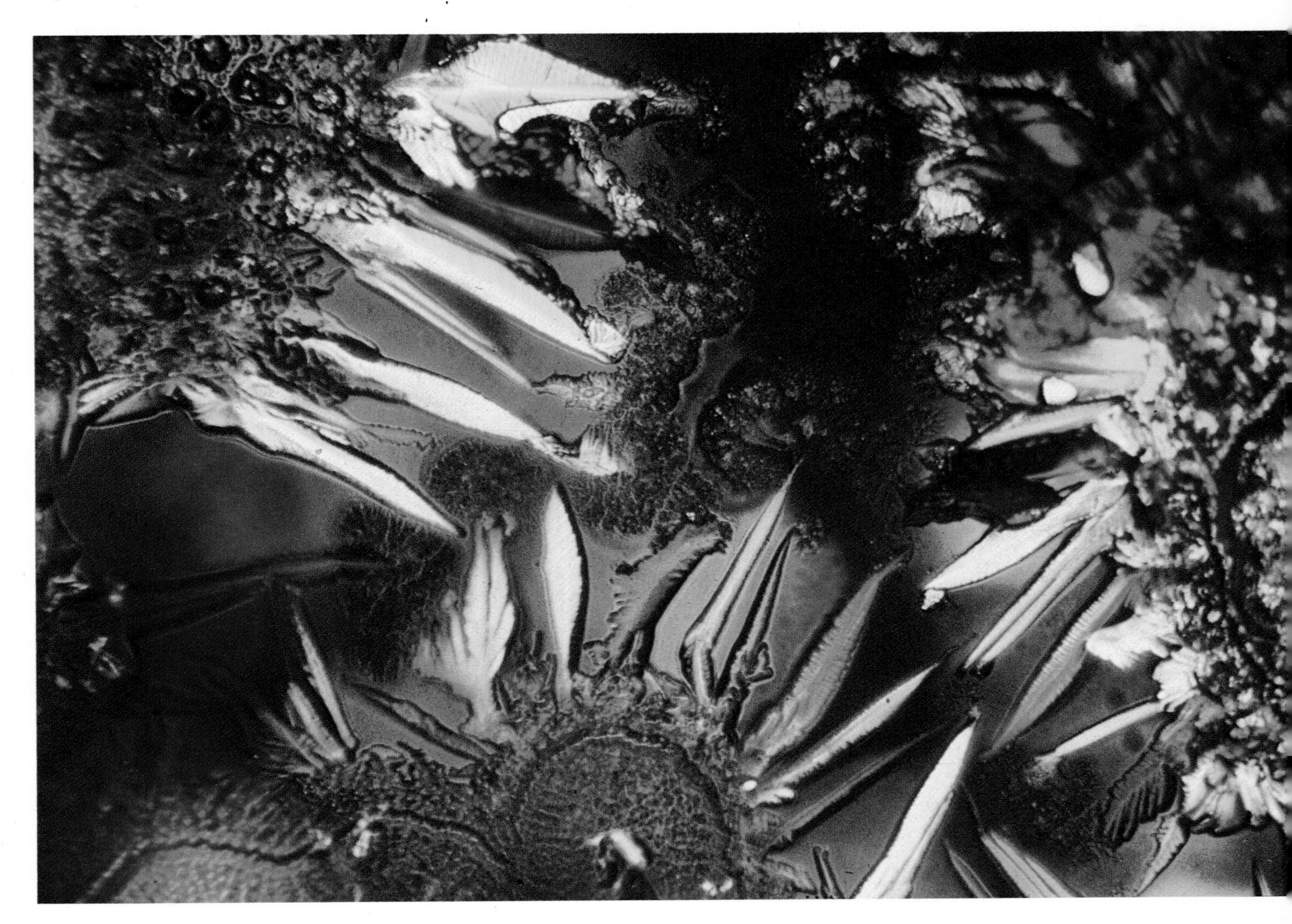

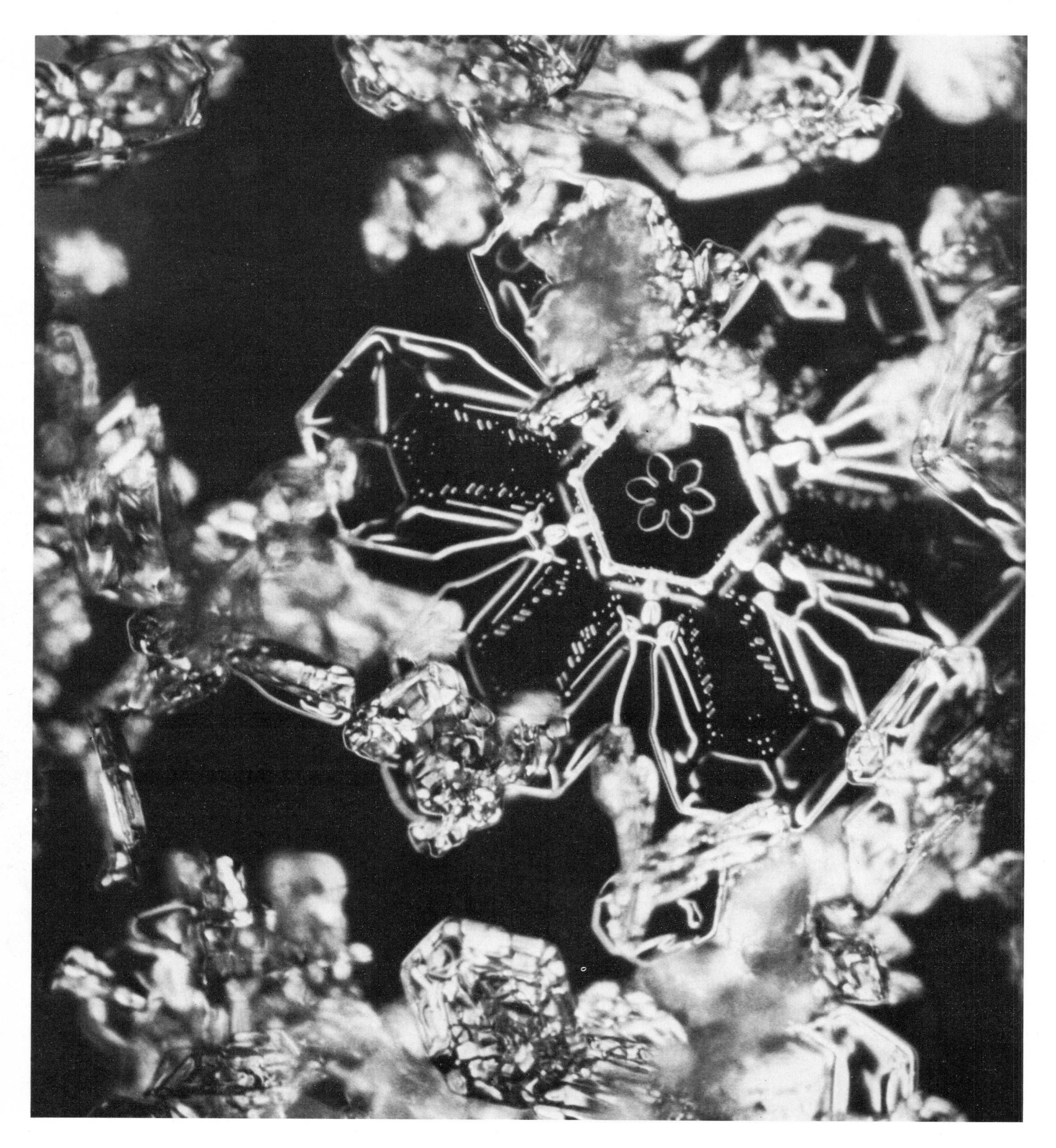

SNOWFLAKE
When drops of water freeze and turn to snowflakes, their atoms reorganize themselves into the infinitely varied patterns of an ice crystal—no two of which are exactly alike. Magnification: × 300.

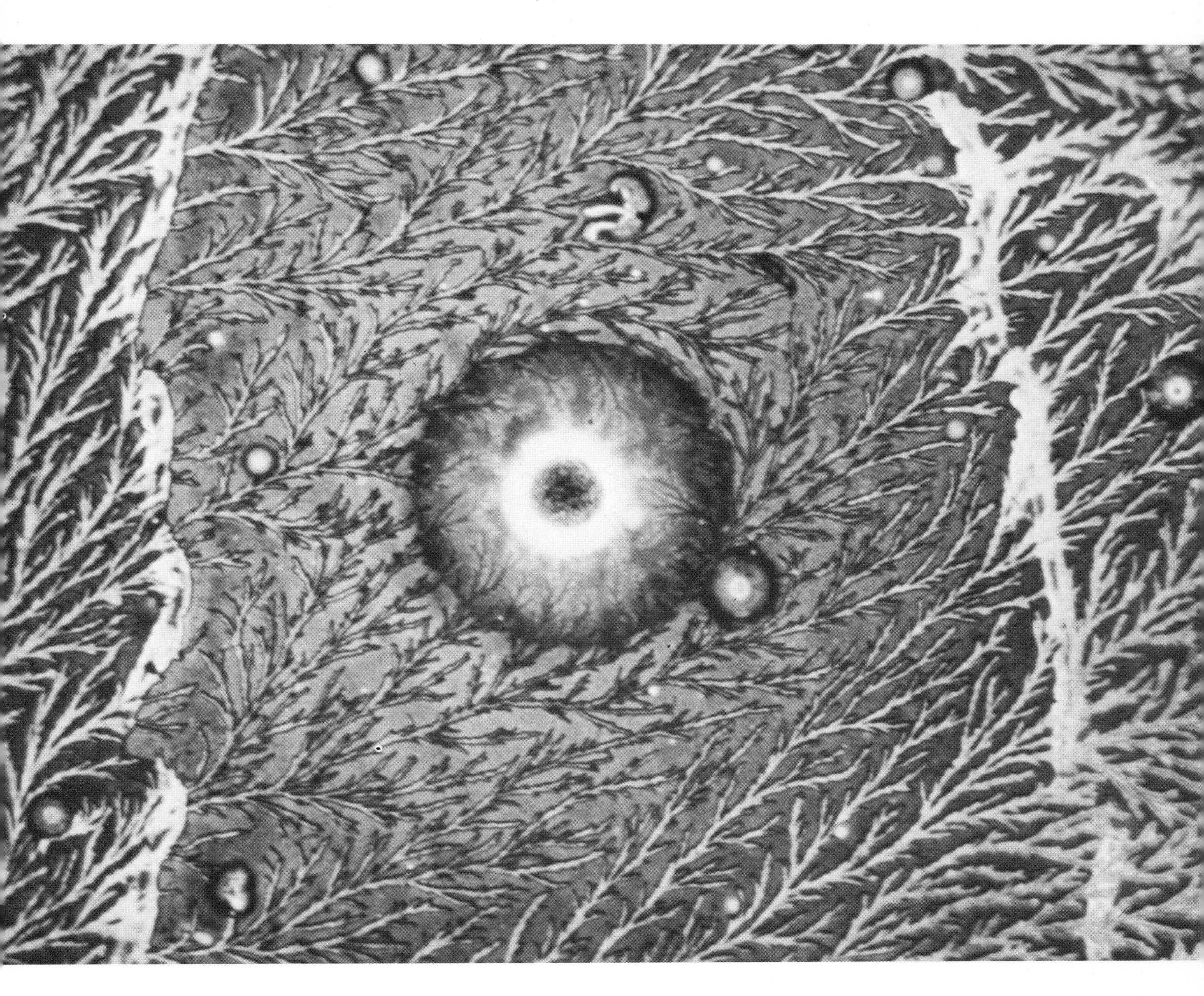

CRYSTAL EYE
A crystallized copper sulfate electroplating solution on a sheet of copper, magnified 25 times.

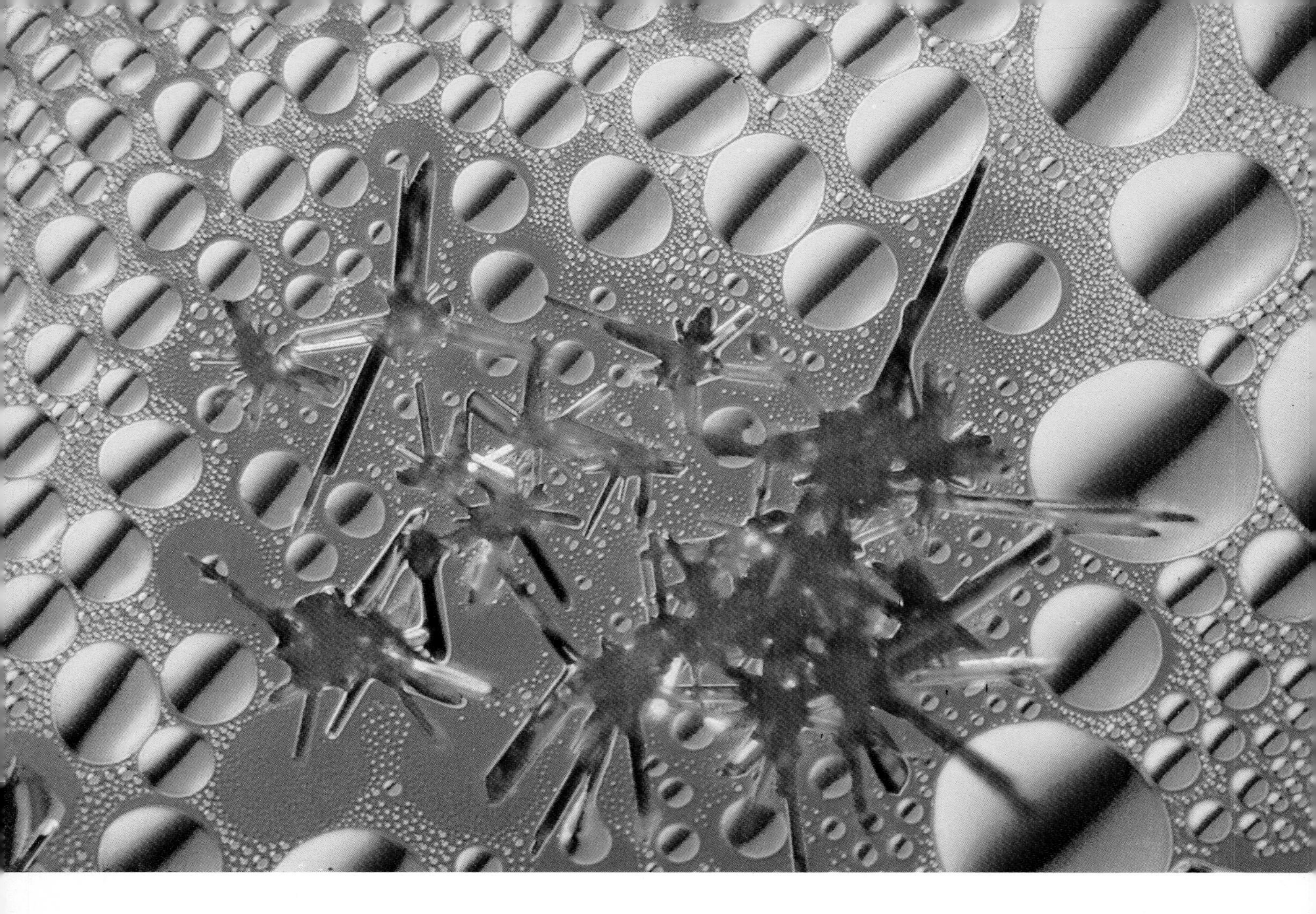

FLUORESCEIN
Doctors often use this crystalline dye to help make minute scratches on the surface of the human eye visible. Magnification: $\times$ 75.

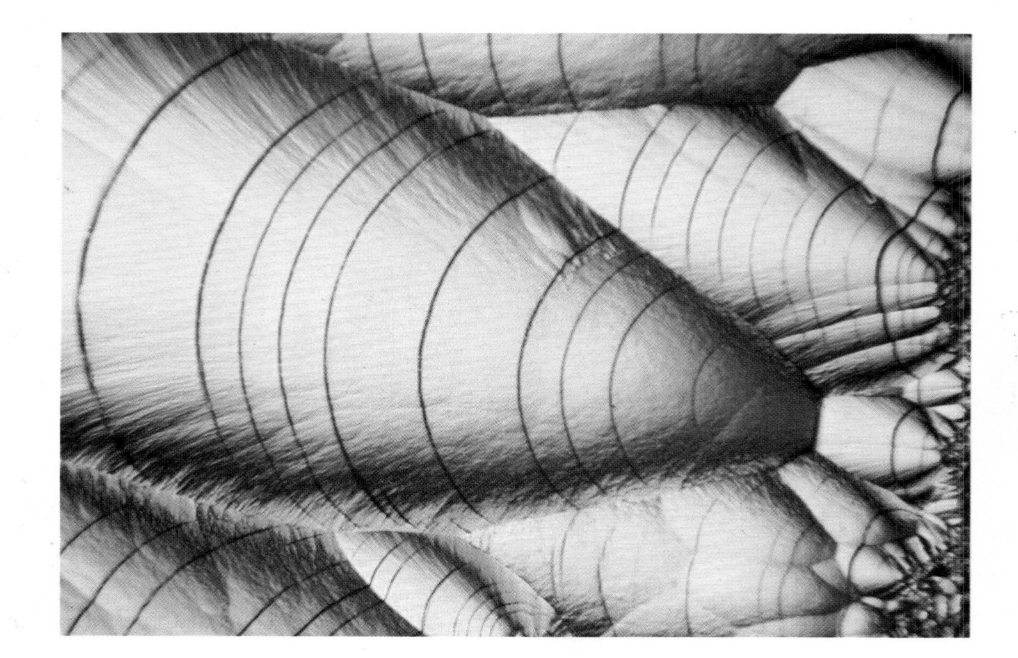

PYROLYTIC GRAPHITE
Graphite is a crystal form of carbon. Its crystals take on hexagonal shapes. If the crystals formed into cubes, a diamond would result. Magnification: $\times$ 75.

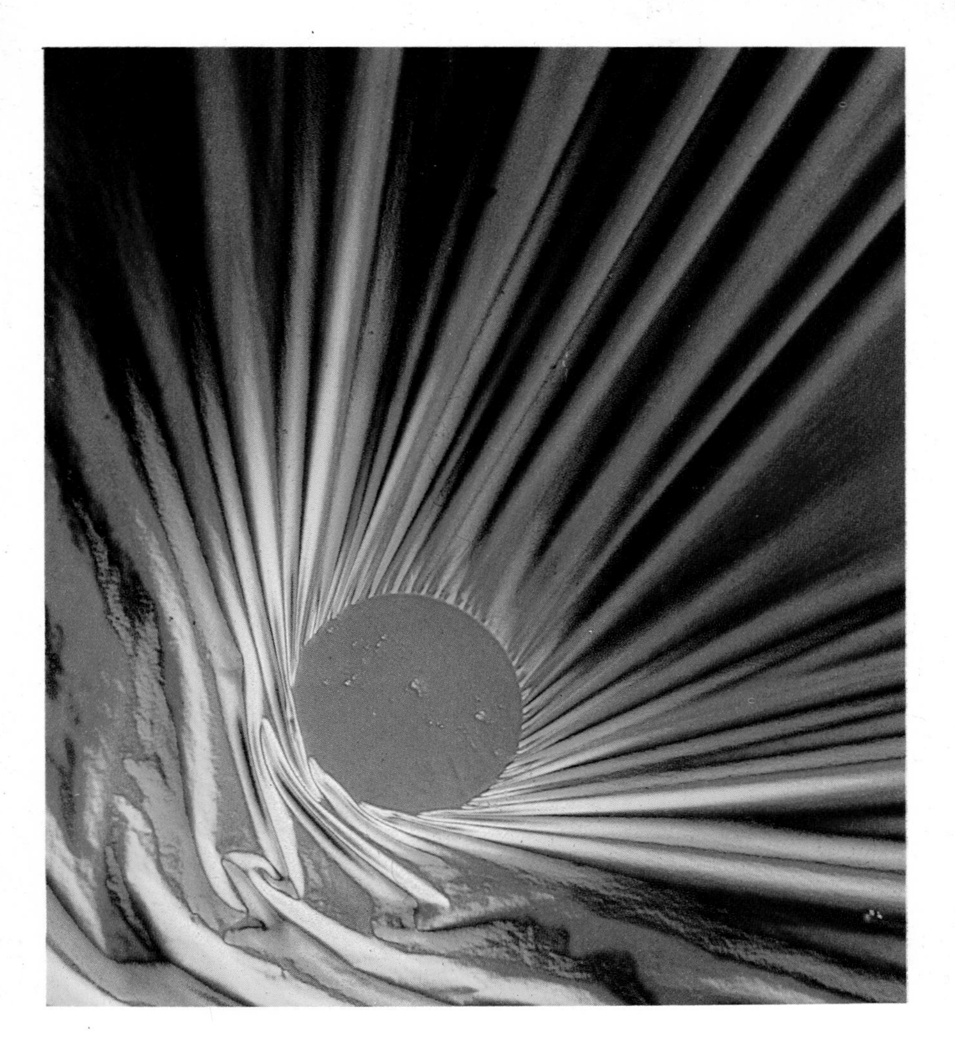

MICRODRUG
This colorful crystal is an antibiotic called doxycycline. It's commonly used as a cure for infections. Magnification: × 25.

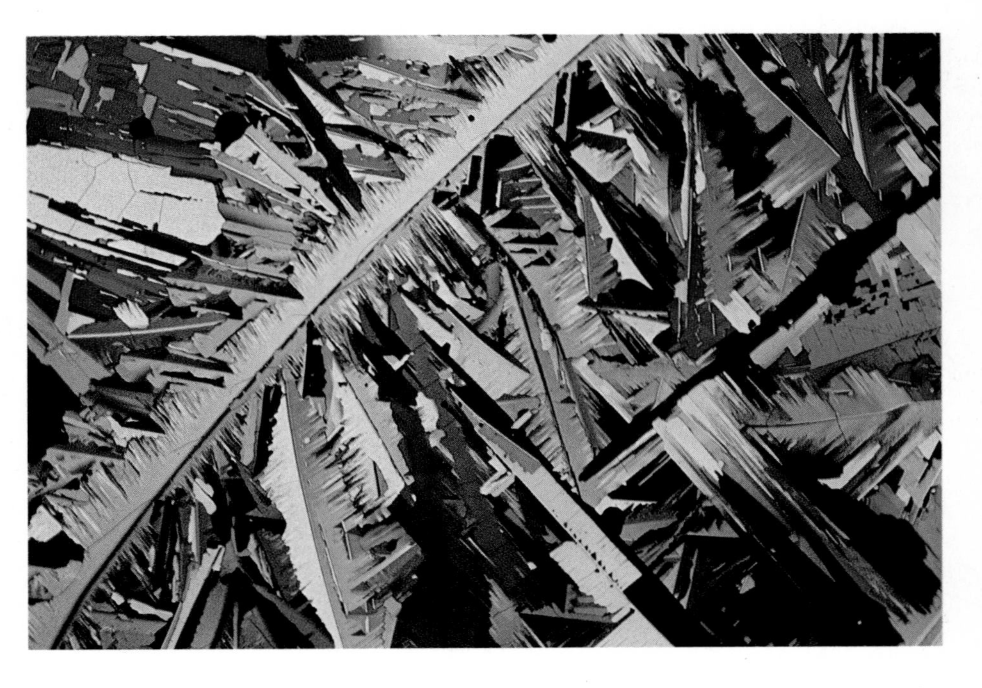

SULFUR
Humans have been aware of sulfur since prehistoric times. It burns naturally near volcanoes, and probably was instrumental in teaching man how to use fire. Ancient Egyptians used it as a medicine and a cosmetic. Today this tasteless and odorless chemical crystal is absolutely essential to modern life. Magnification: × 100.

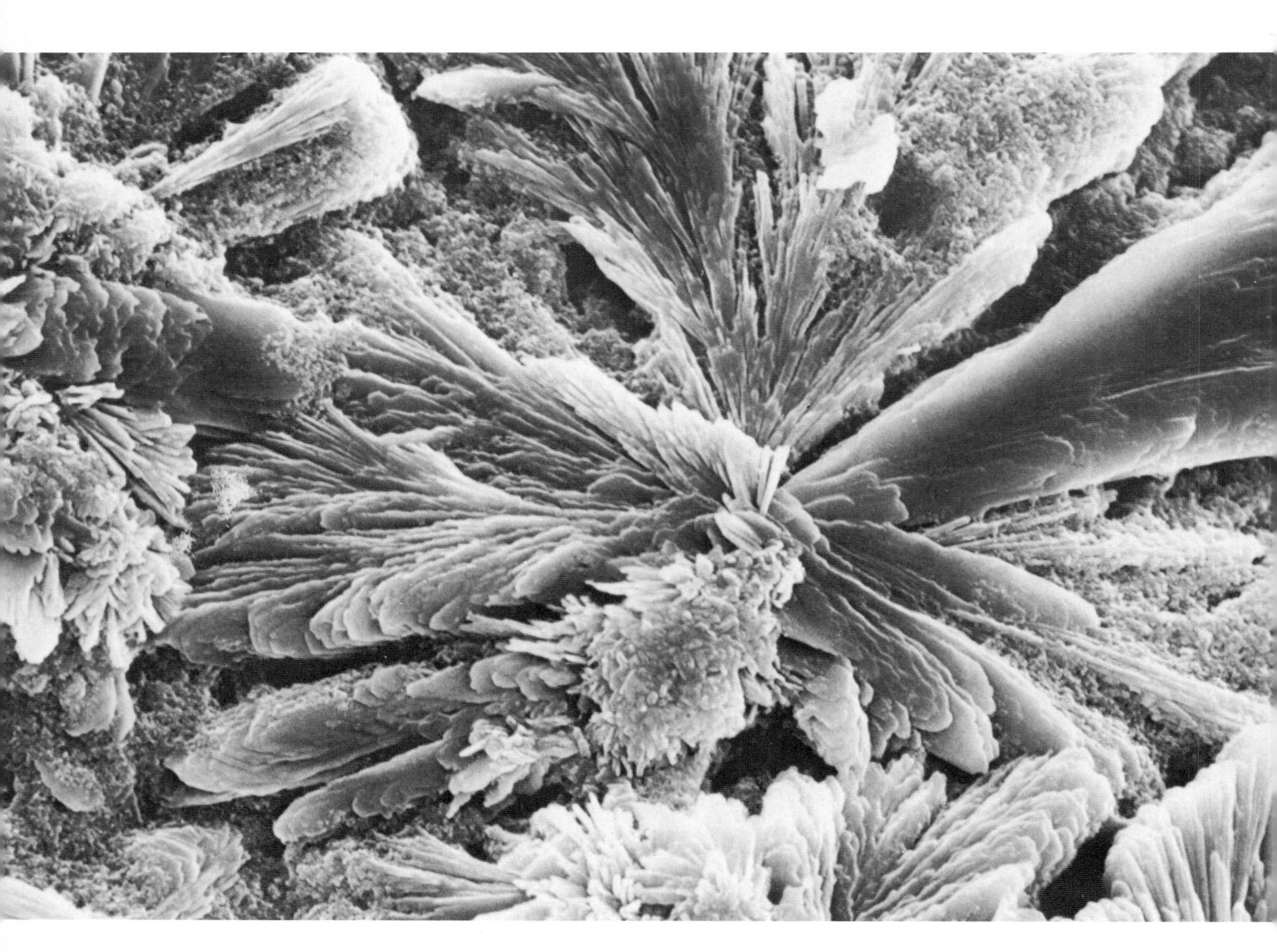

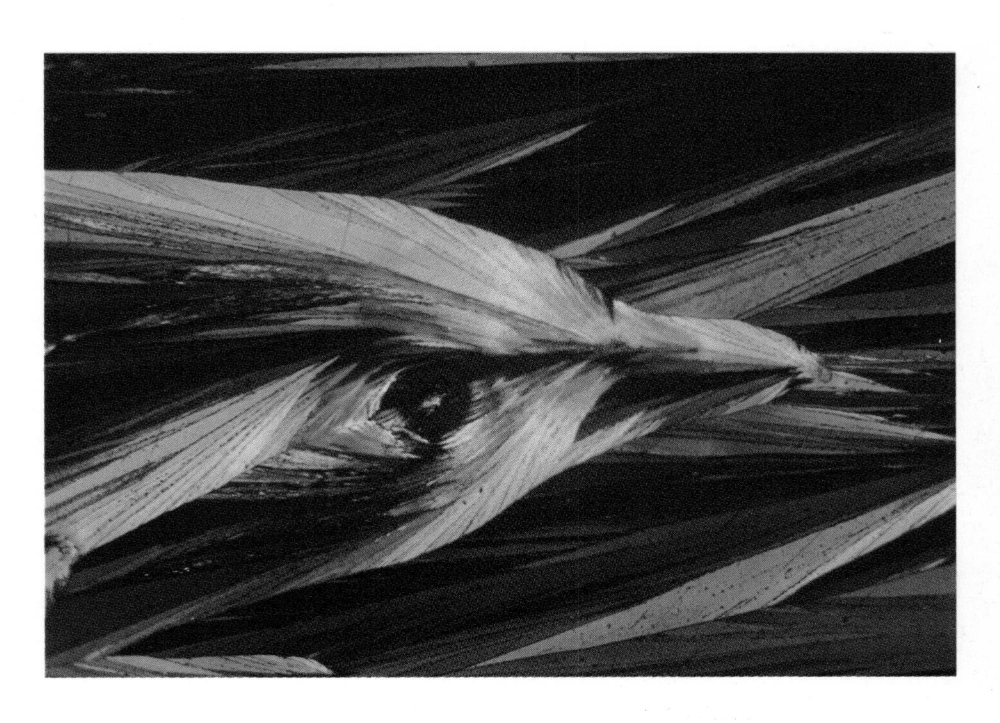

PONTOCAINE
This abstract bird is actually an anesthetic often used during surgery.
Magnification: × 80.

◁ **SWEET TOOTH**
A graphic example of what happens when you eat too many sweets: Calcium crystals attach themselves to the surfaces of your teeth.
Magnification: × 2000.

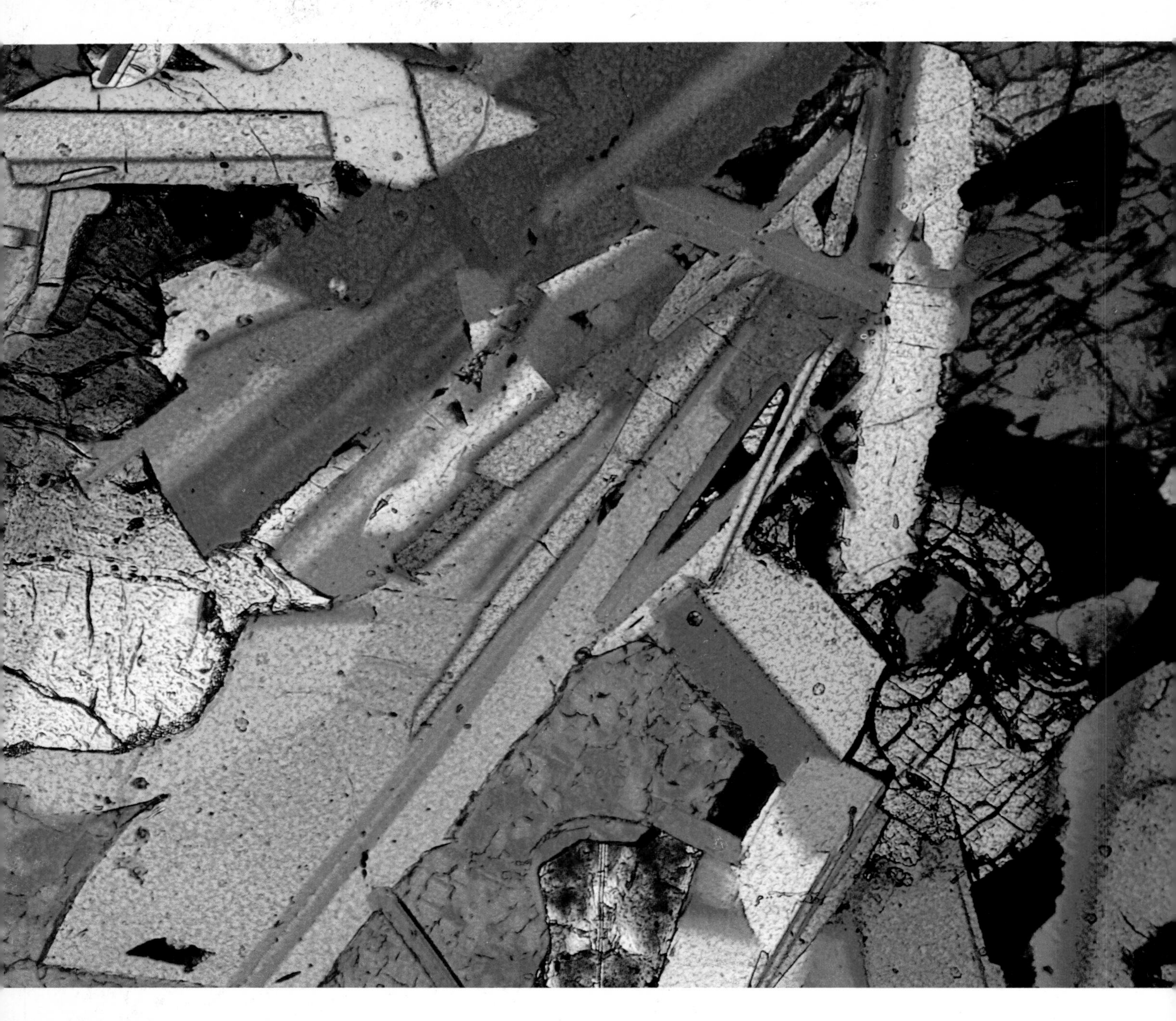

MOON ROCK
This tiny section of moon rock, magnified 50 times, reveals a lunar beauty that could never be seen through a telescope.

SPOT REMOVER ▷
This chemical crystal, hydroquinone, is often used in beauty products. It bleaches out skin blemishes. Magnification: × 75.

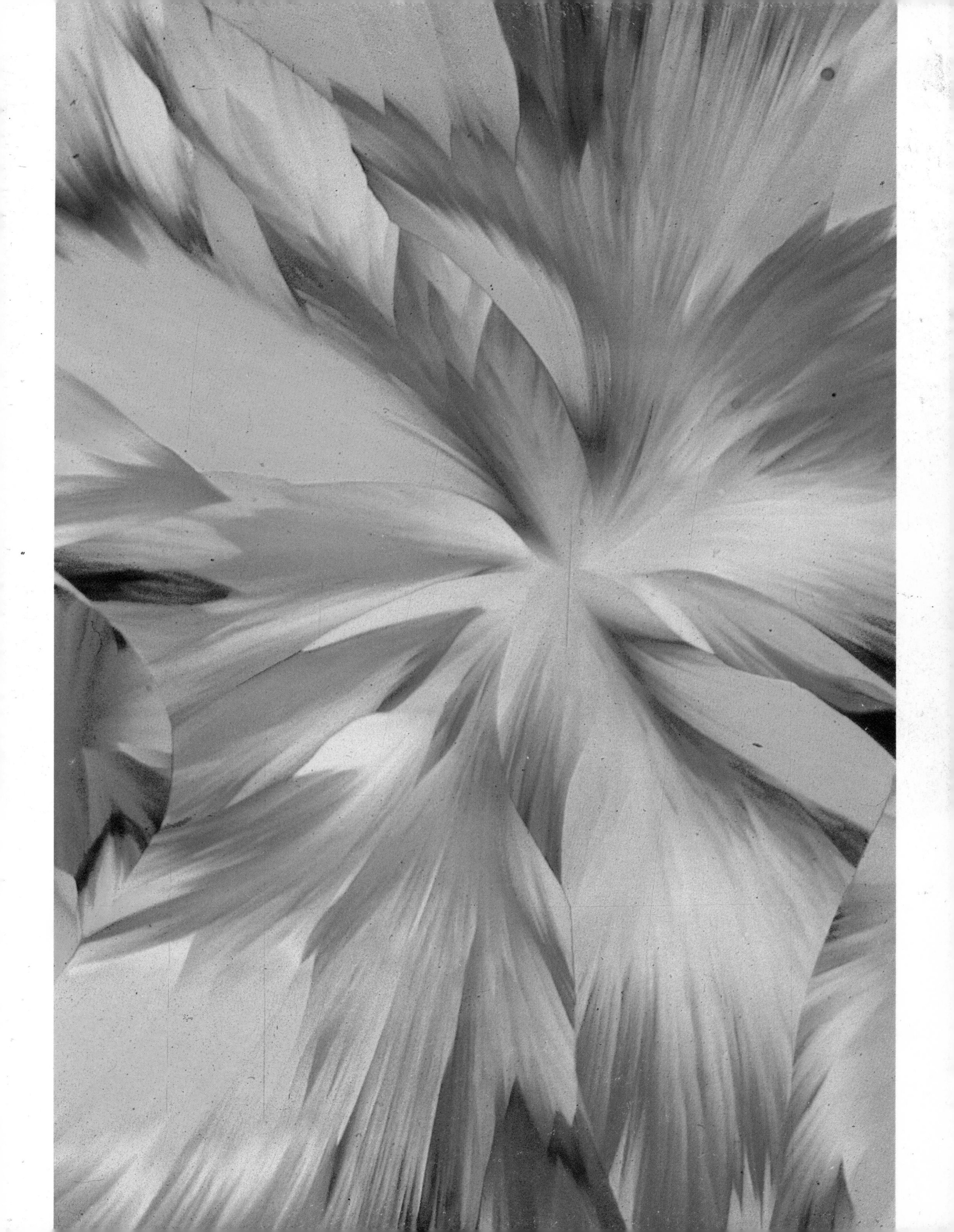

MICROSEX

The miraculous process of reproduction has given up some of its secrets to the probing eye of the microscope. Yet, when seen in the detail of super-high magnification, the re-creative power of life seems all the more magical and awesome.

BUTTERFLY SPERM

Magnified more than 30,000 times, the delicate structure of a butterfly's reproductive cells is strikingly revealed. The tiny flagella provide the means of locomotion. Hundreds of thousands of sperm cells are regularly produced by a single butterfly.

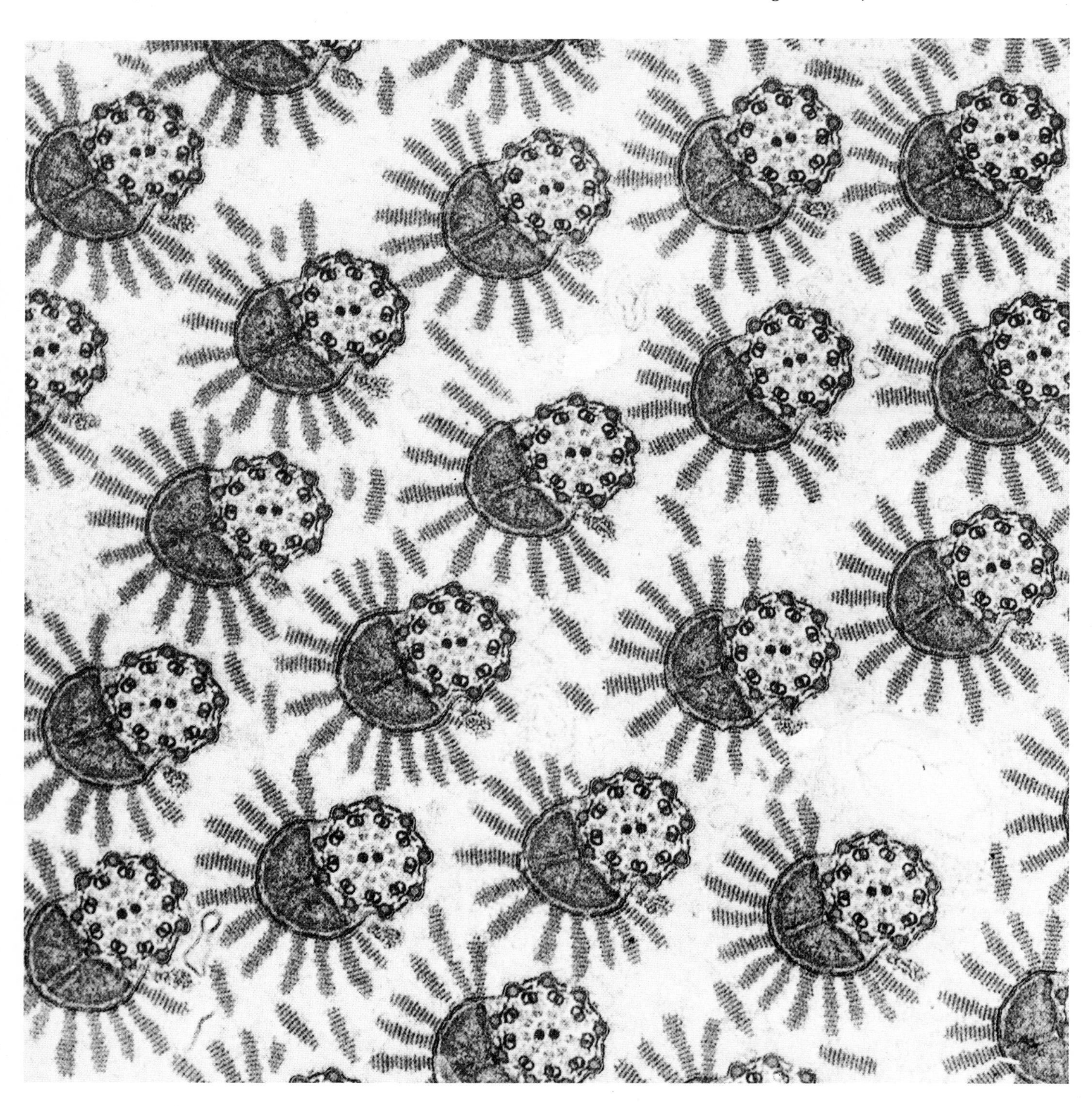

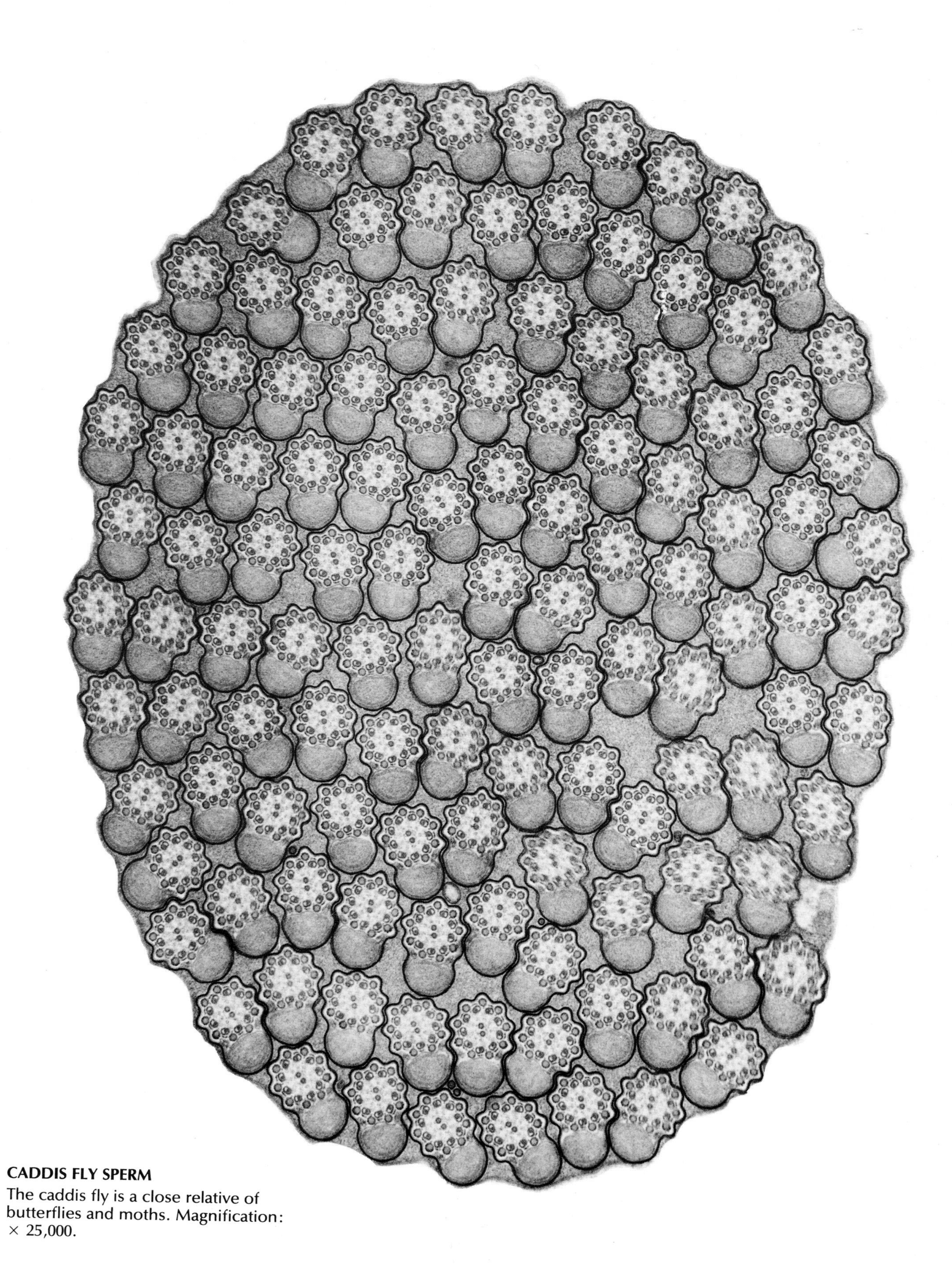

CADDIS FLY SPERM

The caddis fly is a close relative of butterflies and moths. Magnification: × 25,000.

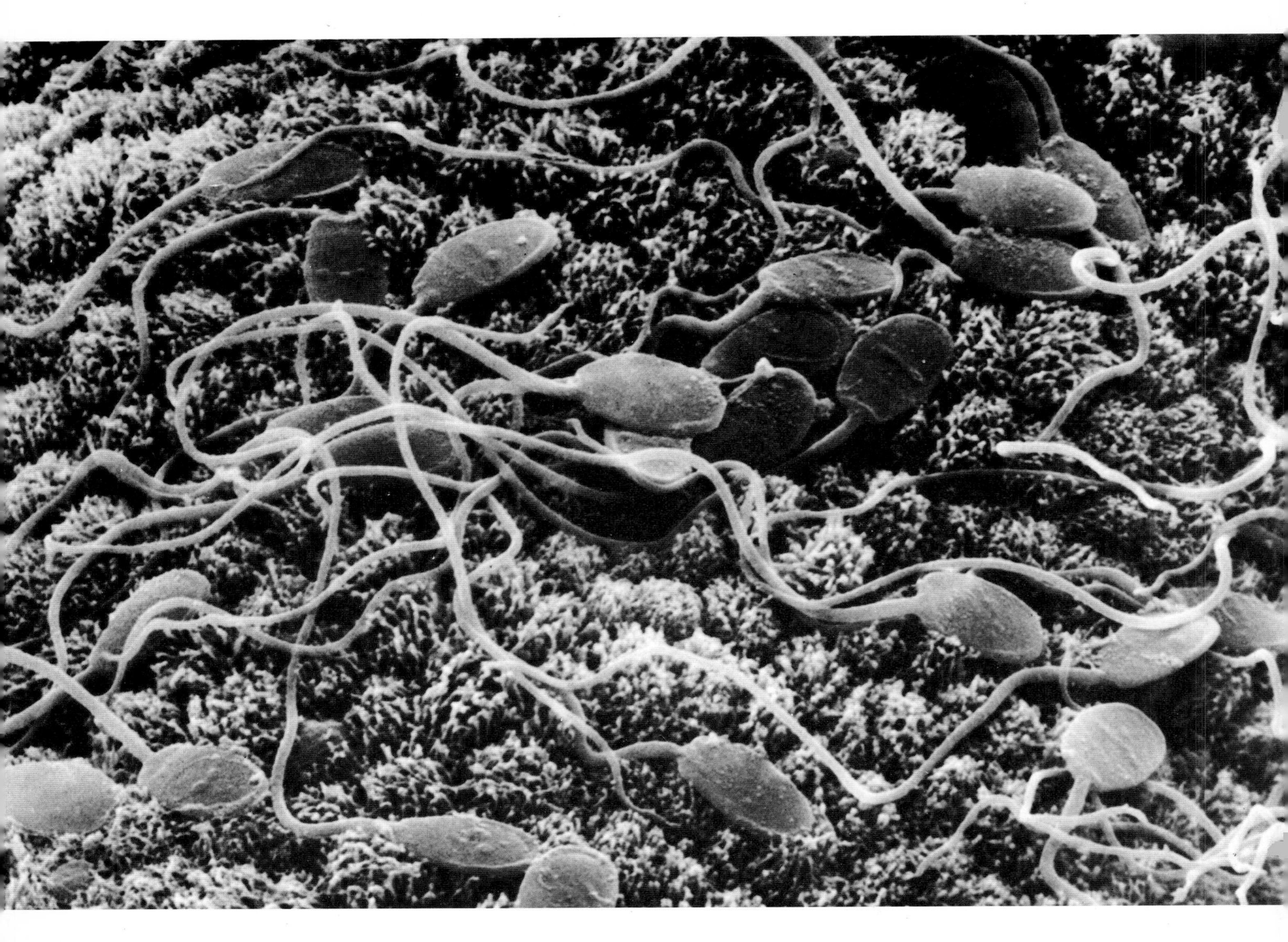

RABBIT SPERM IN VAGINA

An average male rabbit usually has about a million sperm cells available for mating. Only a few of the sperm will survive the perilous journey through the vagina to the egg. Magnification: × 1000.

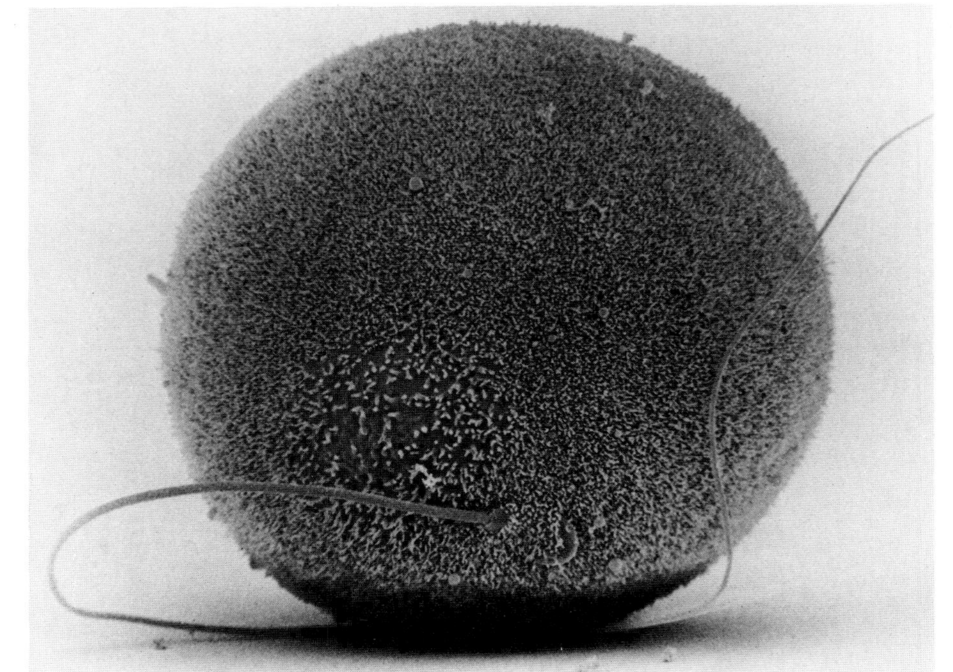

BEGINNING OF A HAMSTER

One sperm cell out of millions has just fertilized a hamster's egg. In three weeks a new life will be born. Magnification: × 5000.

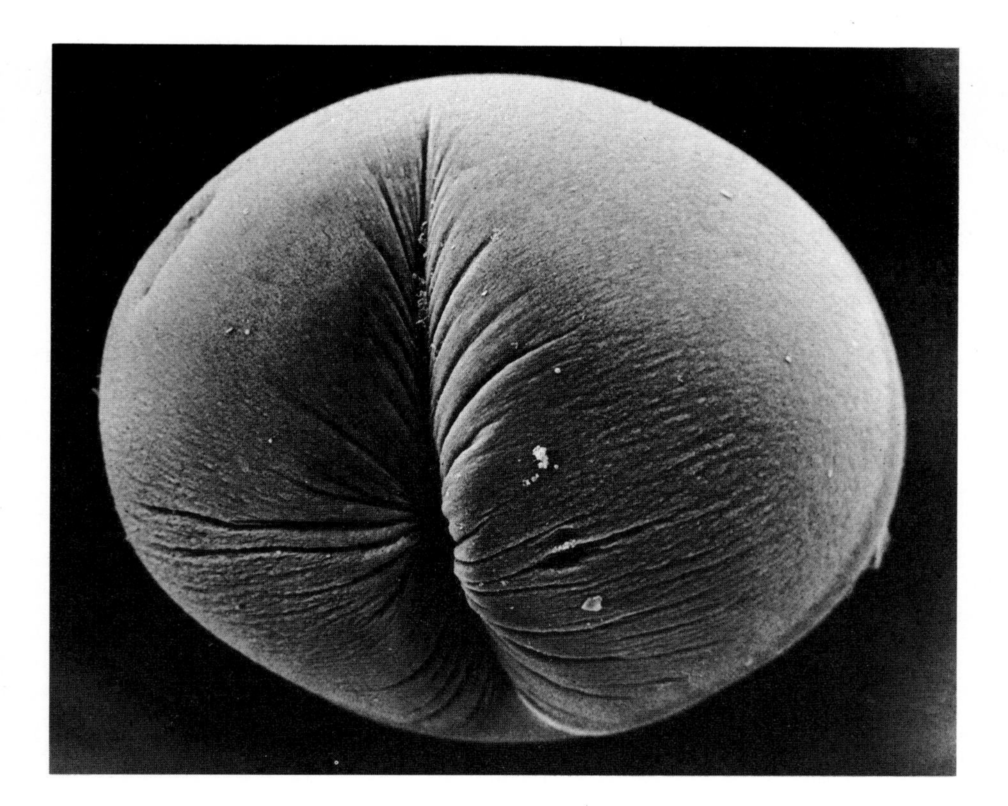

FROG TO BE

A frog's egg begins dividing eighty minutes after fertilization. In several weeks it will be a free-swimming tadpole. Magnification: $\times$ 350.

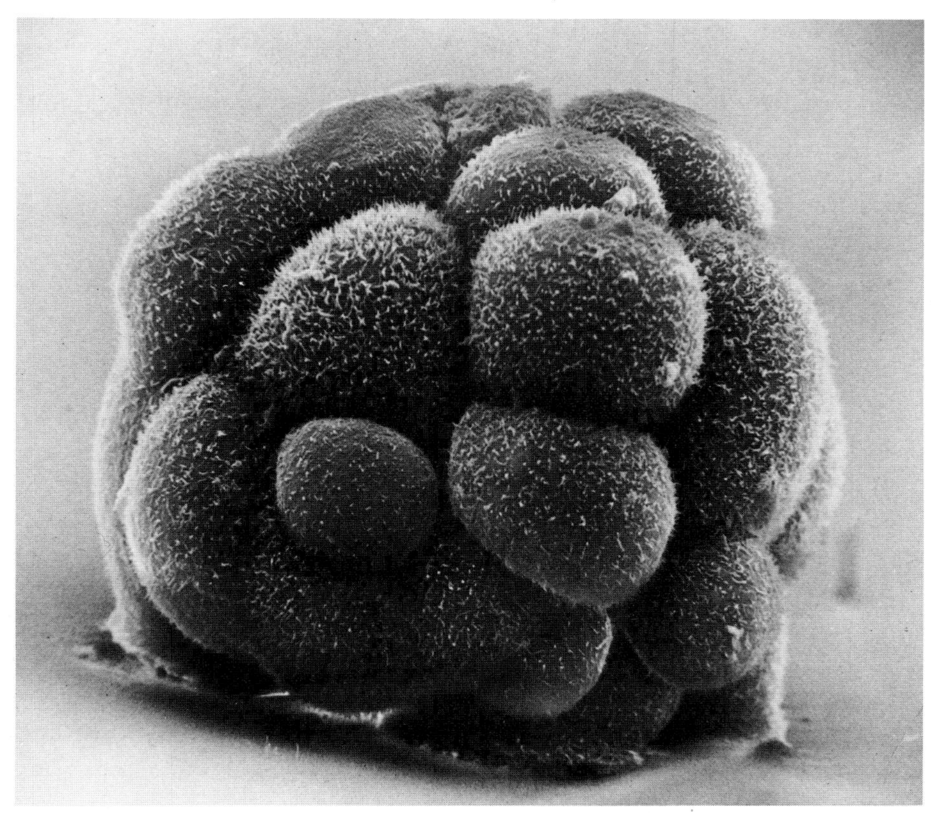

MINIMOUSE

A mouse embryo, magnified 400 times. It will be fully developed in about three weeks.

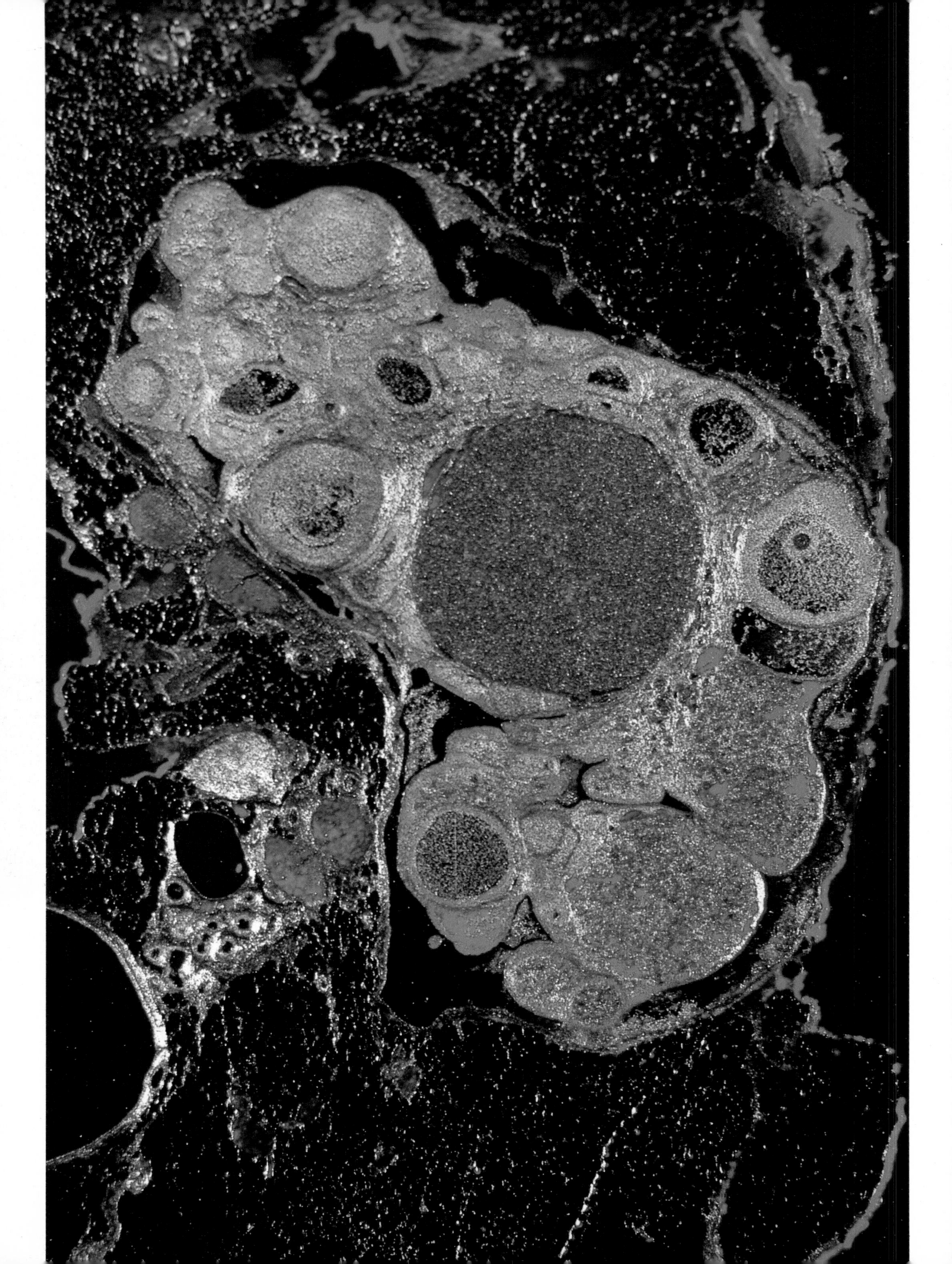

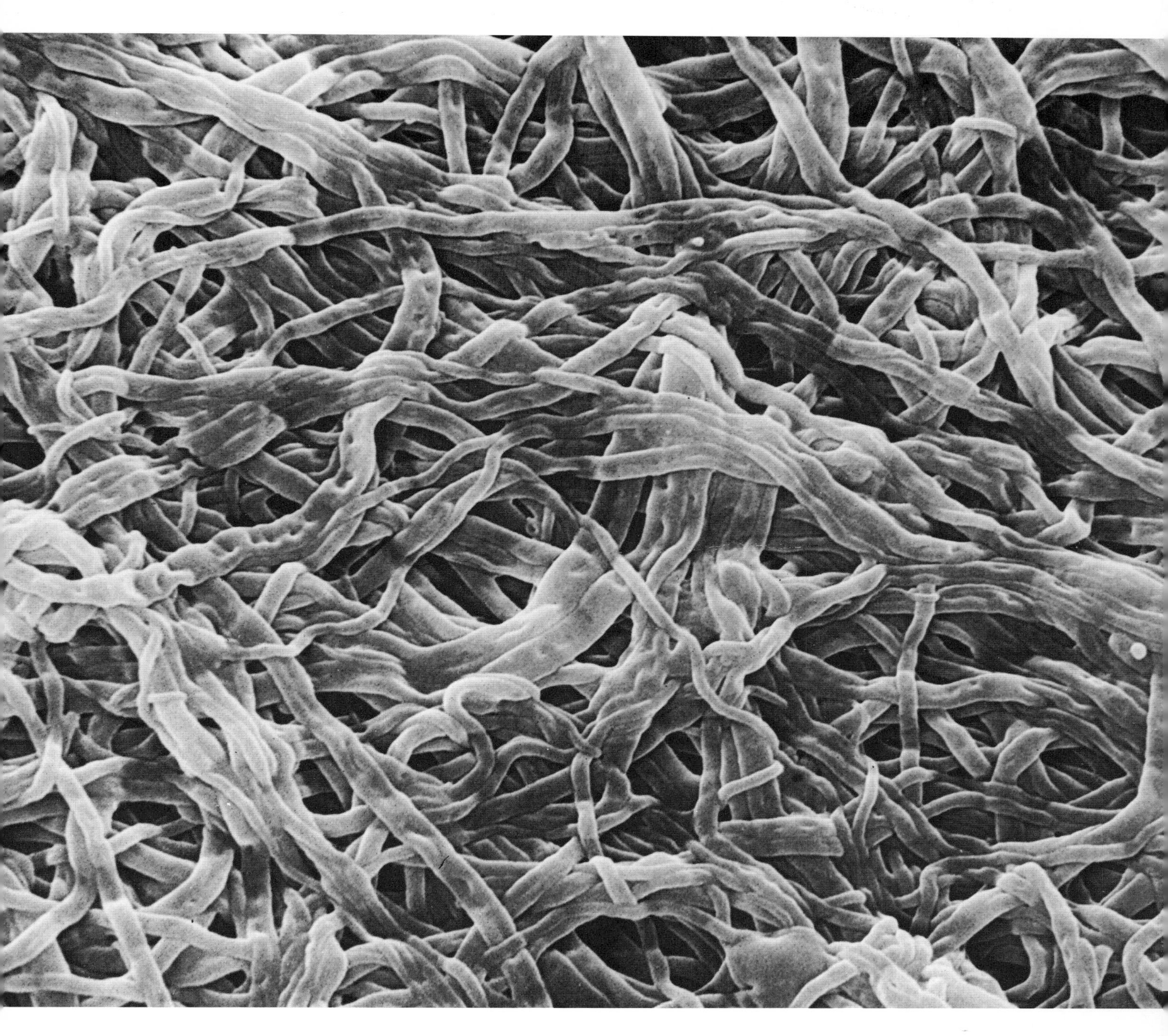

LIZARD EGG

The exterior of a developing lizard egg is protected by a relatively thick woven net, magnified here 1500 times.

◁ **EGGS**

A rat's ovary containing several eggs, each in a different stage of growth. Magnification: × 500.

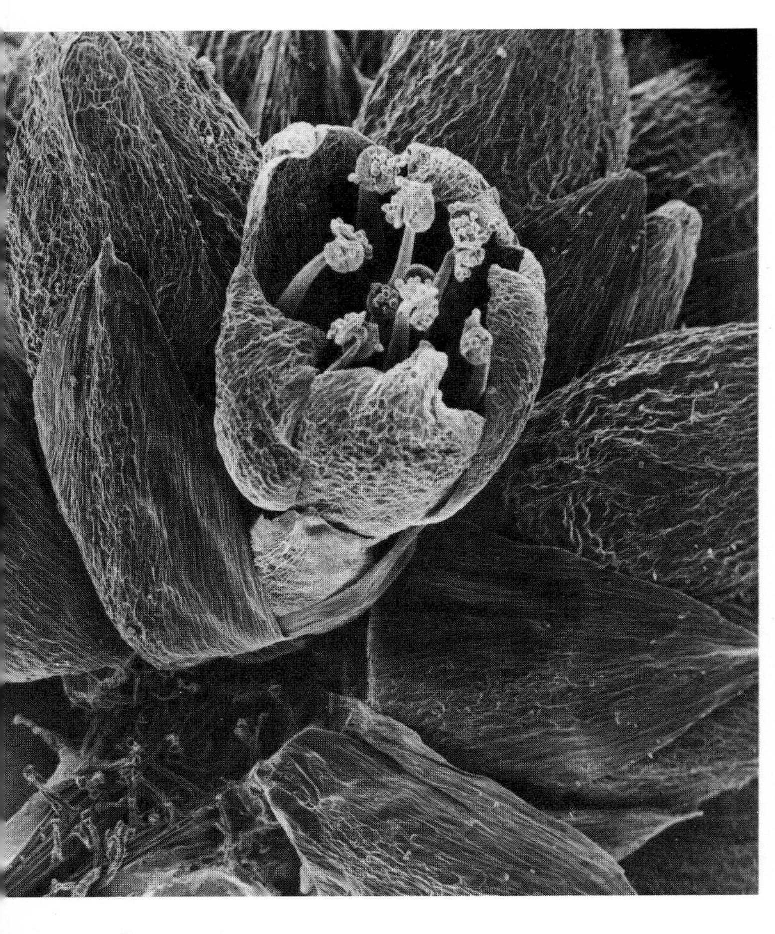
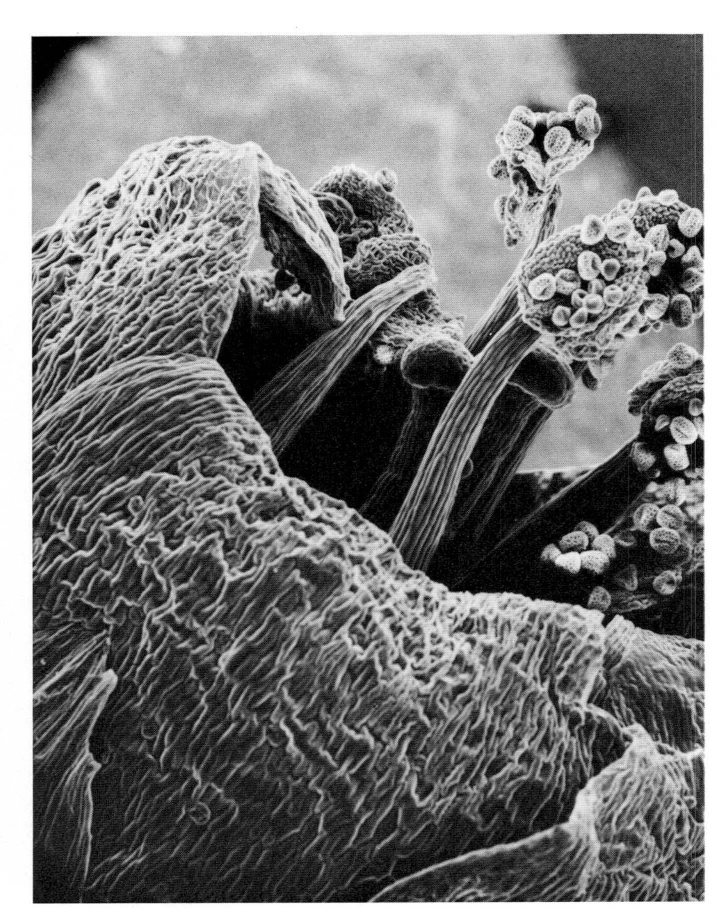
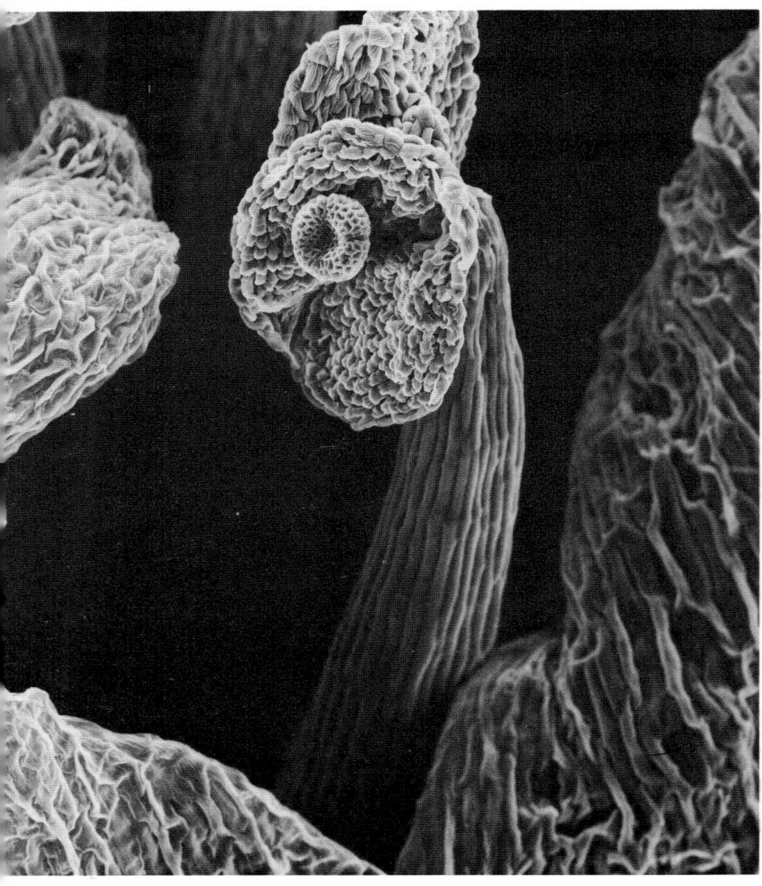
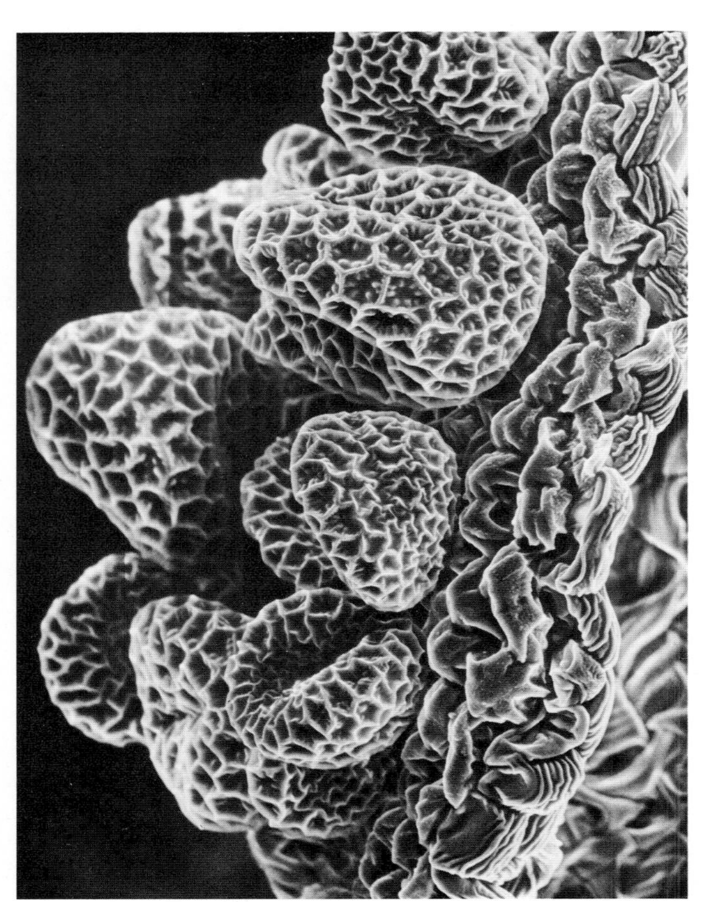

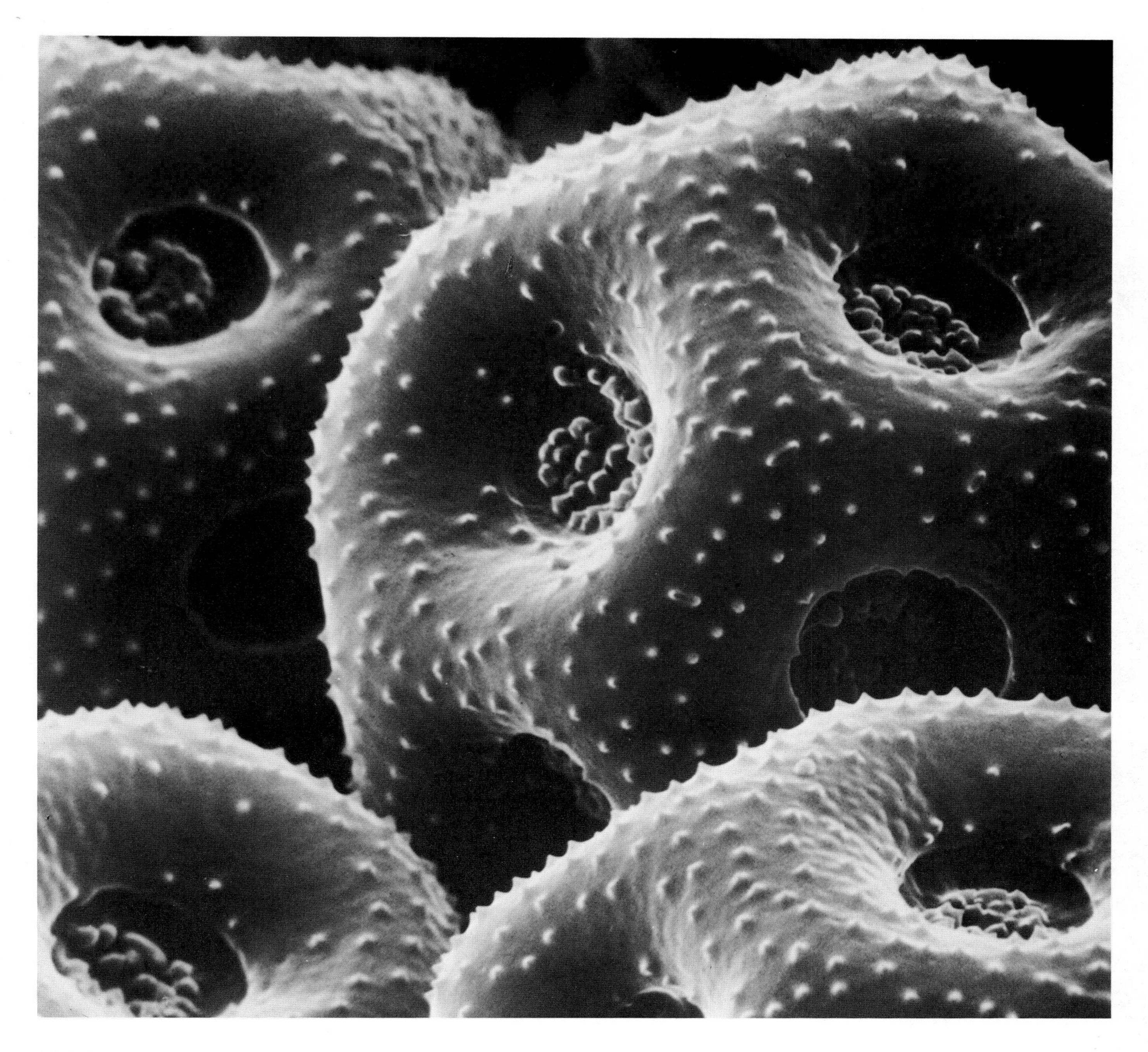

POLLEN

Until the invention of the microscope, pollen was visible only as a fine dust. Today, a scanning electron microscope can reveal the structure of a single grain in incredible detail. Pollen is the male sex cell of seed-bearing plants. It is carried by wind, water, or insects to the pistil of female plants, where fertilization takes place. Pollen is so abundant that it is a significant component of the earth's atmosphere . . . as people with allergies will attest. Magnification: × 400.

◁ **SEX AMONG THE FLOWERS**

Increasingly greater magnifications of a knotweed flower reveal the tiny grains of pollen that will create a new generation of flowers . . . and allergies in sensitive humans.
Magnifications: × 200, × 400, × 600, × 800.

MINIATURE GARDENS

We may marvel at the beauty of a flower or a leaf, but a closer look at the world of plants reveals a highly intricate microstructure impossible to imagine.

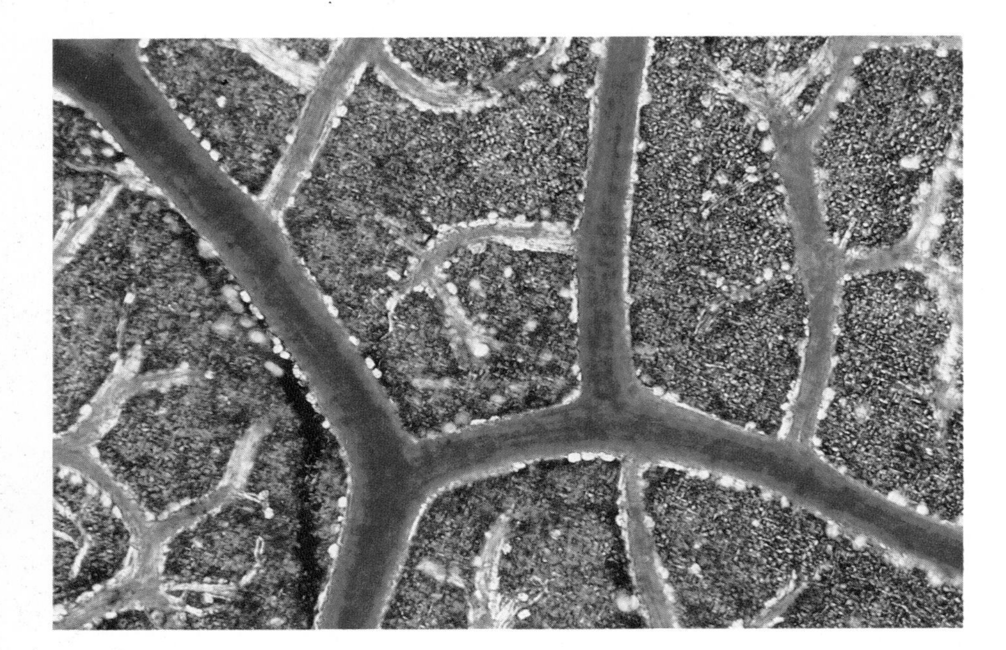

WOOD ▷
The body of a tree, like our own bodies, contains a vast circulatory system that provides the vital nutrients essential for survival. A cross-section of pine wood reveals this intricate internal structure. Magnification: × 100.

LEAF VEINS
When magnified 31 times, the leaf of a pittosporum plant shows its otherwise invisible vascular system. The veins serve both to strengthen the leaf's structure and to conduct the water and minerals that keep the plant alive.

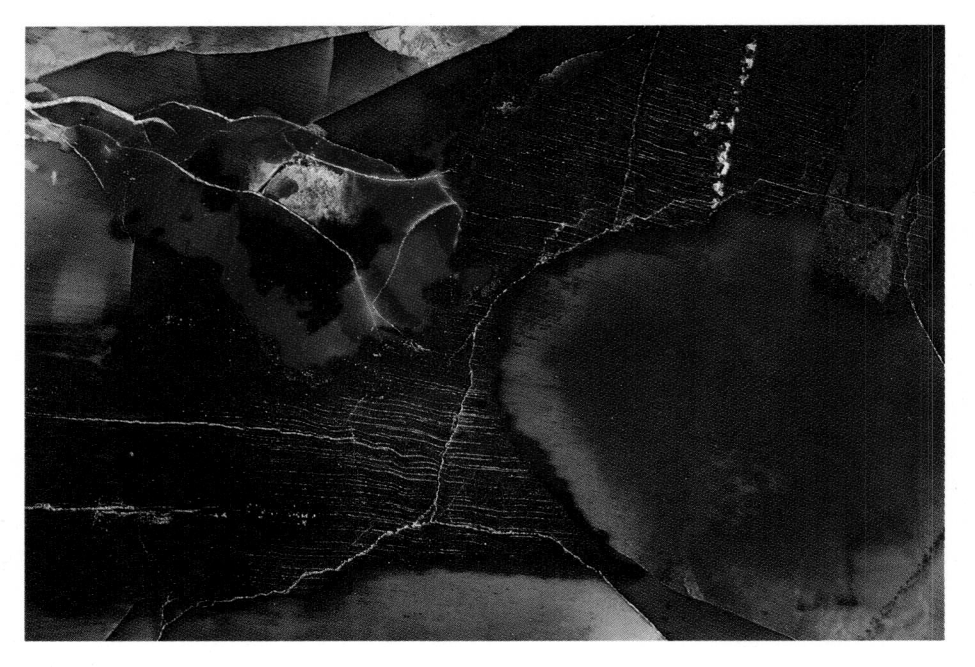

PETRIFIED WOOD
Millions of years of heat, pressure, and chemical leaching can transform a common piece of wood into a colorful crystalline stone. Magnification: × 25.

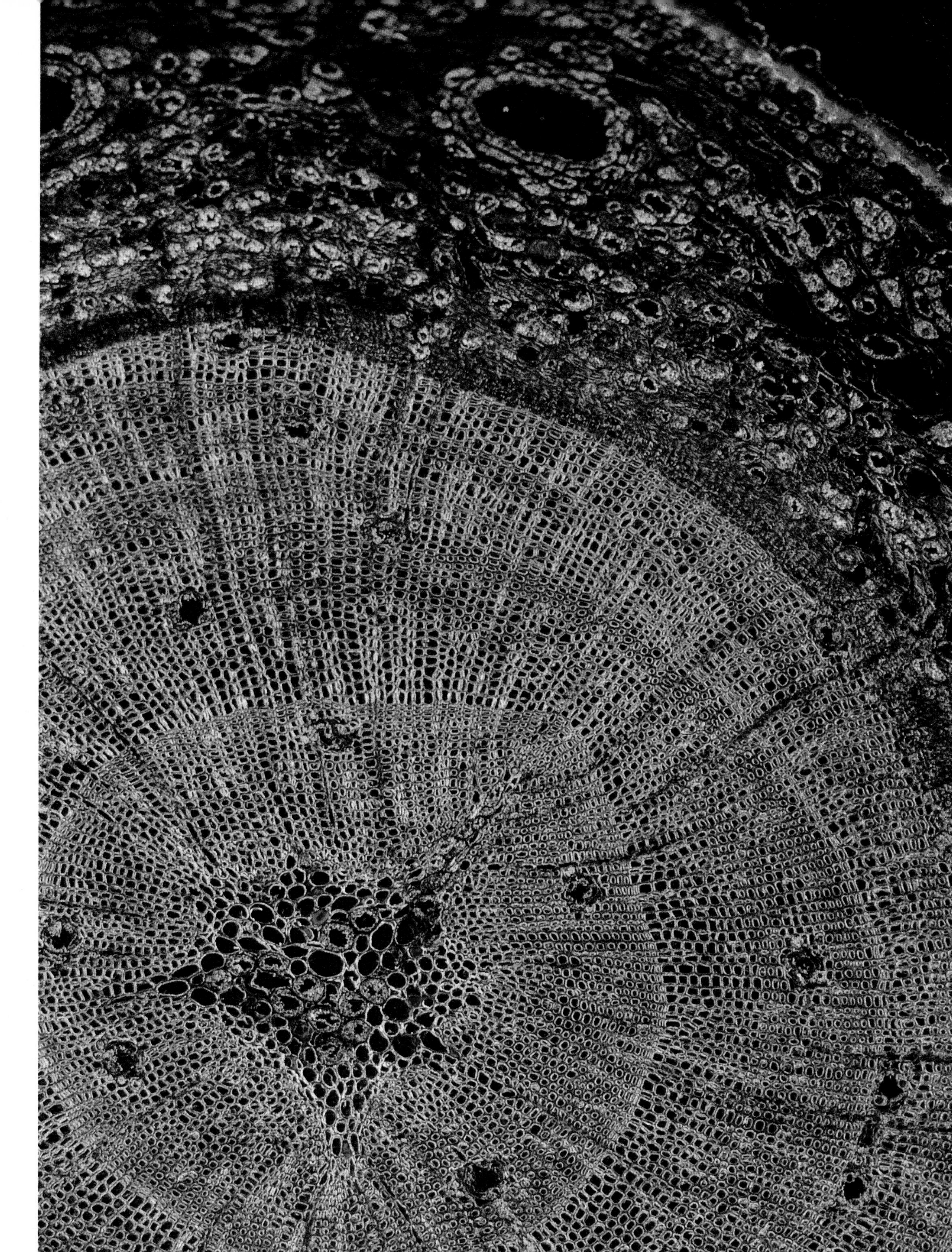

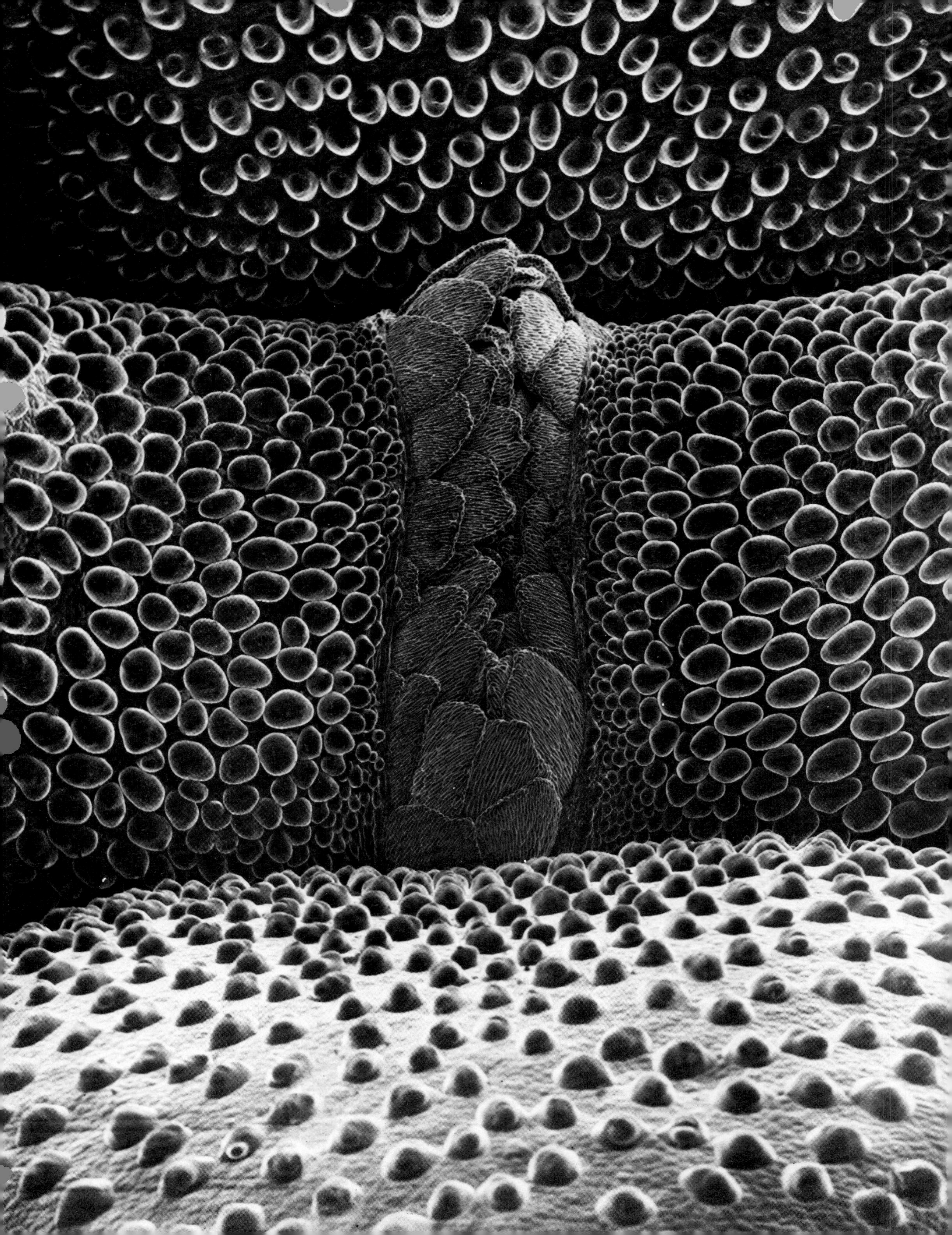

◁ **BABY'S-TEARS**

When magnified 33 times by a scanning electron microscope, this common houseplant takes on an otherworldly appearance. A tiny emerging bud is surrounded by larger, mature leaves.

MARIJUANA MONSTER

Tiny spider mites are frequent visitors on the leaves of marijuana plants. This mite is unable to leave. It has become stuck to one of the leaf's resin nodules, which contain the plant's hallucinogenic chemicals. Magnification: × 600.

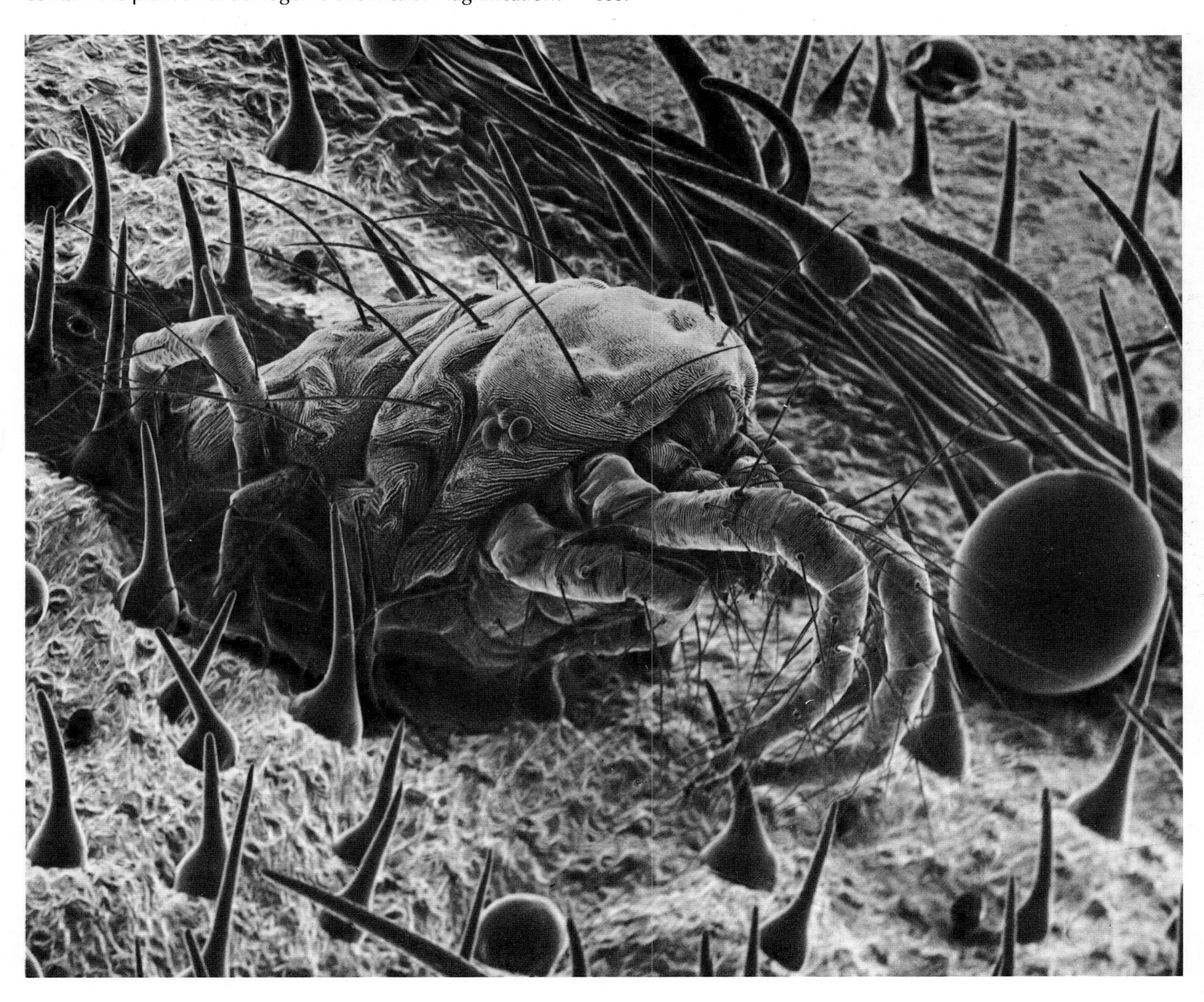

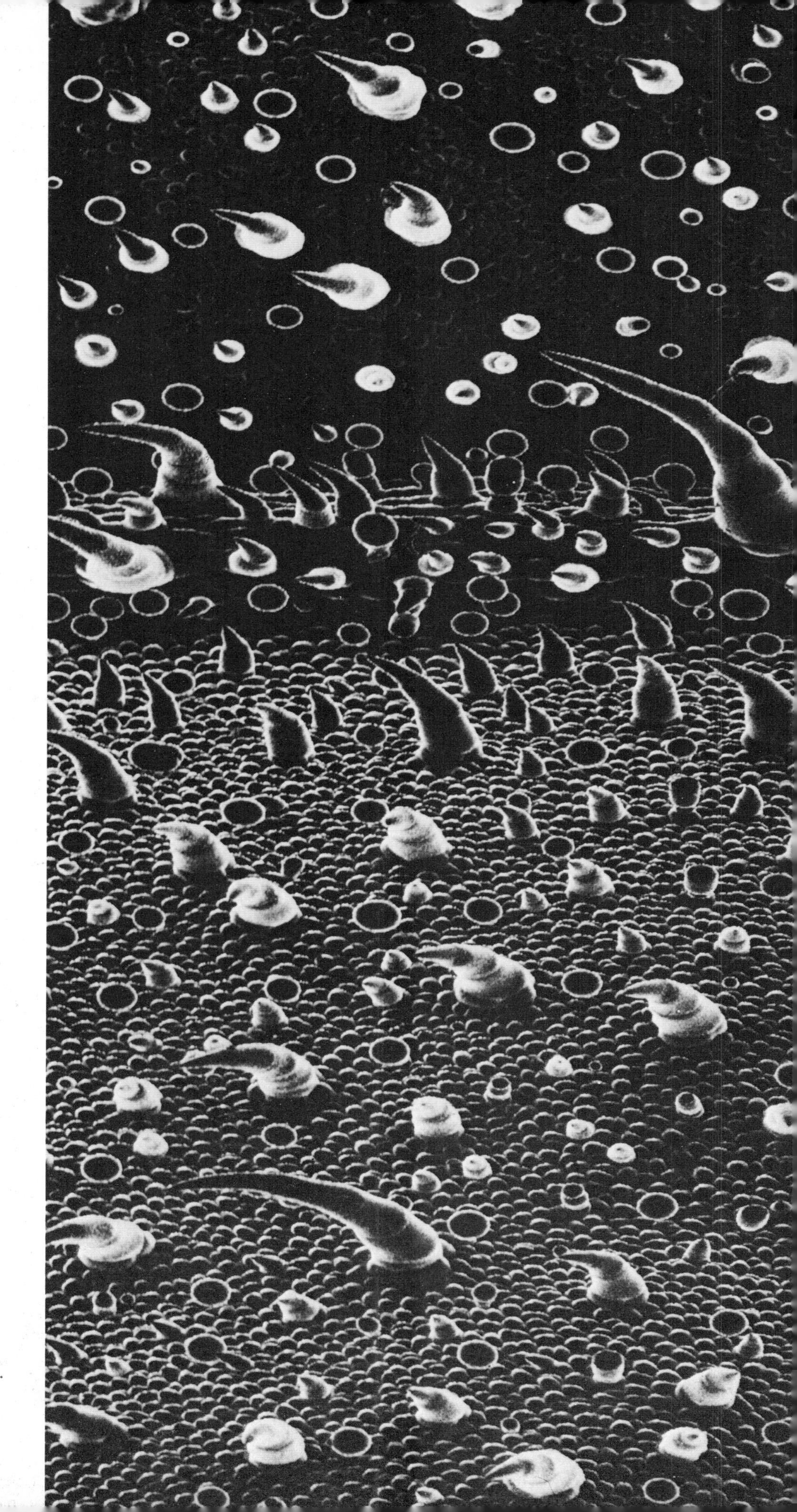

COLEUS LEAF

The smooth leaf of a coleus plant is really a vast barbed jungle, which protects the plant from harmful insects. Magnification: × 360.

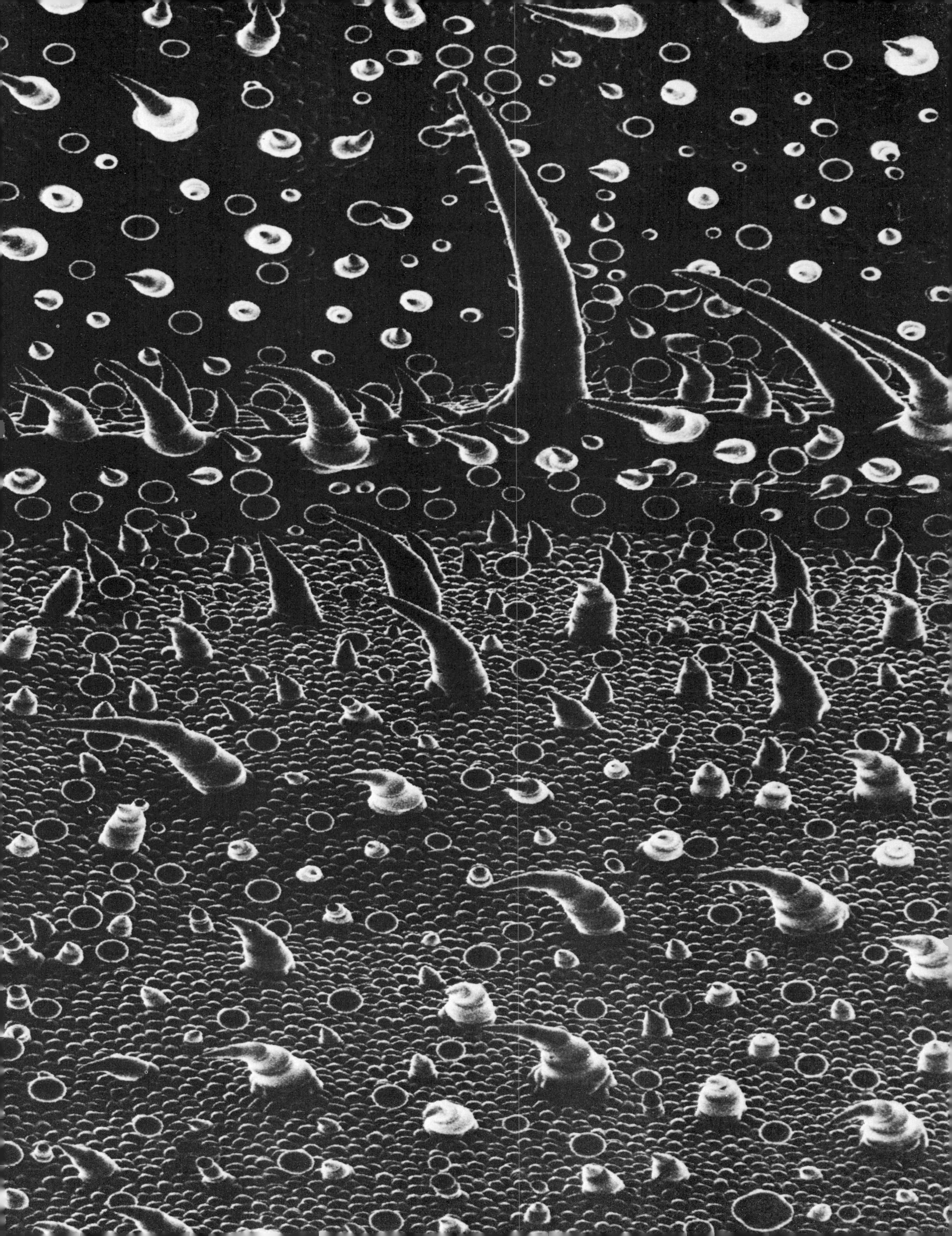

CLOSE-UPS

If we look a little closer at familiar everyday things, we might come to feel like strangers in our own world. Through the powerful eyes of microscopes, common objects show us hidden textures and structure, and unexpected complexity . . .

BLEACH
Magnification: × 75.

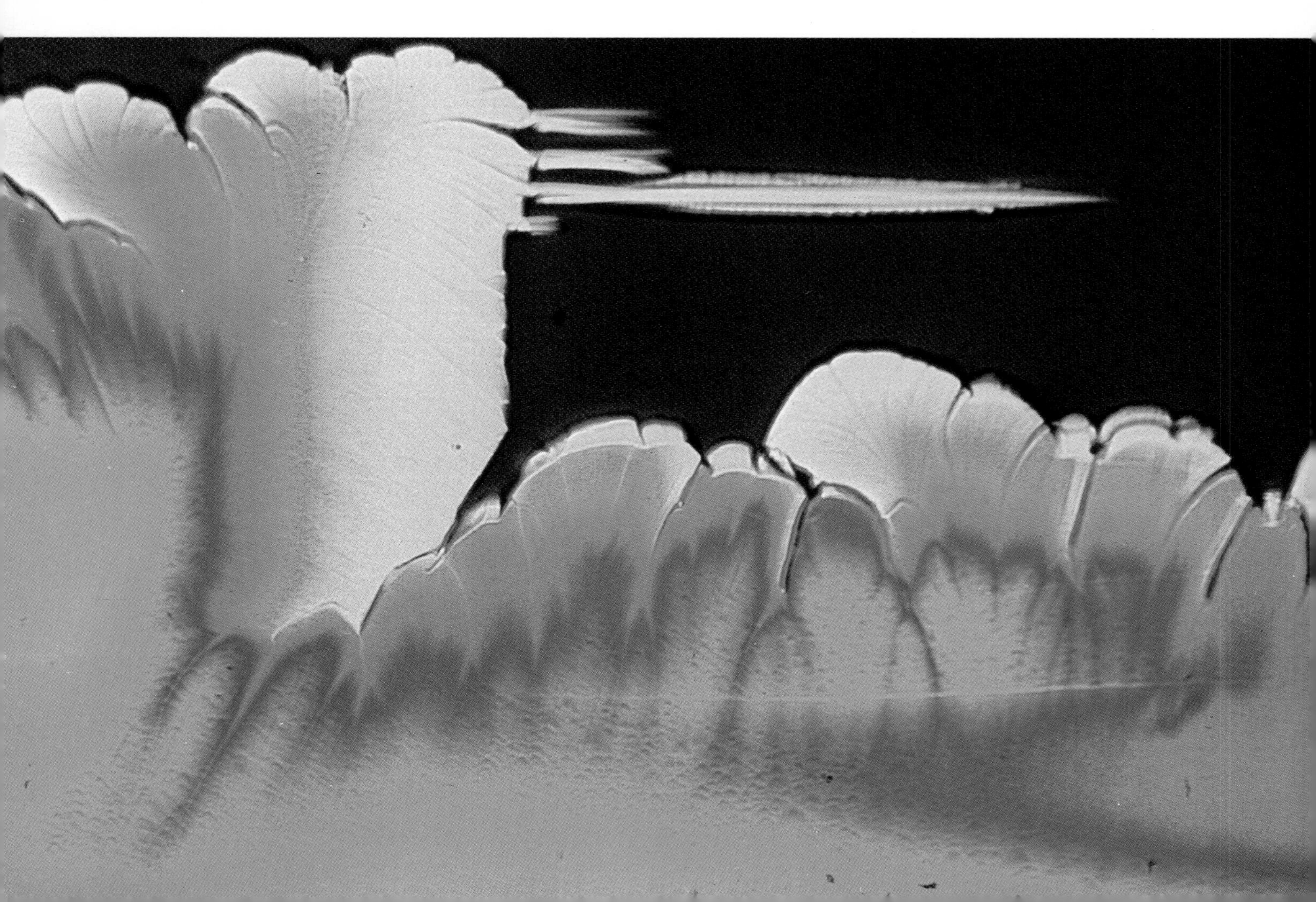

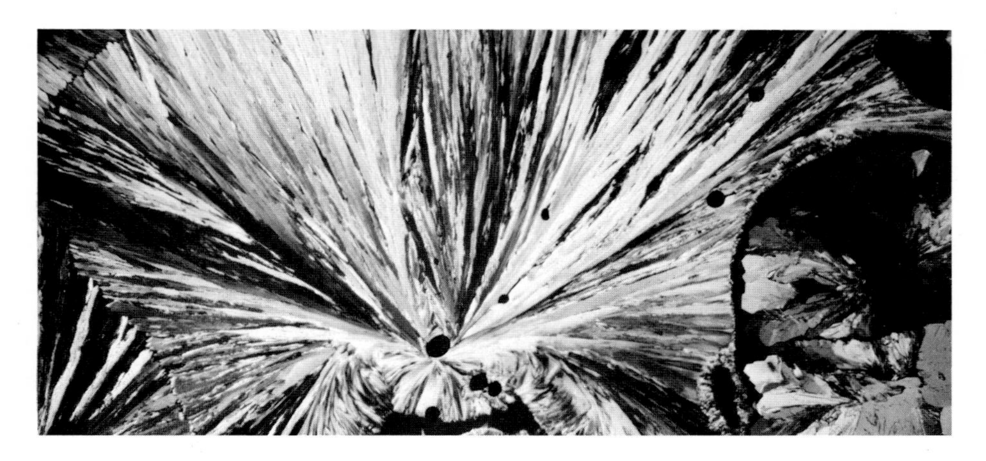

VITAMIN C
Magnification: × 100.

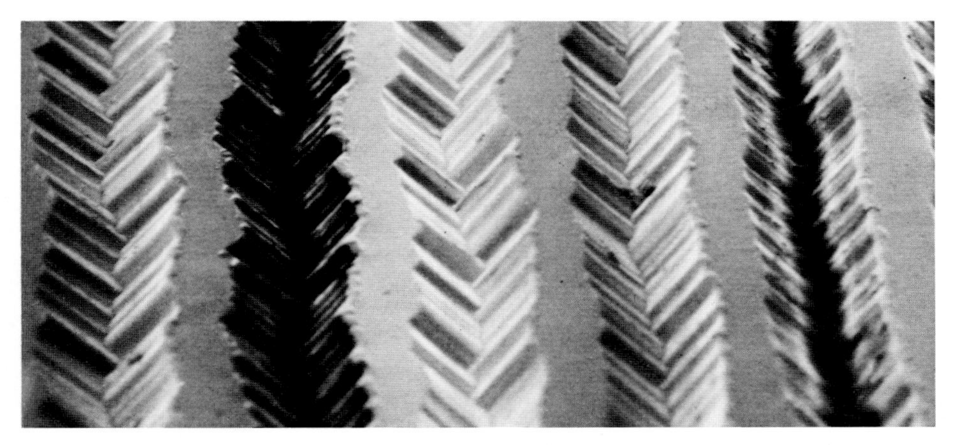

RECORD GROOVES
Magnification: × 300.

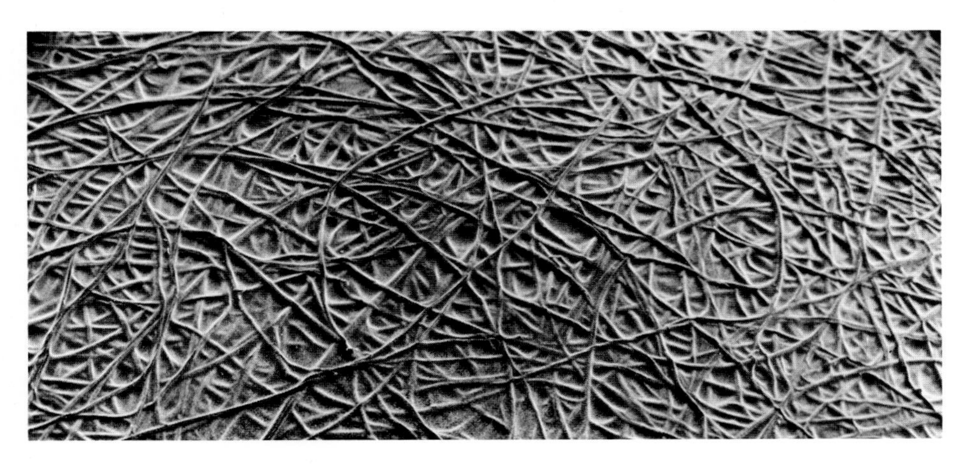

PAPER
Magnification: × 100.

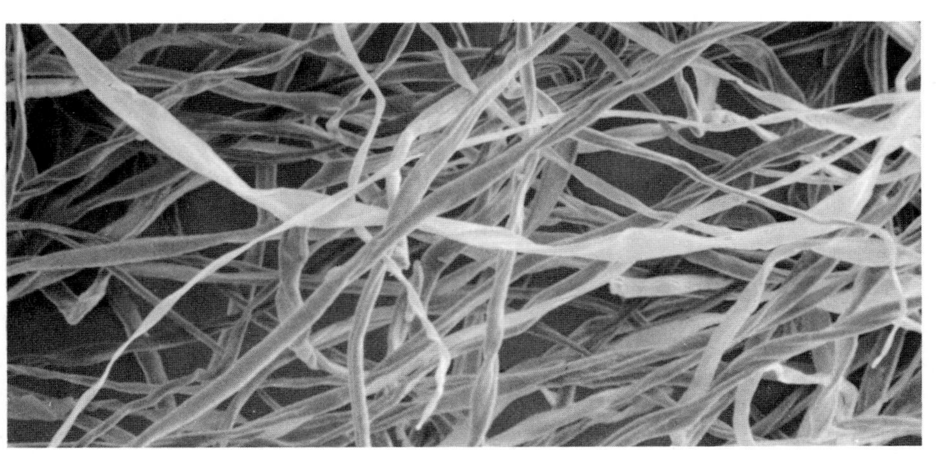

COTTON
Magnification: × 150.

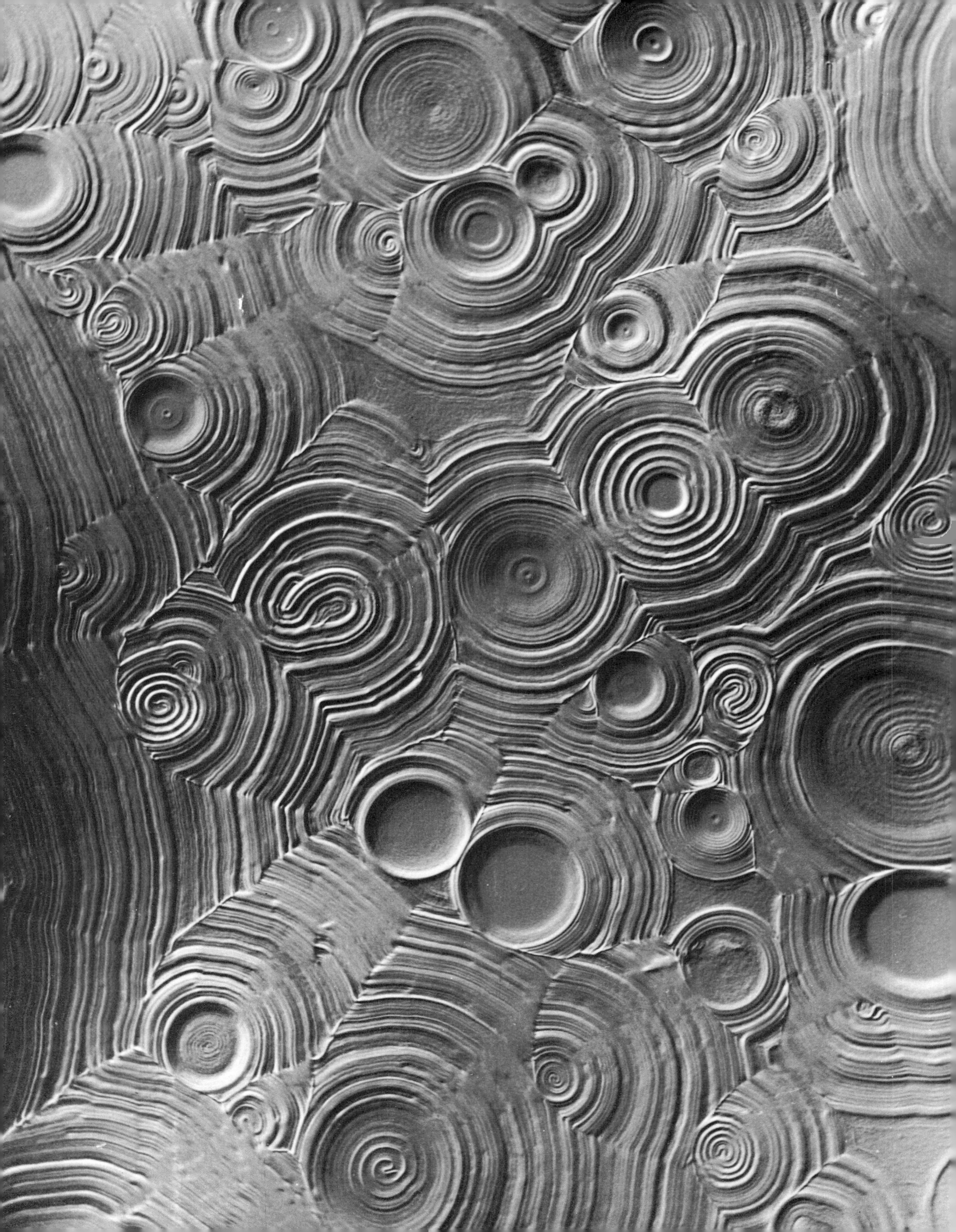

◁ **SOAP**
Magnification: × 200.

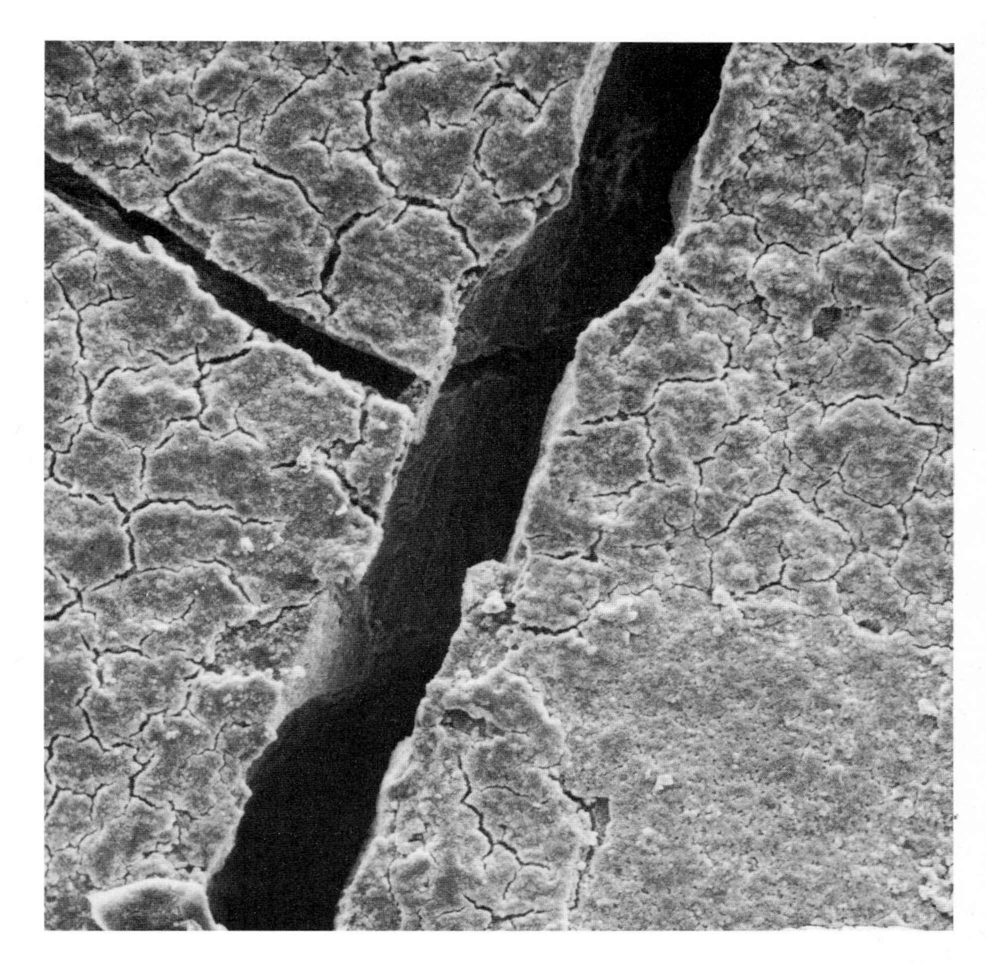

CRACK IN EGG
Magnification: × 1000.

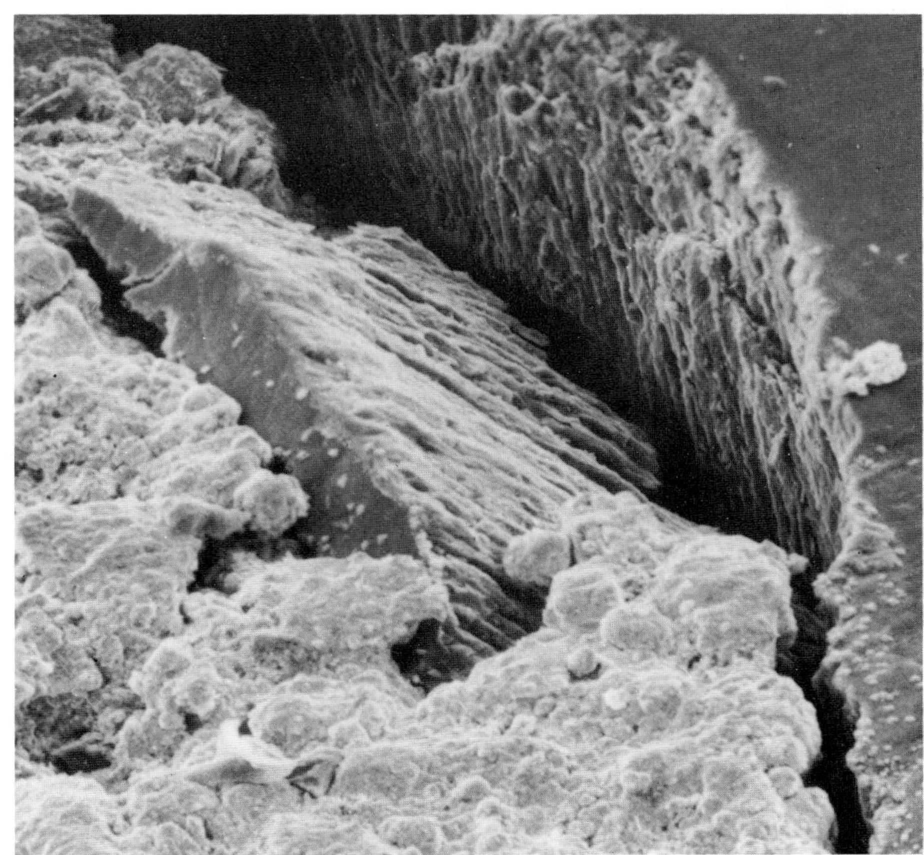

BROKEN TOOTH
Magnification: × 500.

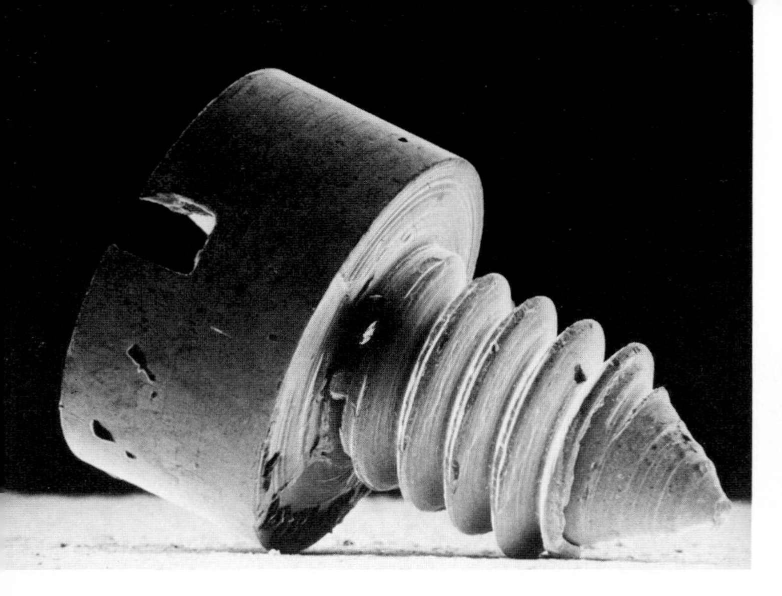

BALANCE SCREW OF A WRISTWATCH
Magnification: × 300.

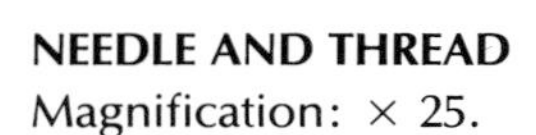

NEEDLE AND THREAD
Magnification: × 25.

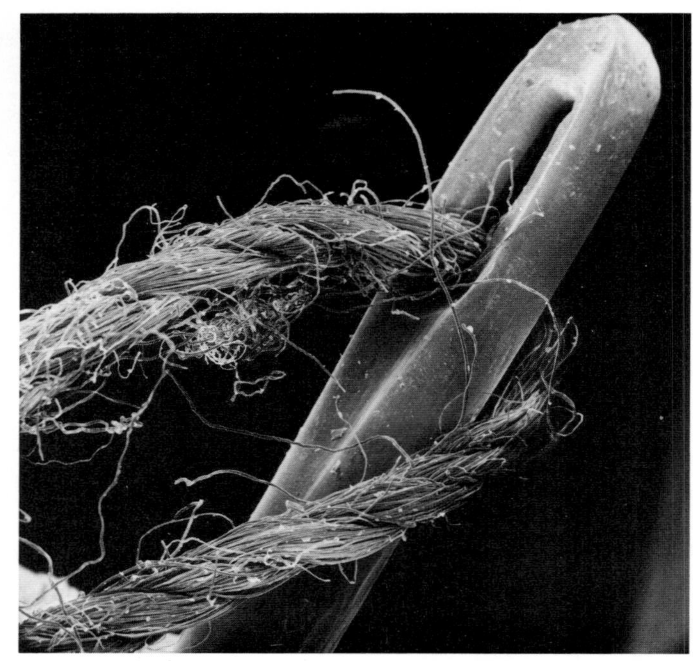

HONEYBEE STINGER
Magnification: × 1500.

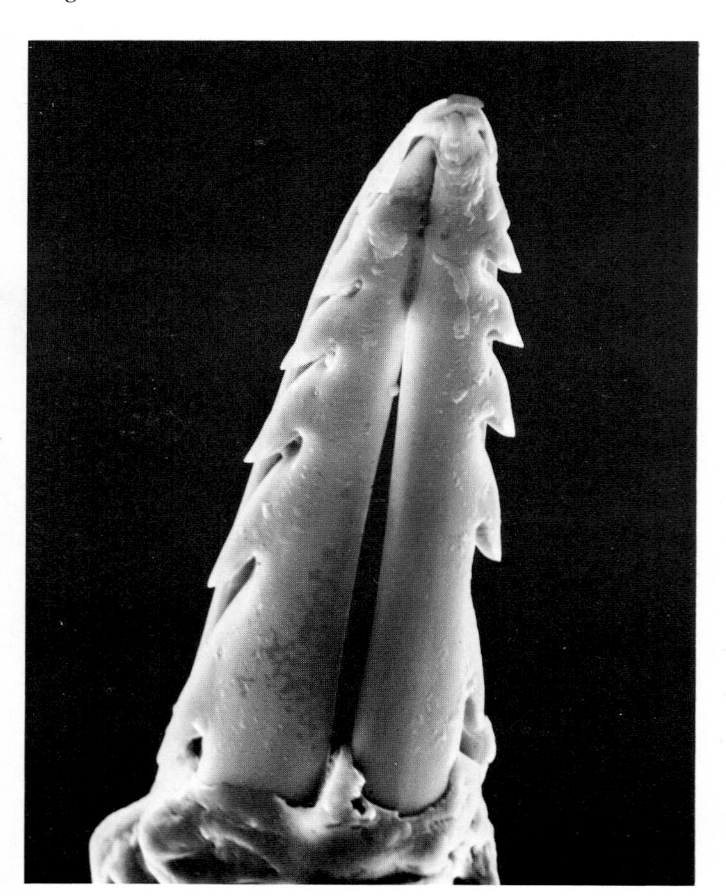

DIAMOND-STUDDED DENTIST'S DRILL
Magnification: × 250.

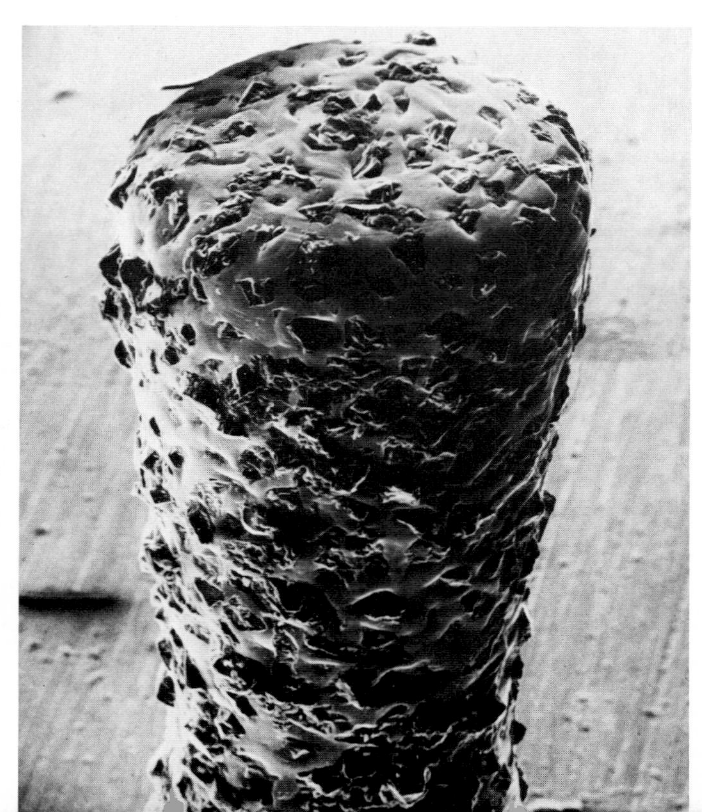

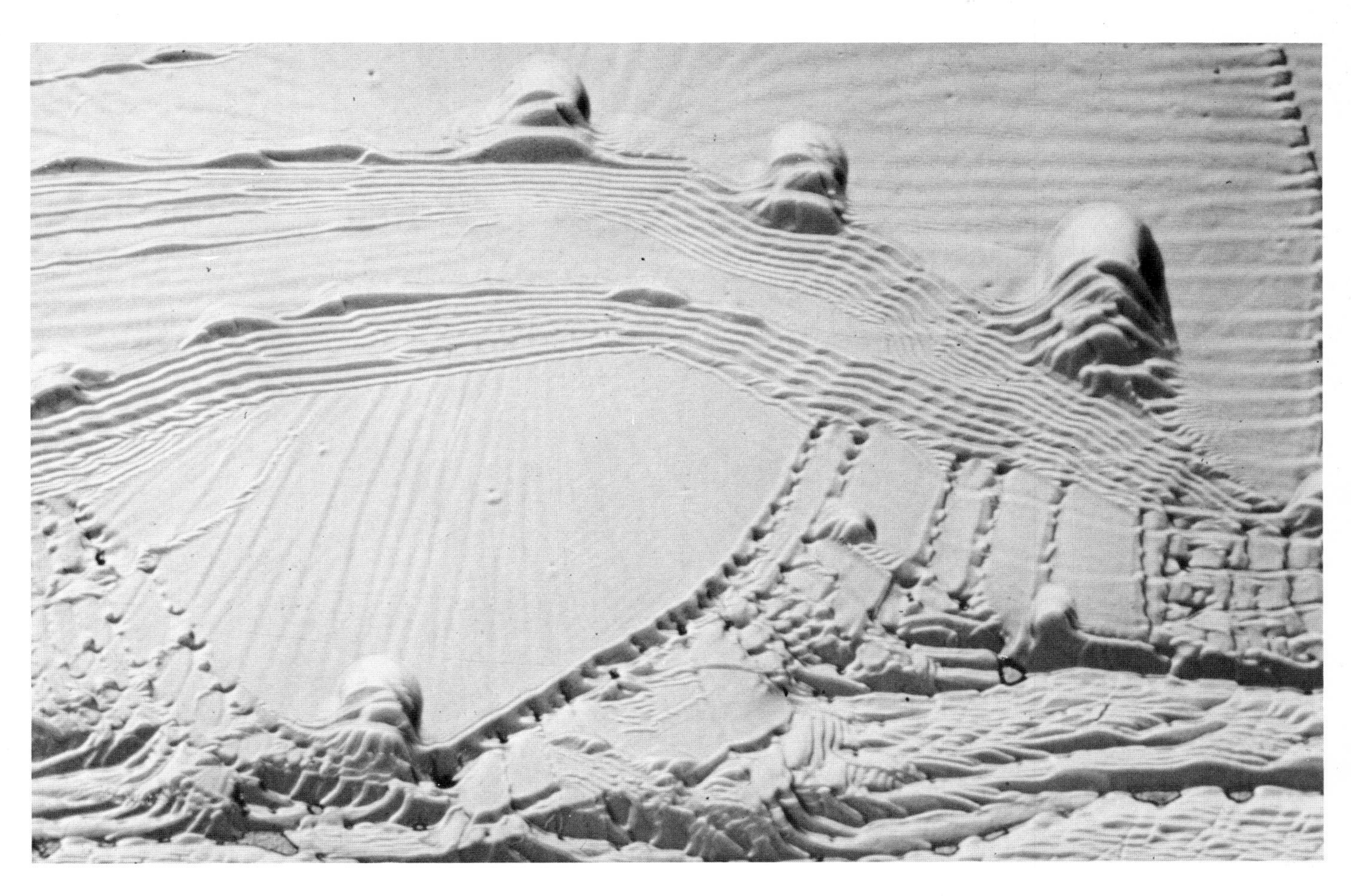

GOLD
Magnification: × 55.

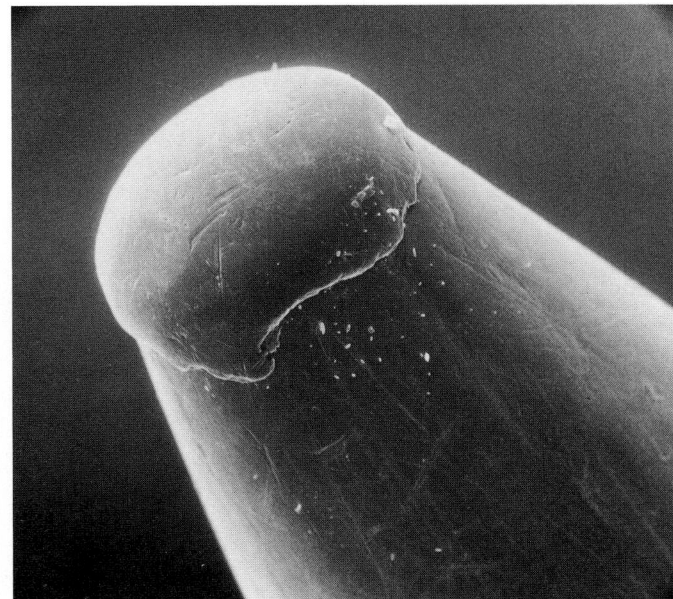

DULL PIN TIP
Magnification: × 40.

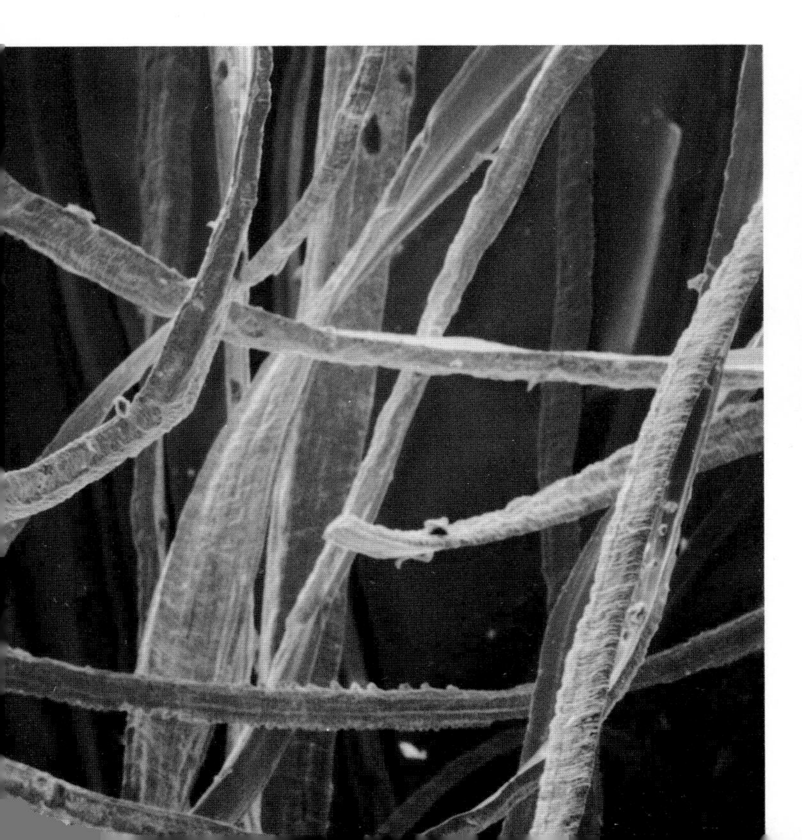

STEEL WOOL
Magnification: × 150.

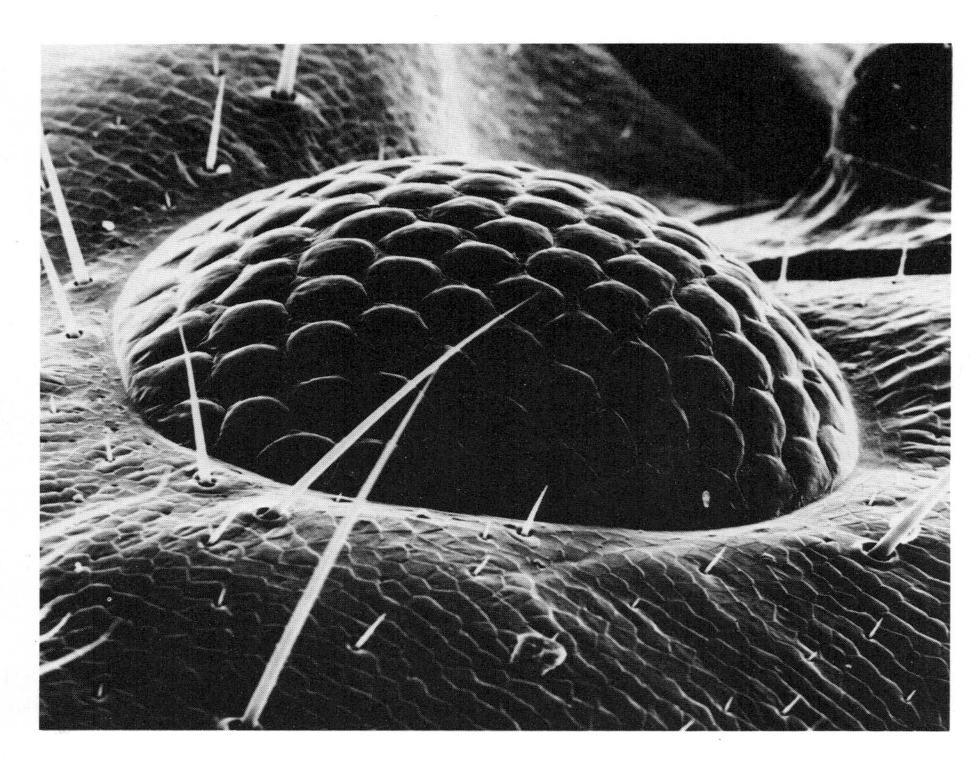

ANT EYE
Magnification: × 250.

ANT
Magnification: × 200.

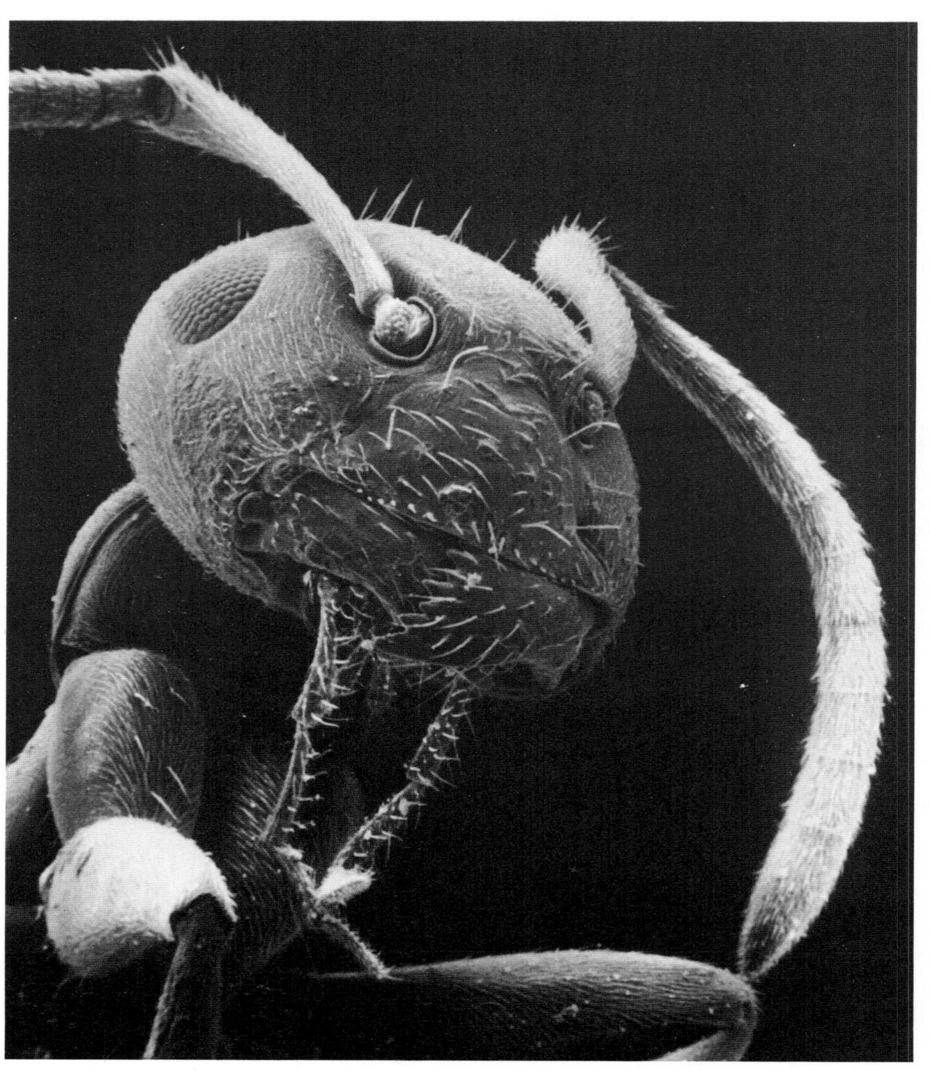

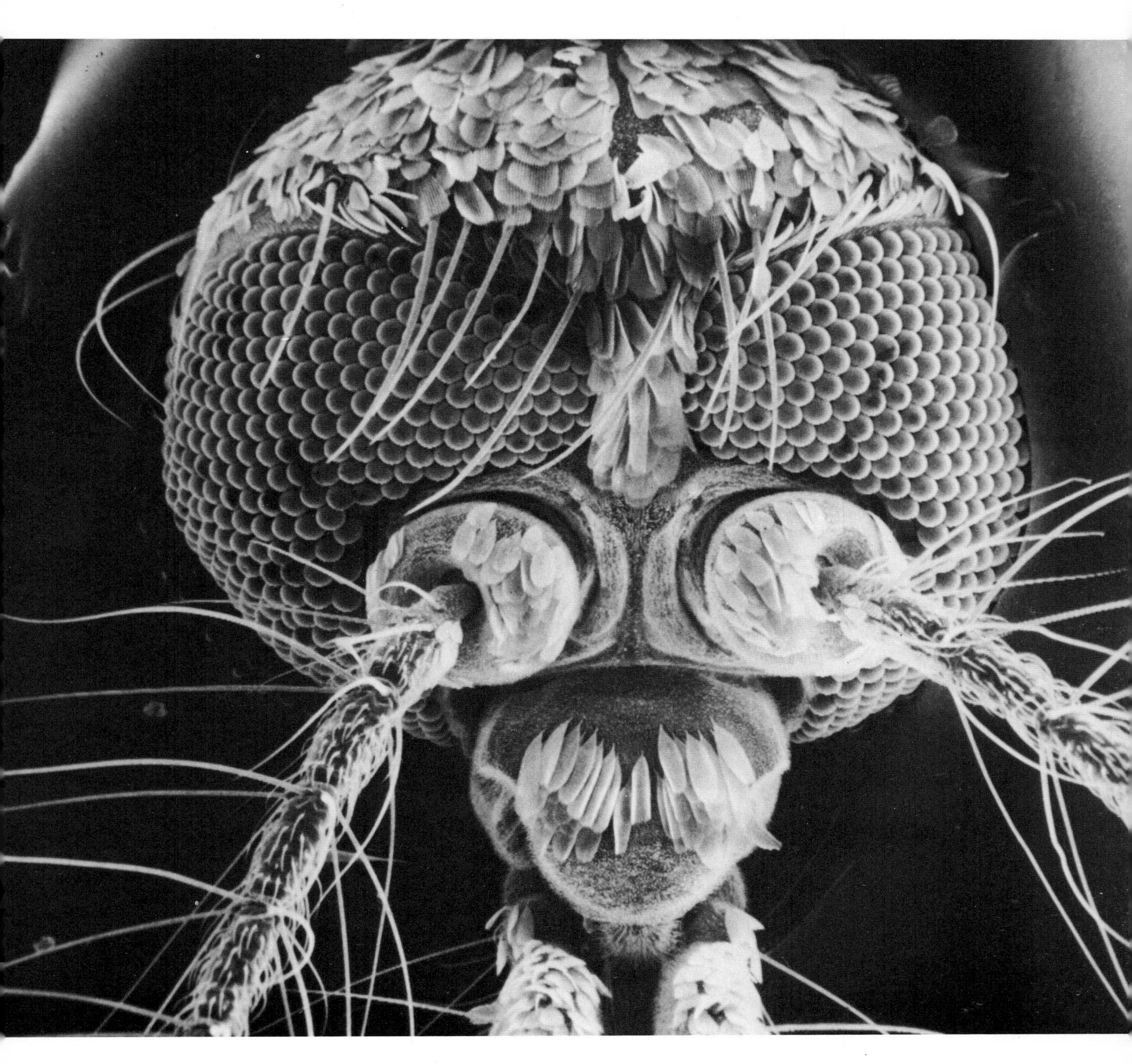

MOSQUITO
Magnification: × 200.

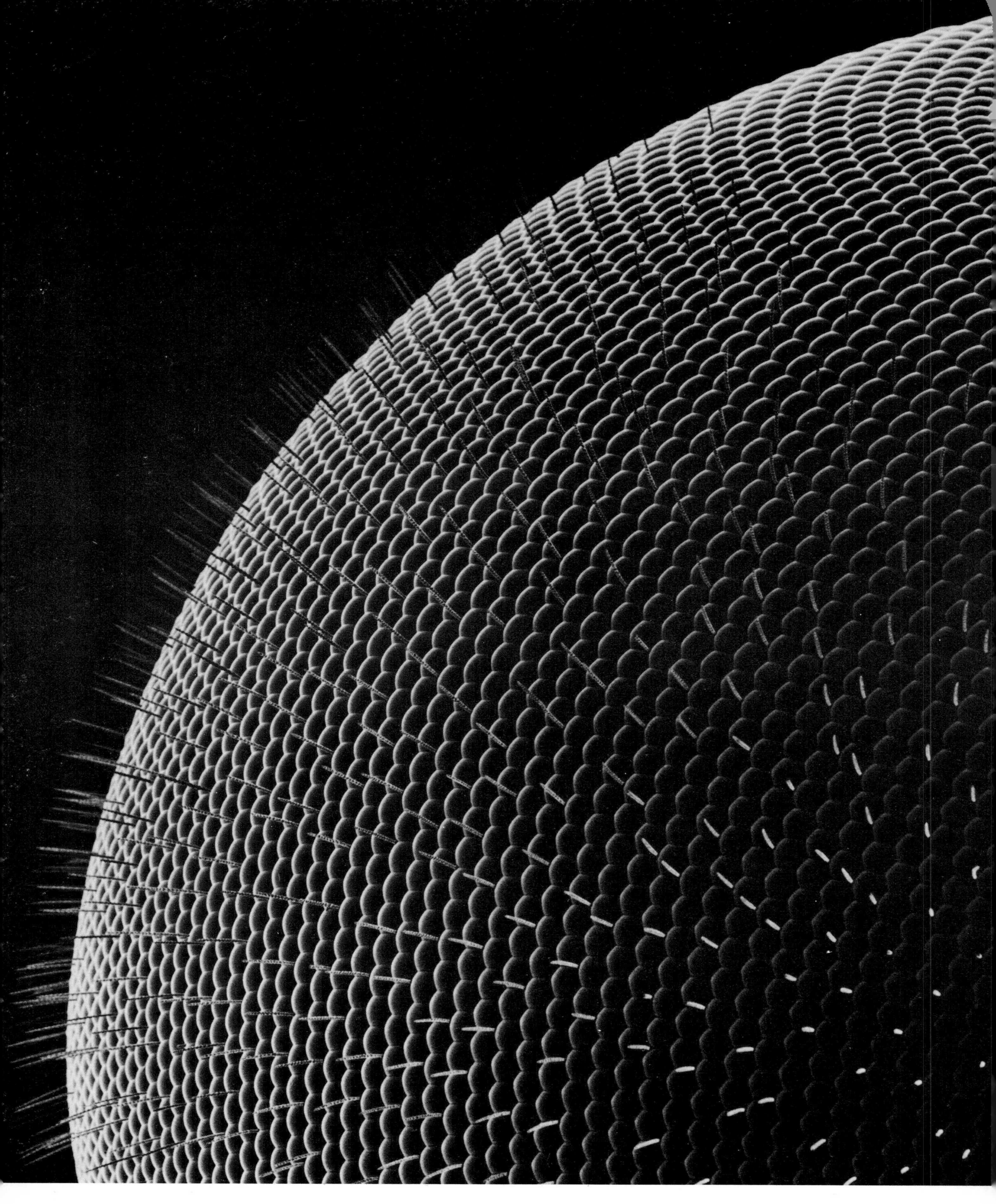

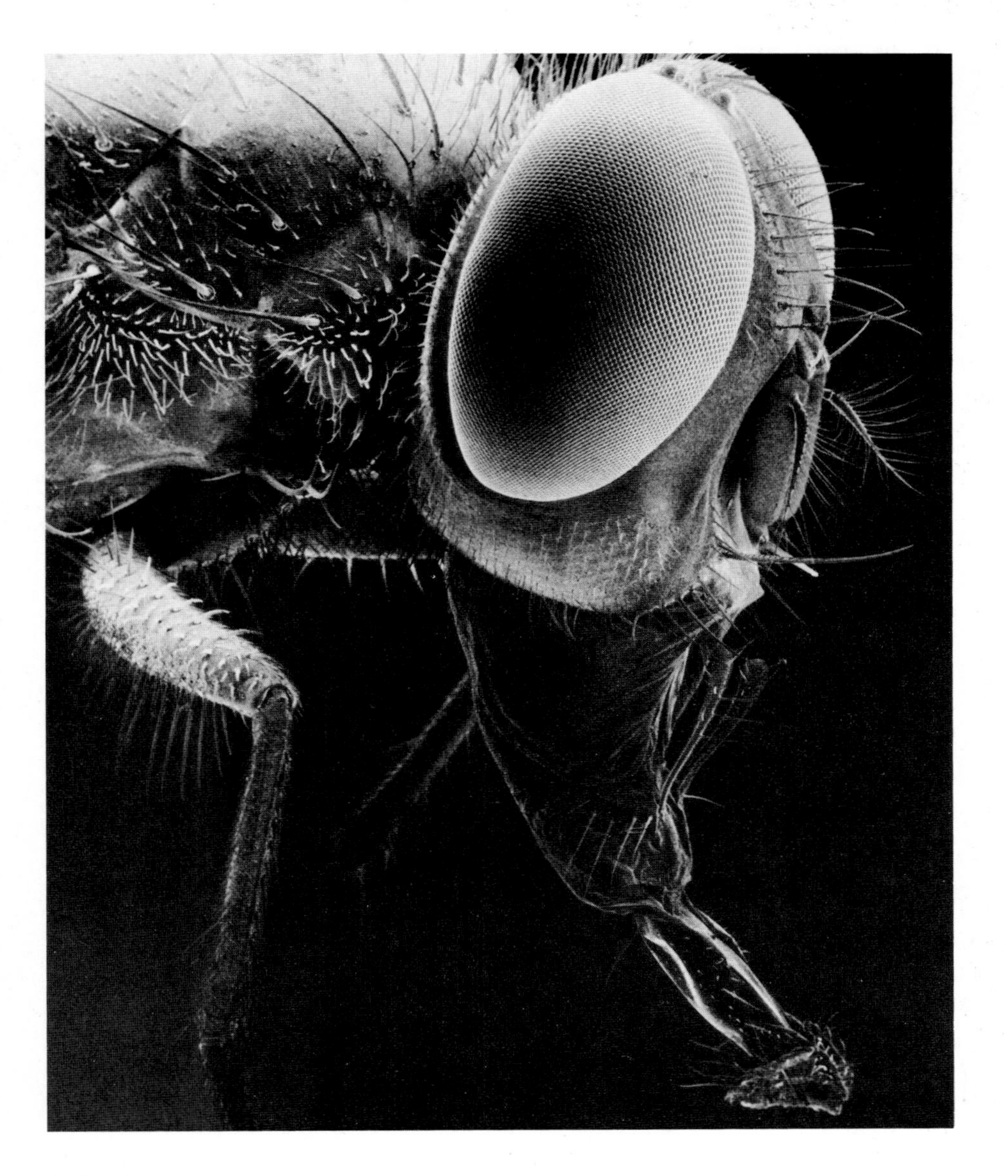

GREENBOTTLE FLY
Magnification: × 20.

FLY TONGUE ▷
Magnification: × 30.

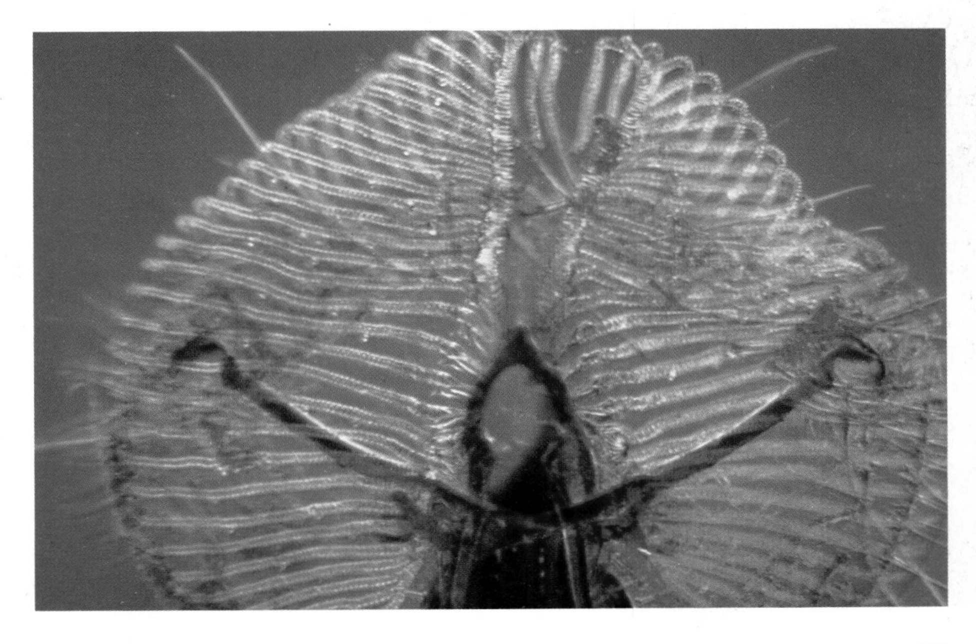

◁ **FLY EYE**
Magnification: × 400.

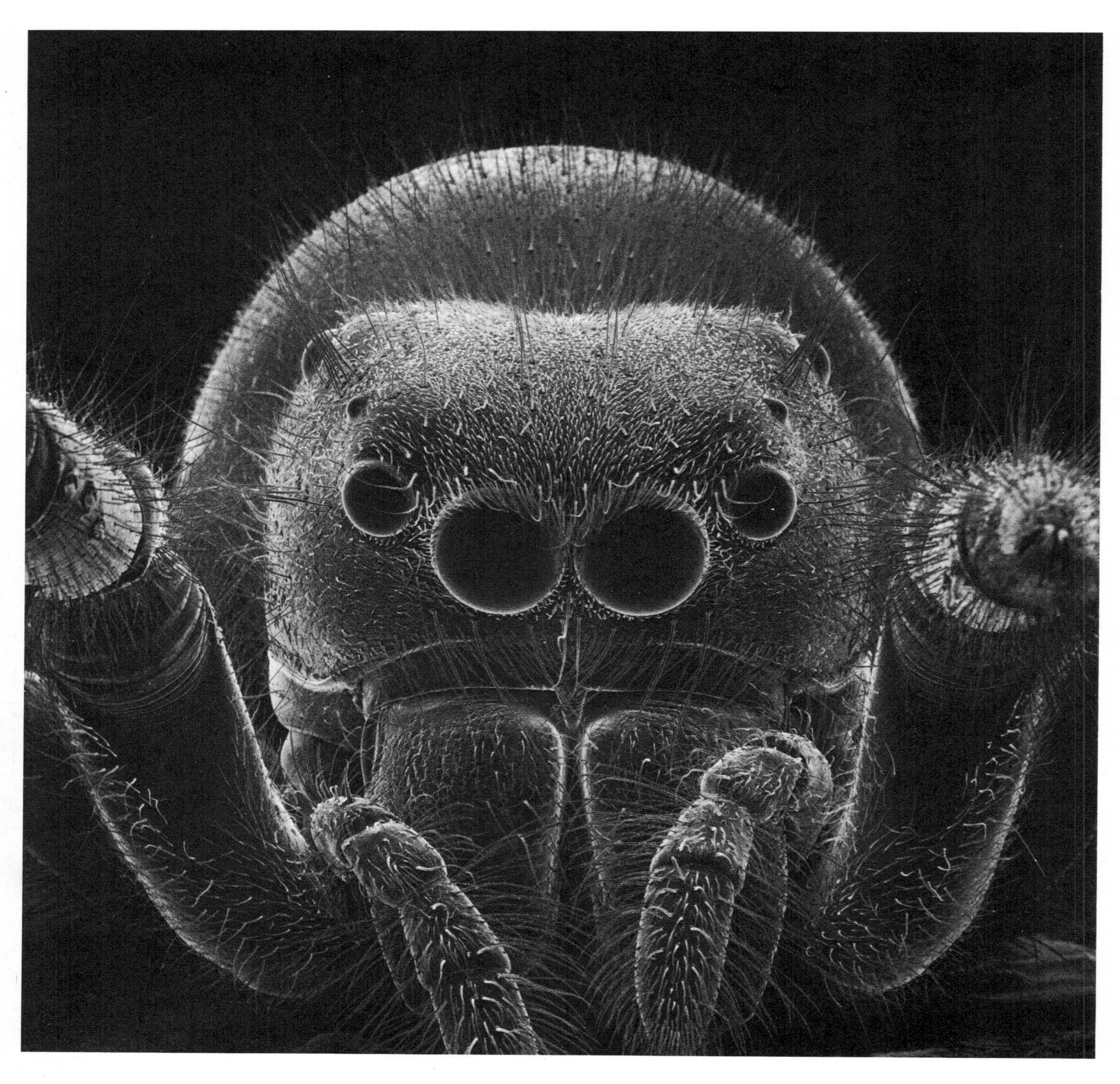

JUMPING SPIDER
Magnification: × 50.

BABY STRAWBERRY ▷
Magnification: × 80.

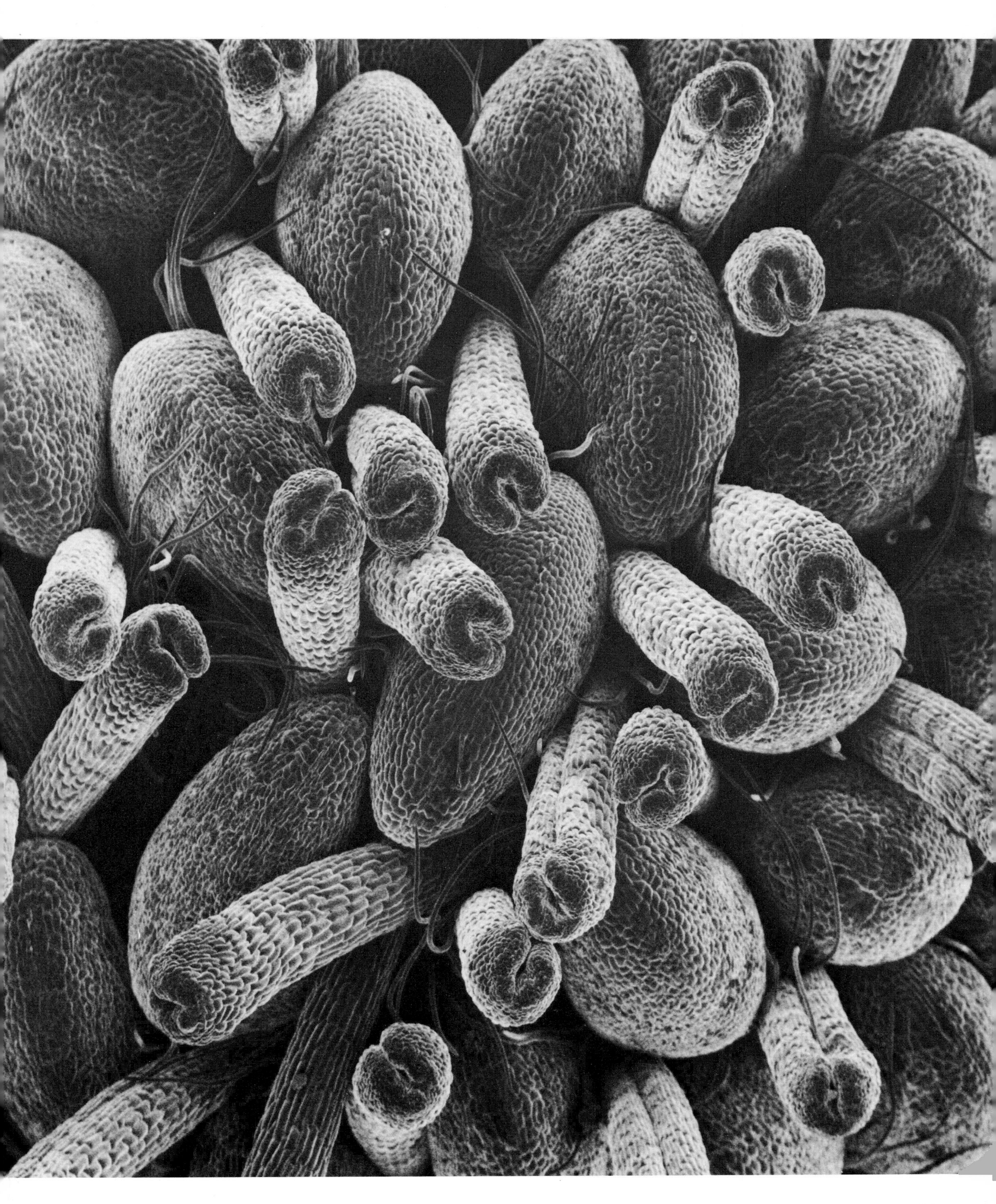

MICROSCAPES

Similar patterns and forms seem to repeat themselves throughout every scale of existence. Hidden within the realm of things that are too small for the naked eye to see lie miniature landscapes that seem to mimic geographies that we know.

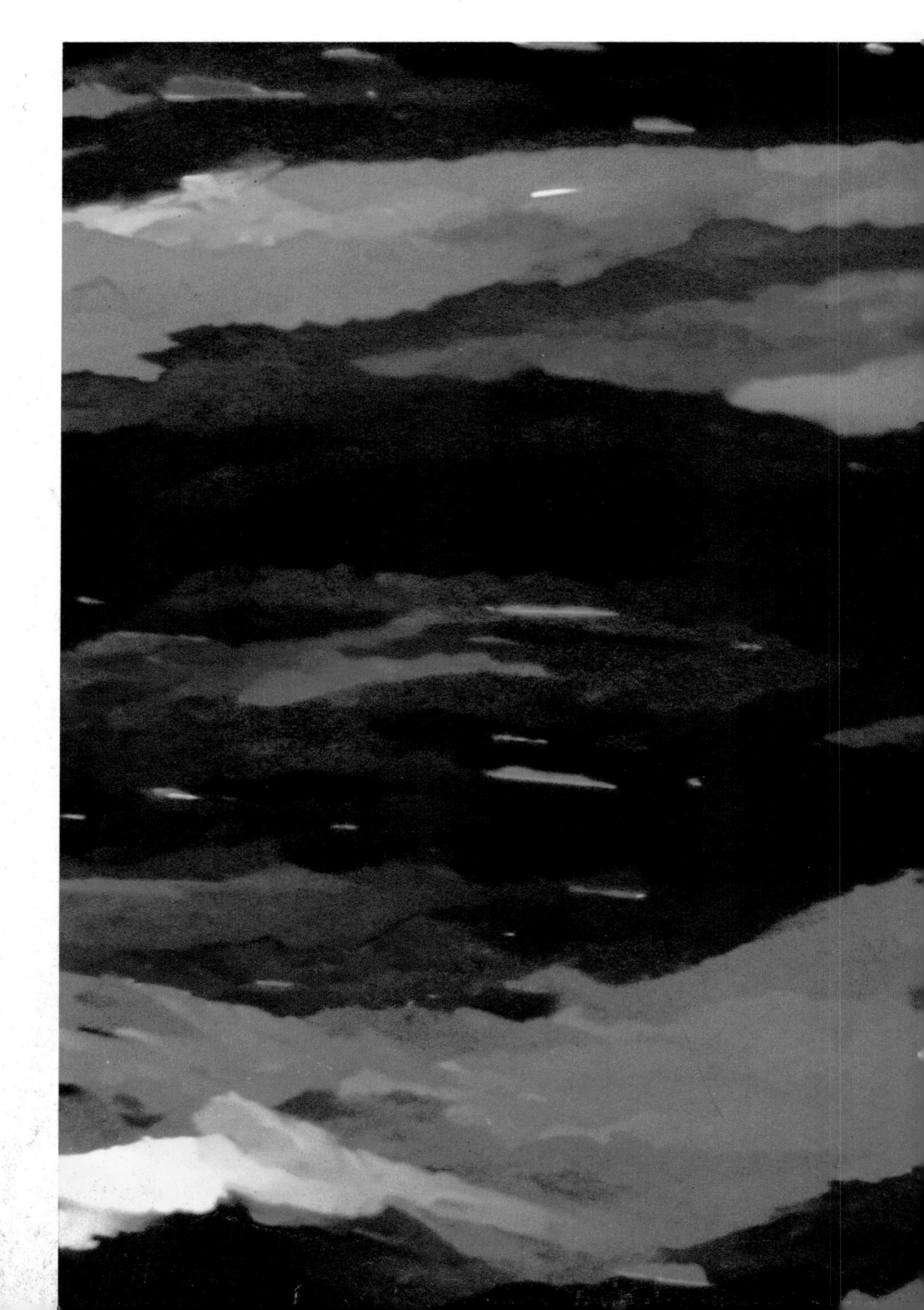

PAINTED DESERT
What appears to be an abstract desert landscape is actually a crystal of sulphonal—a sleeping pill—magnified 40 times.

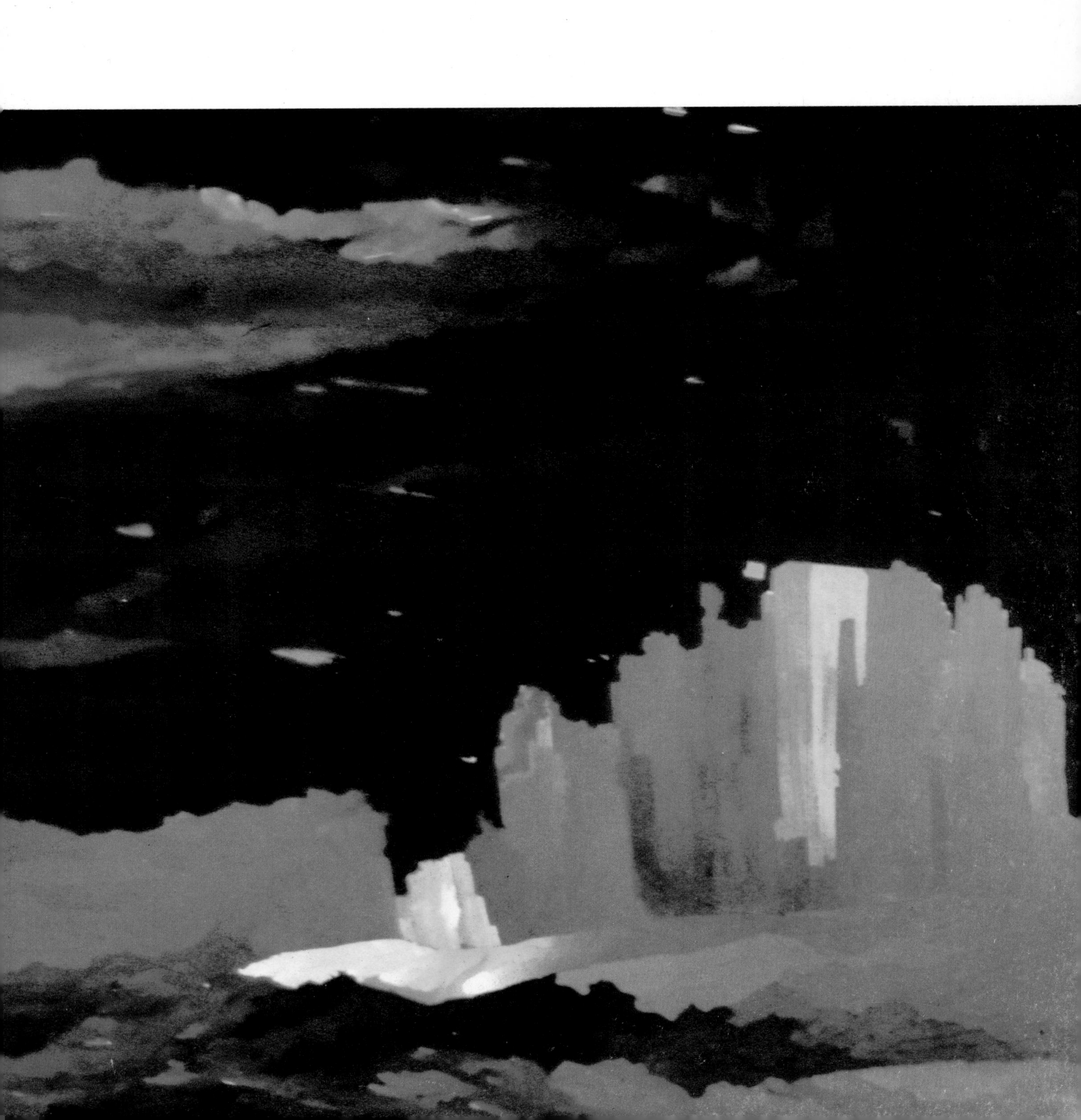

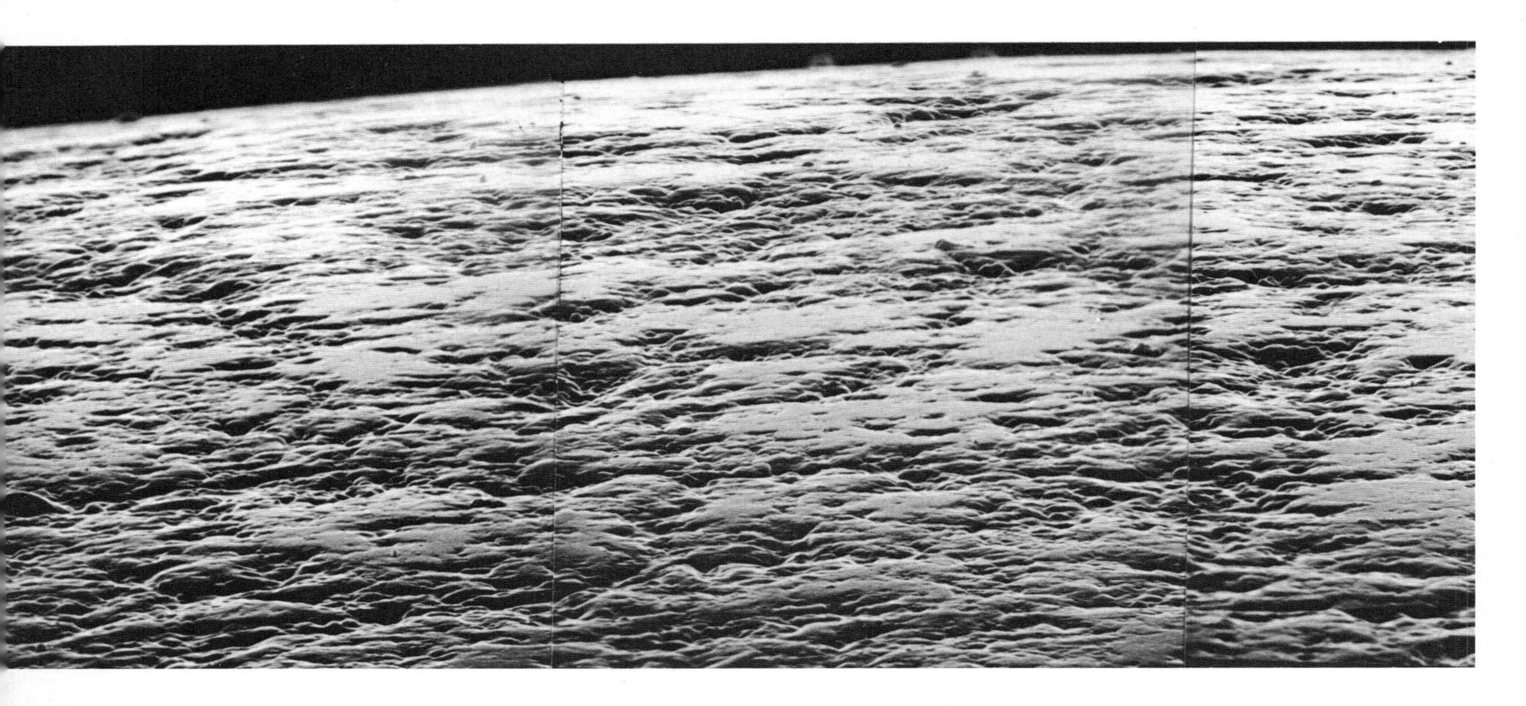

MOON
When the tip of a ballpoint pen is enlarged 5150 times, a barren lunarscape appears.

MIRAGE
Migrating cells moving across a layer of gold appear to be a strange desert sand dune. Magnification: × 1580.

ROCKS ▷
This pile of boulders is really common table salt, magnified 50 times by a scanning electron microscope.

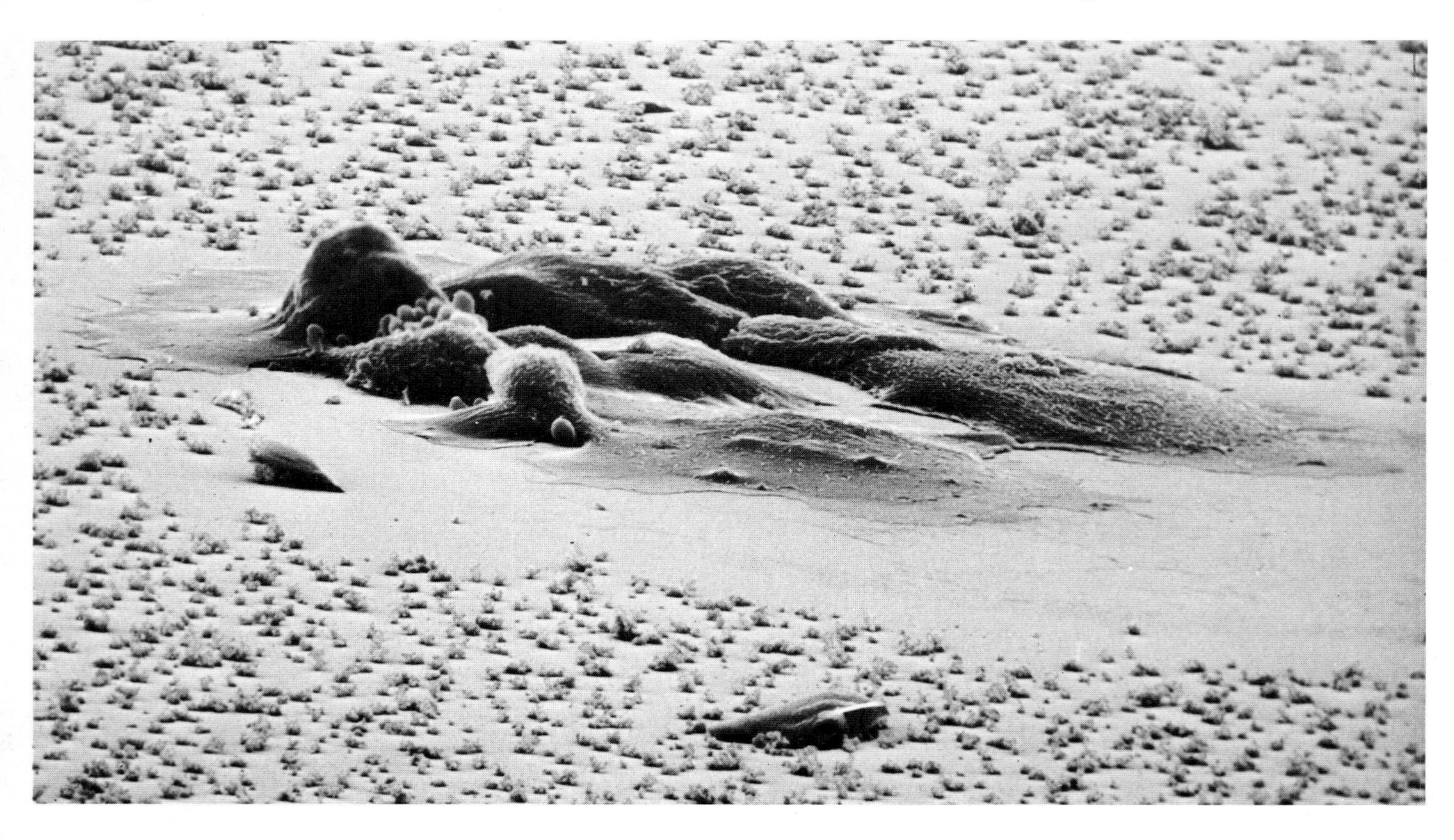

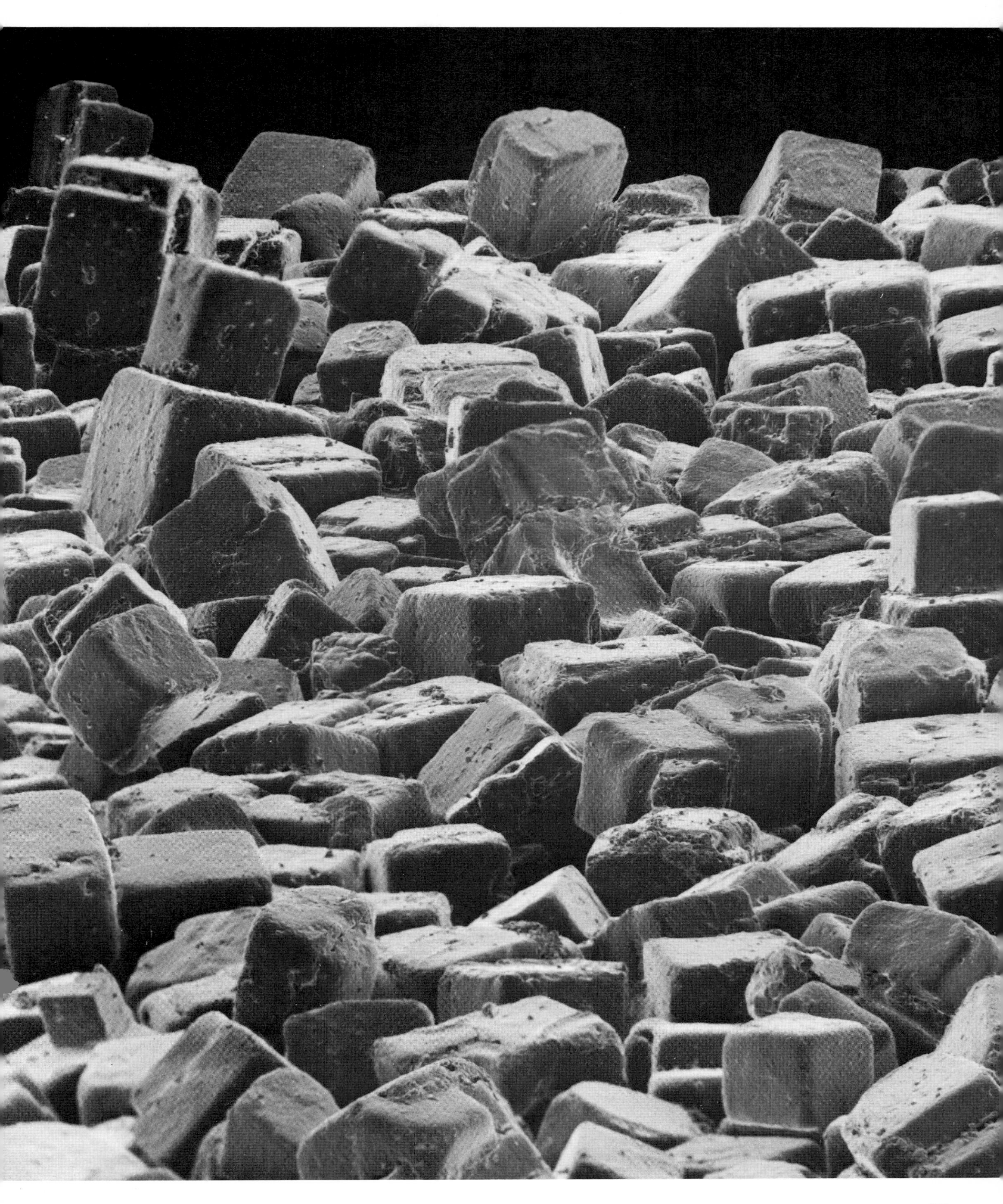

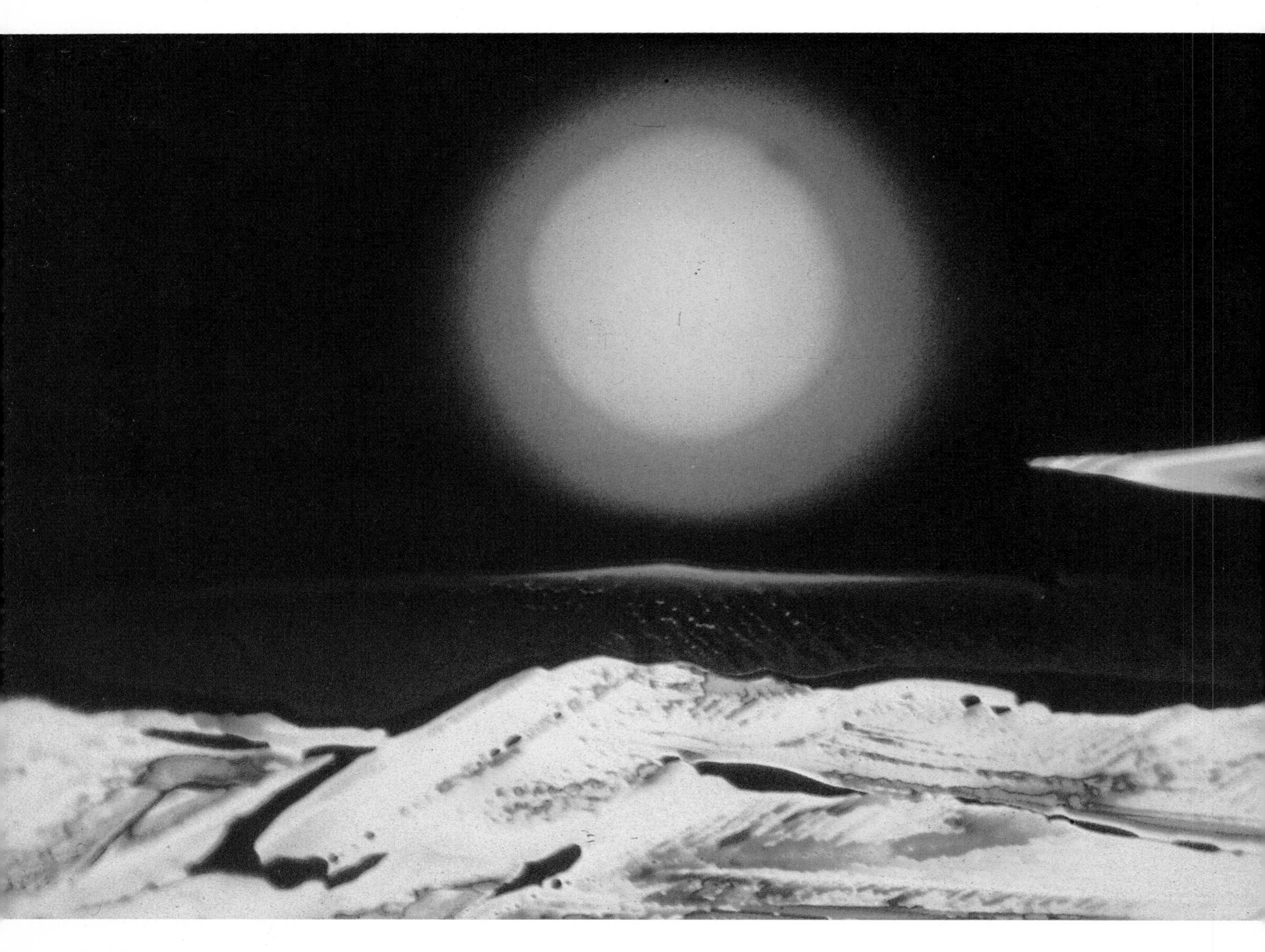

SUNRISE
What might be a dawn in some faraway world is actually a dye called aceto-toluidine. Magnification: × 100.

MOUNTAIN
This jagged geological formation is a crystallized form of methyl alcohol, magnified 175 times.

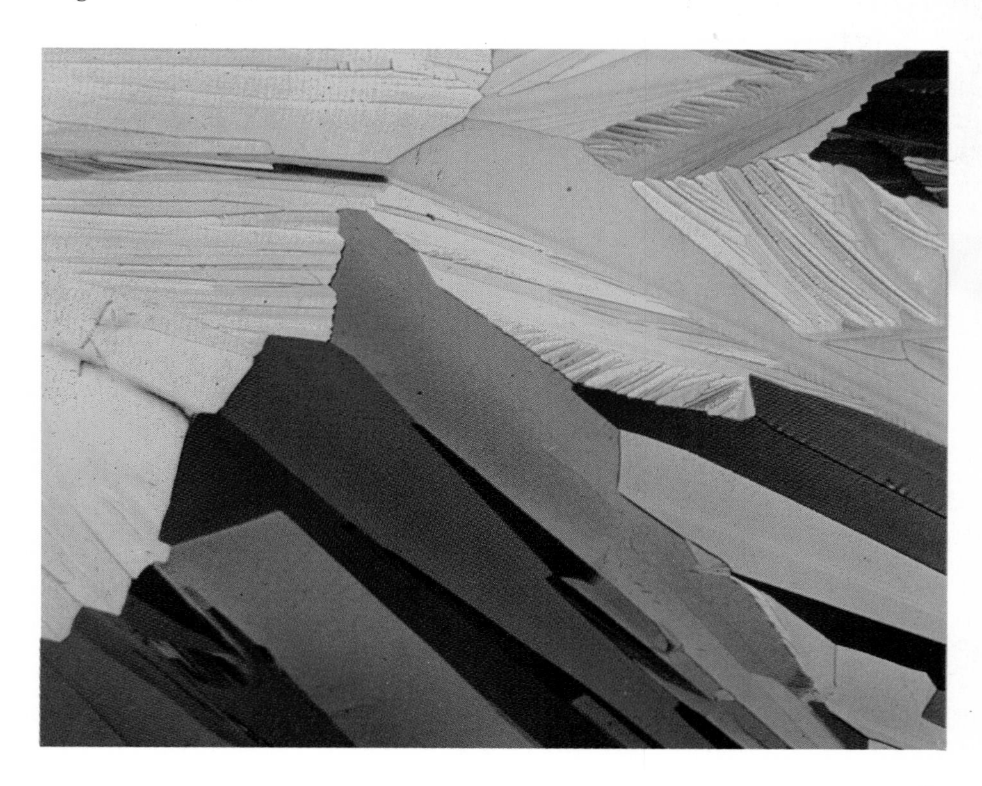

CLIFF
Not the white cliffs of Dover, but an electron micrograph of a fractured eggshell.
Magnification: × 1200.

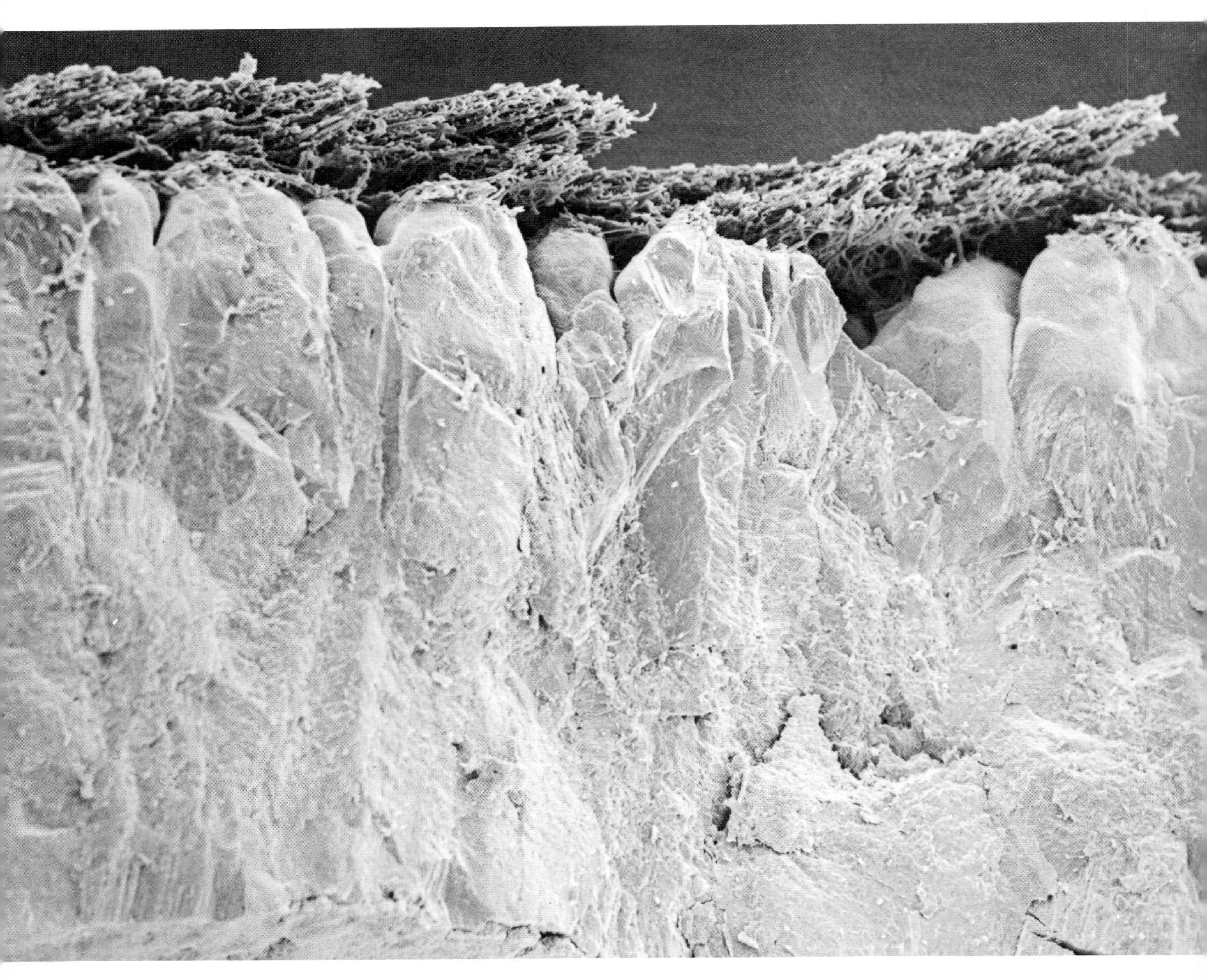

RIVERBED

What looks like an aerial photograph of a dry desert riverbed is, in fact, a piece of liver tissue magnified 100,000 times. The meandering channel is the thin membrane between two cells.

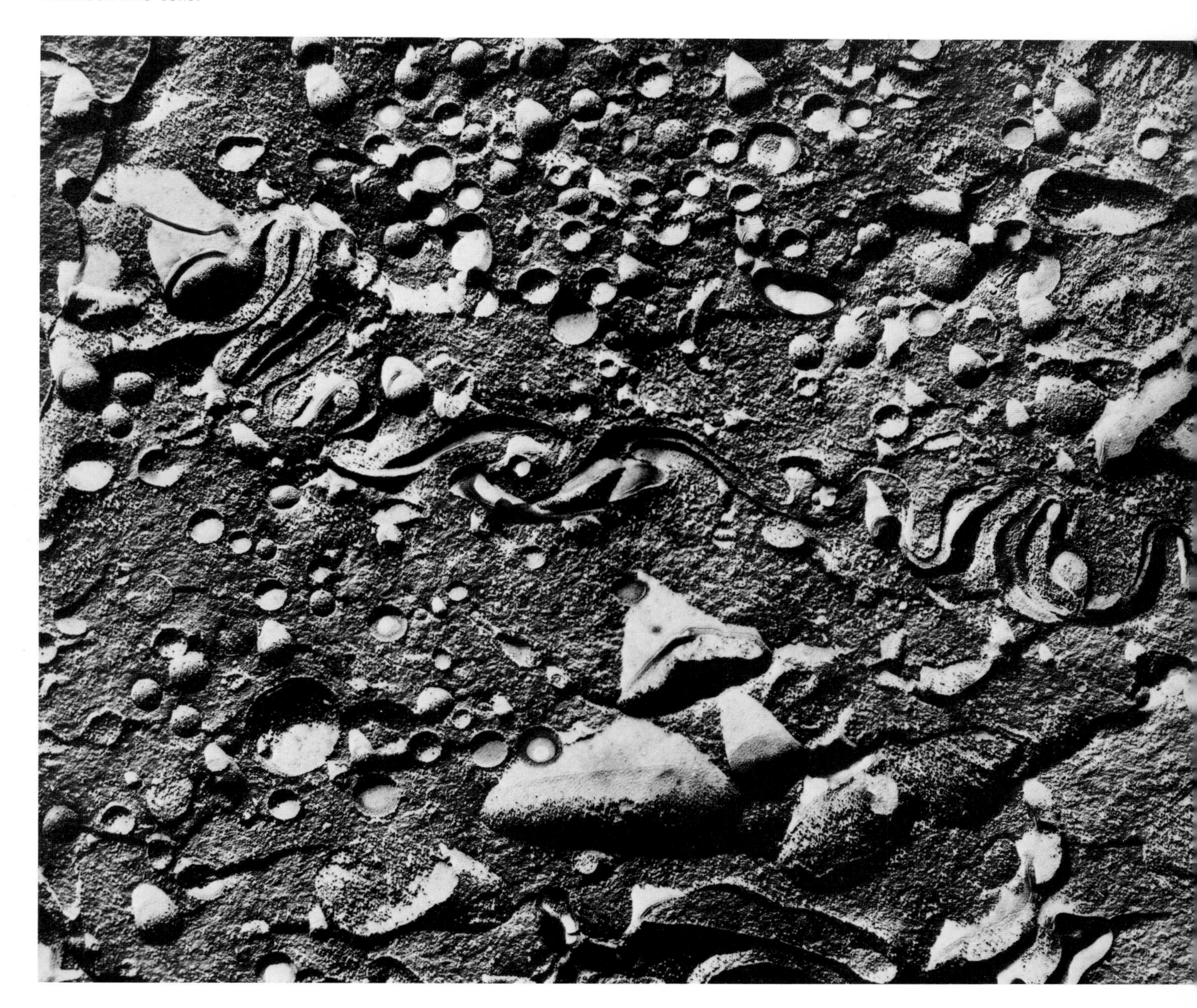

WILDLIFE . . . AT HOME

In our sofas and beds, on our floors and carpets, even in our food, millions of microscopic creatures quietly live their lives.

Though some may look like miniature dinosaurs from a long lost world, their bodies rarely grow large enough for the naked eye to see.

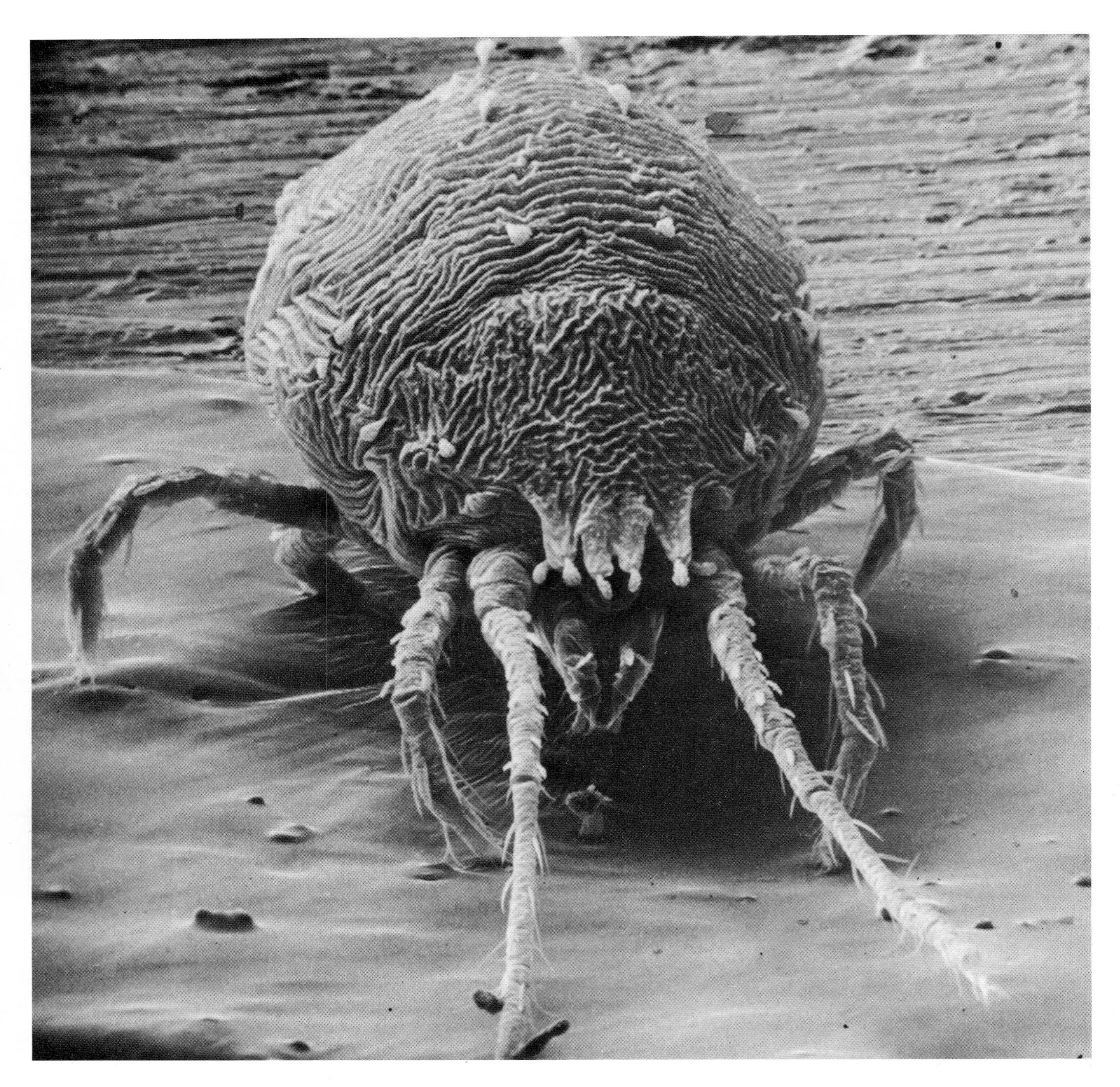

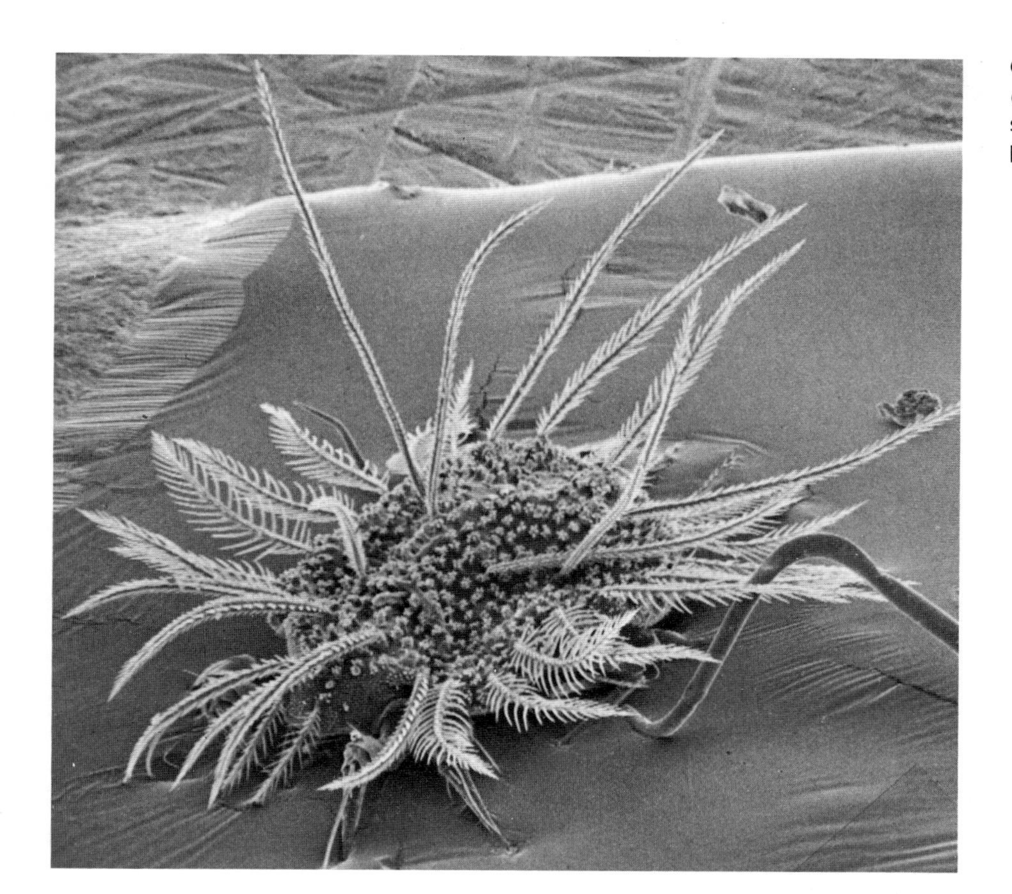

GRAIN MITE

Ctenoglyphus pluminger likes to live in stored cereals, flour, and other grain products. Magnification: × 200.

◁ **BRYOBIA**

This microscopic mite infests the interiors of buildings. Although they are not known to do any damage, large colonies of them have rendered homes unsalable until they were removed. Magnification: × 50.

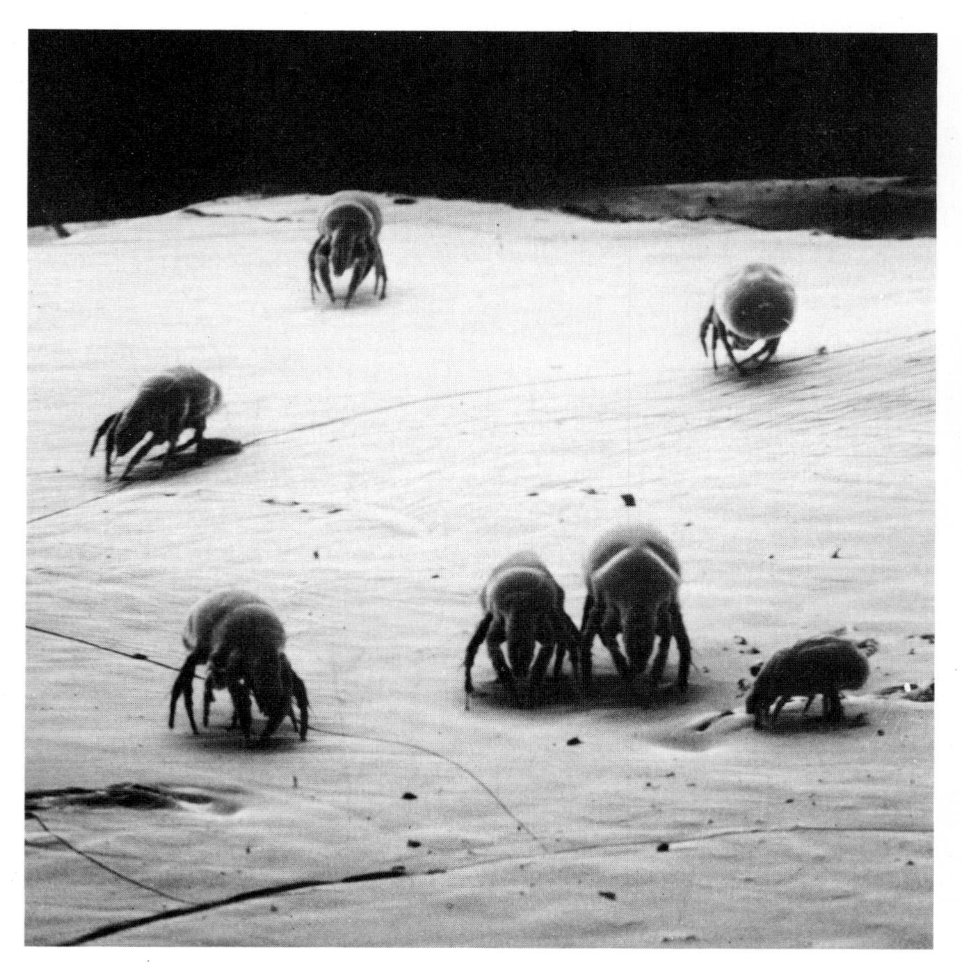

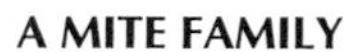

A MITE FAMILY

A family of flour mites, magnified 85 times. These tiny creatures are not insects. They have eight legs and are classified as Arachnids, a group of animals that includes spiders and scorpions. Altogether there are at least a million different species of mites. They have successfully adapted to a wide range of habitats throughout the world. This particular mite is fond of living in flour and other stored grain products. If you look very closely, you may be able to find one in your home.

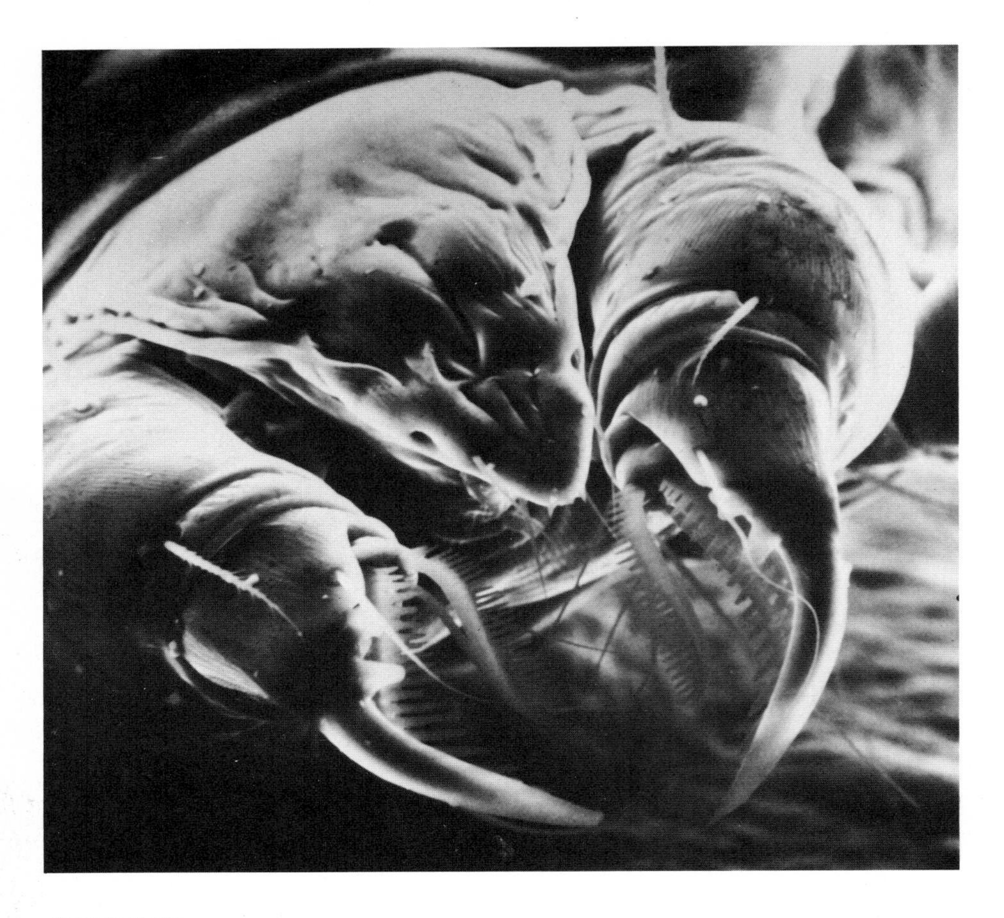

KILLER MITE

The large claws of this predatory mite make it a formidable foe. It attacks and feeds on other mites. Magnification: × 250.

DUST MITES

Dependent on us for survival, invisible dust mites live in our beds and upholstered furniture. They feed primarily on the flakes of dead skin that our bodies constantly shed. Magnification: $\times$ 250.

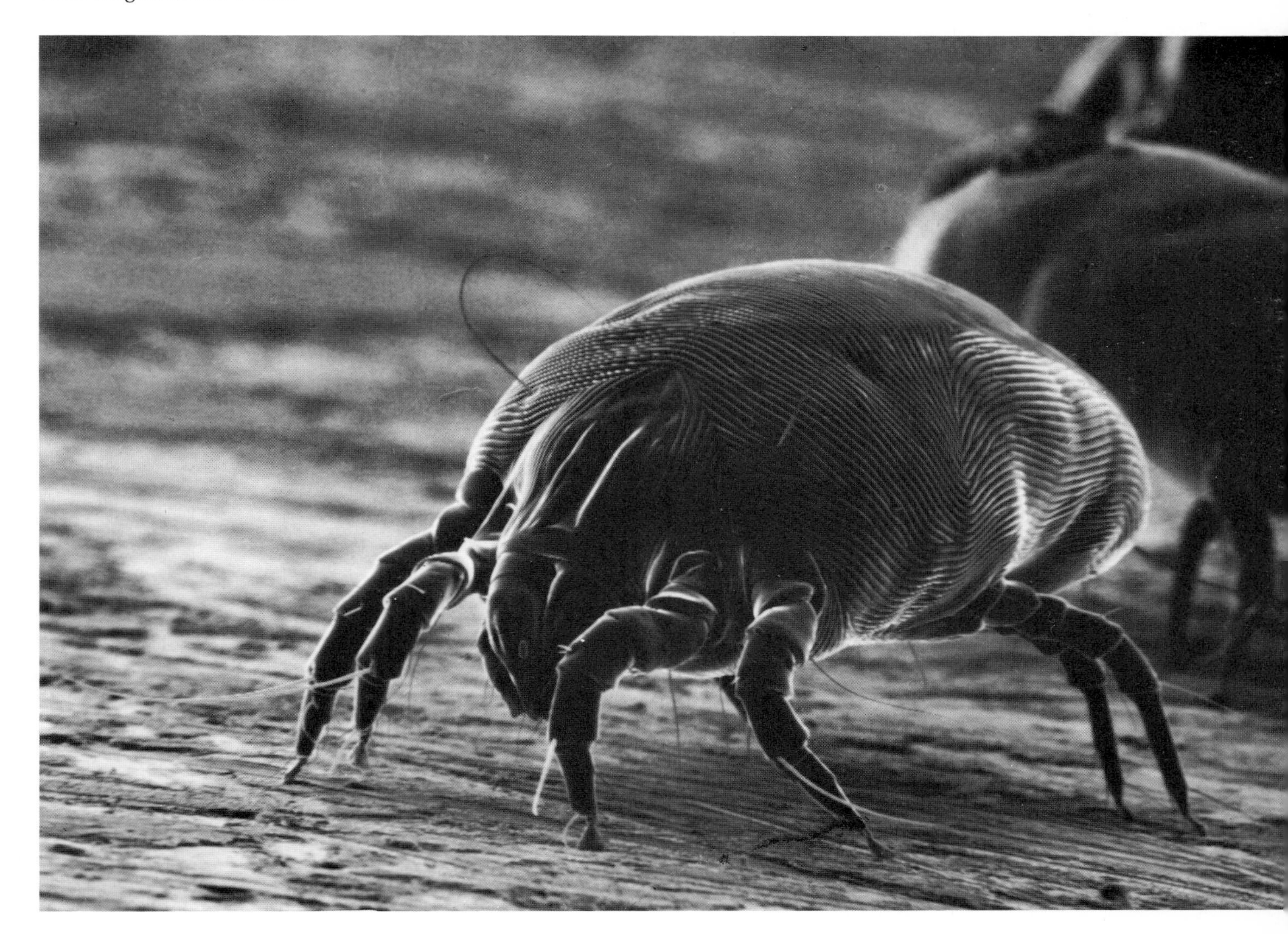

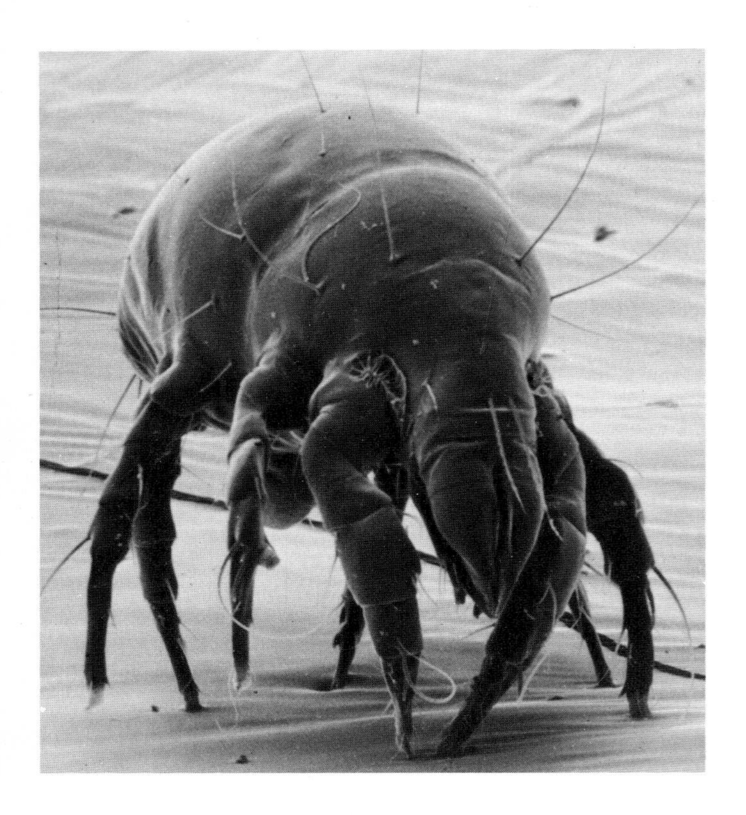

FLOUR MITE
Its scientific name is *Acarus siro* and, like the grain mite, this one also infects flour and other stored products. Magnification: × 250.

FAMILY OF DUST MITES
In this family portrait, mom is the largest. Magnification: × 200.

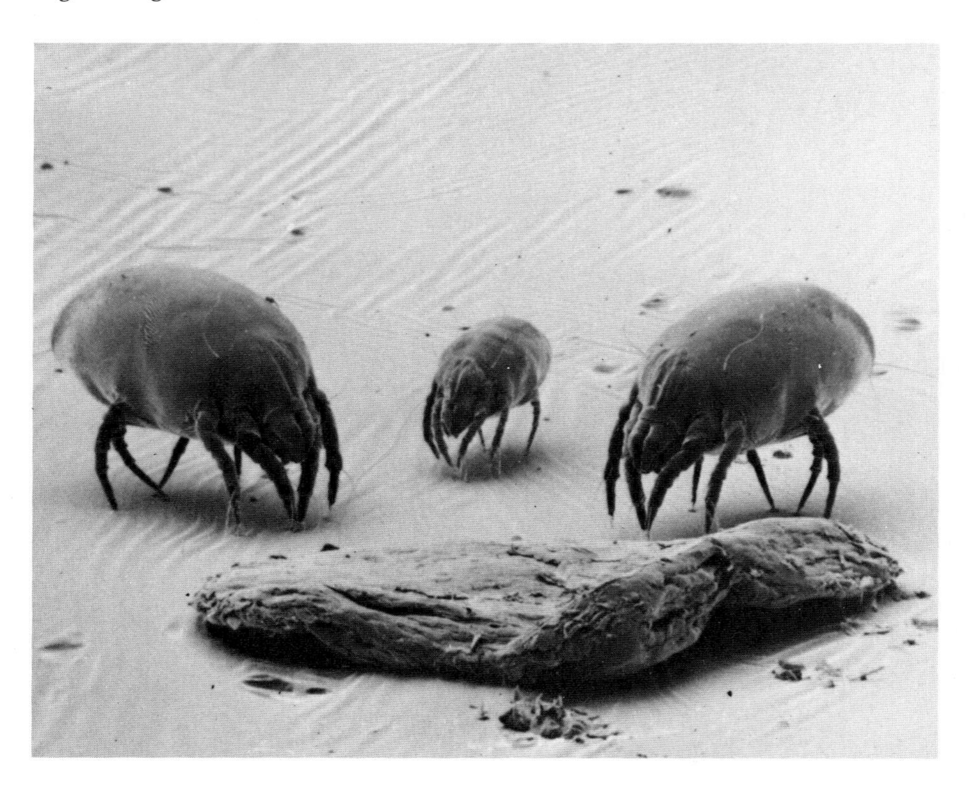

LIFE THAT LIVES ON US

The surface of our skin hides an incredible miniature world from the normal view of our eyes. When seen at high magnification, an alien landscape abundant with life suddenly appears.

Each of us is the keeper of a huge invisible zoo. In fact, at any given time, there are as many creatures living on our bodies as there are people on Earth.

If our numerous companions do not inspire our love, at least we have the consolation of knowing that we are never completely alone.

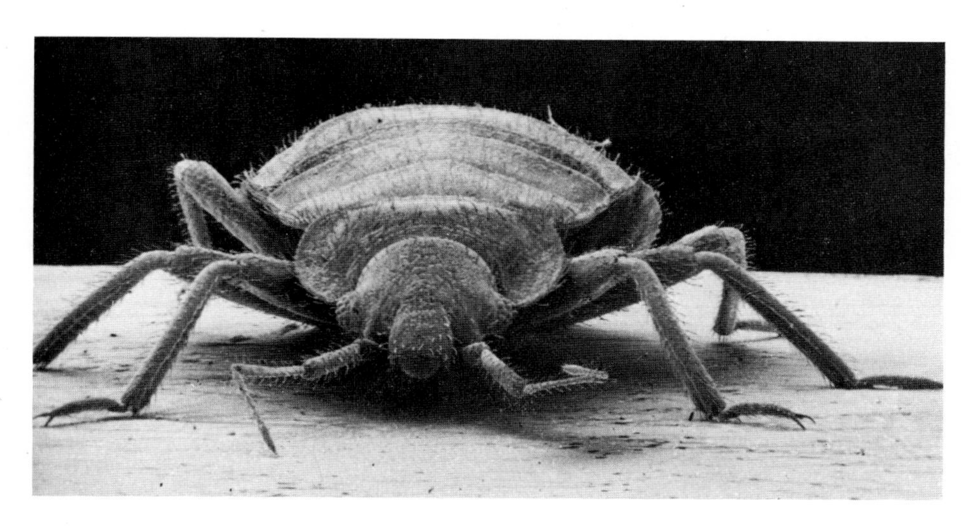

BEDBUG
Cimex lectularius, the bedbug, is most famous for its favorite home—our beds. It can also live in the cracks of walls and in furniture. A single bedbug can live for more than a year. This microvampire survives by piercing our skin and sucking away a few drops of blood per meal. The bedbug can feed on any warm-blooded animal. The most common time for feeding is between 3 A.M. and 6 A.M. Magnification: × 300.

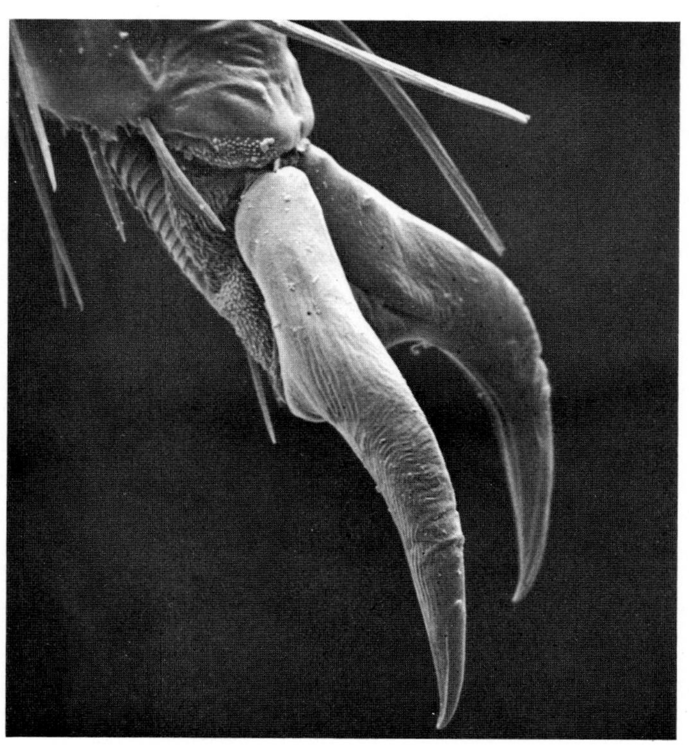

BEDBUG CLAW
The razor-sharp claw of a bedbug, magnified 720 times, gives this aggressive intruder a powerful hold on its victims.

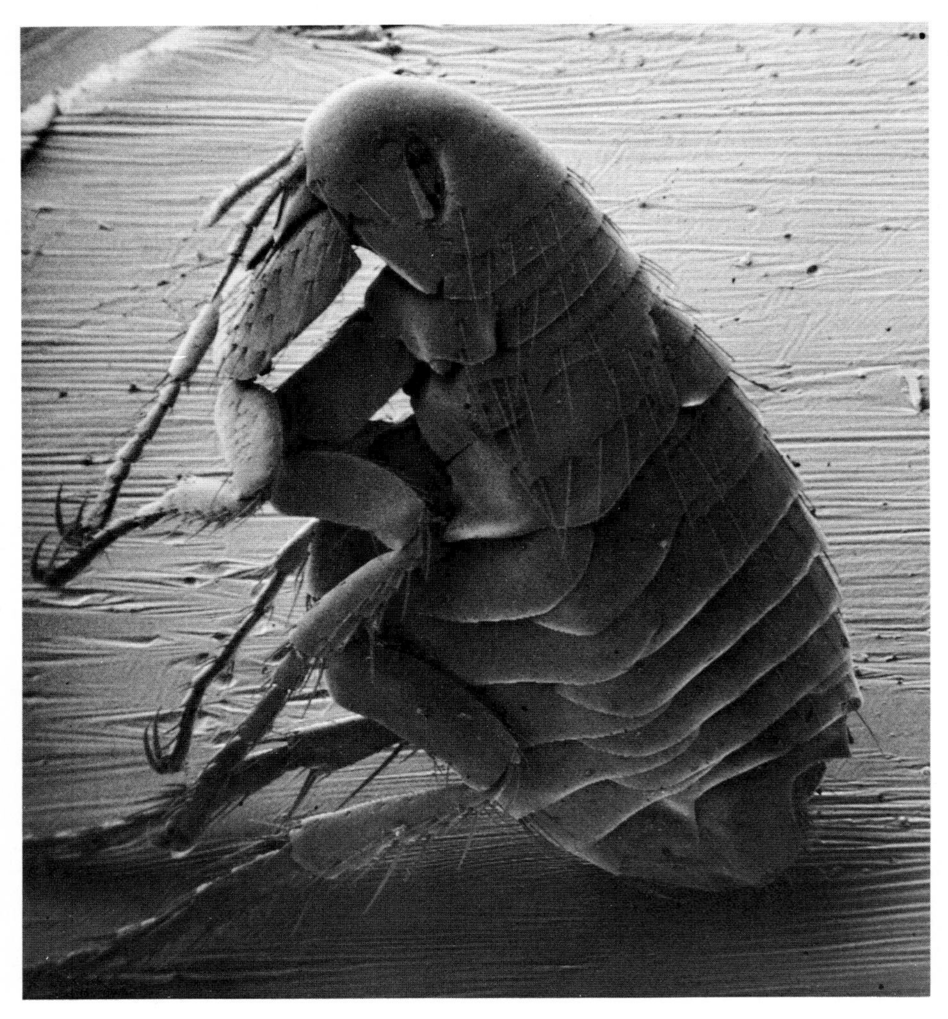

PORTRAITS OF A FLEA

There are over two thousand species of flea. This one—*Pulex irritans*—feeds on humans. Few of us have them nowadays, but they were once as common on man as they now are on our cats and dogs. The profile view of the entire body is magnified 80 times; the head shot 125 times; and the claw 425 times.

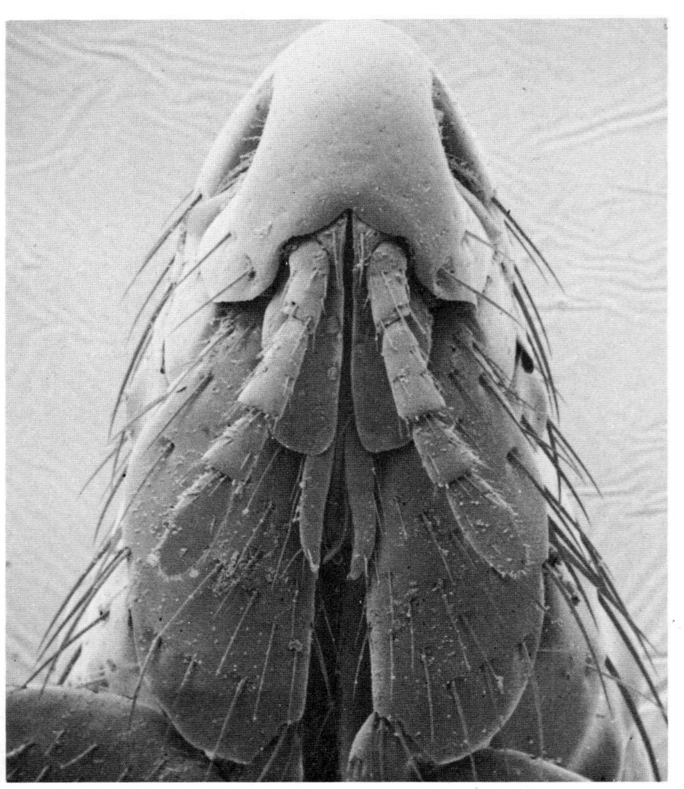

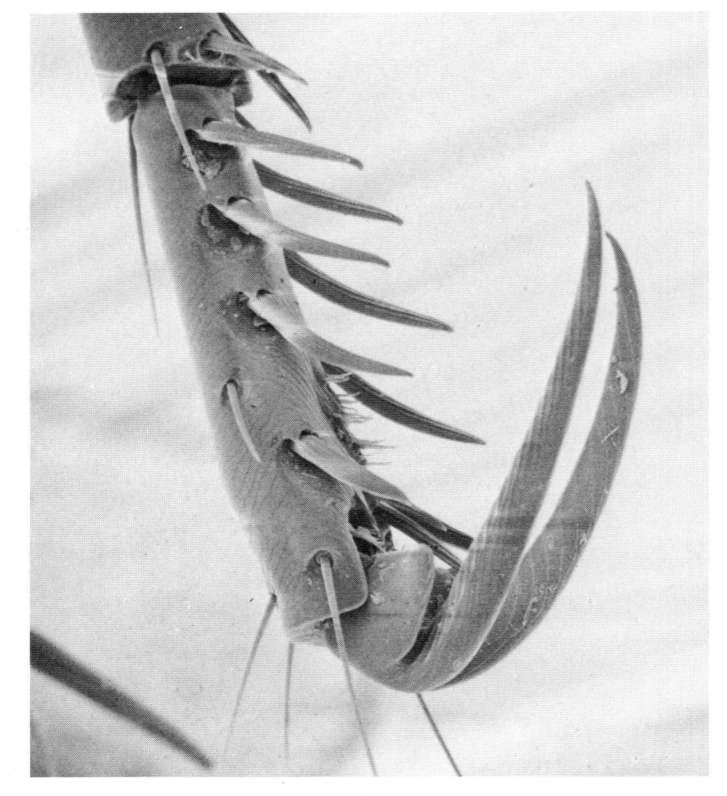

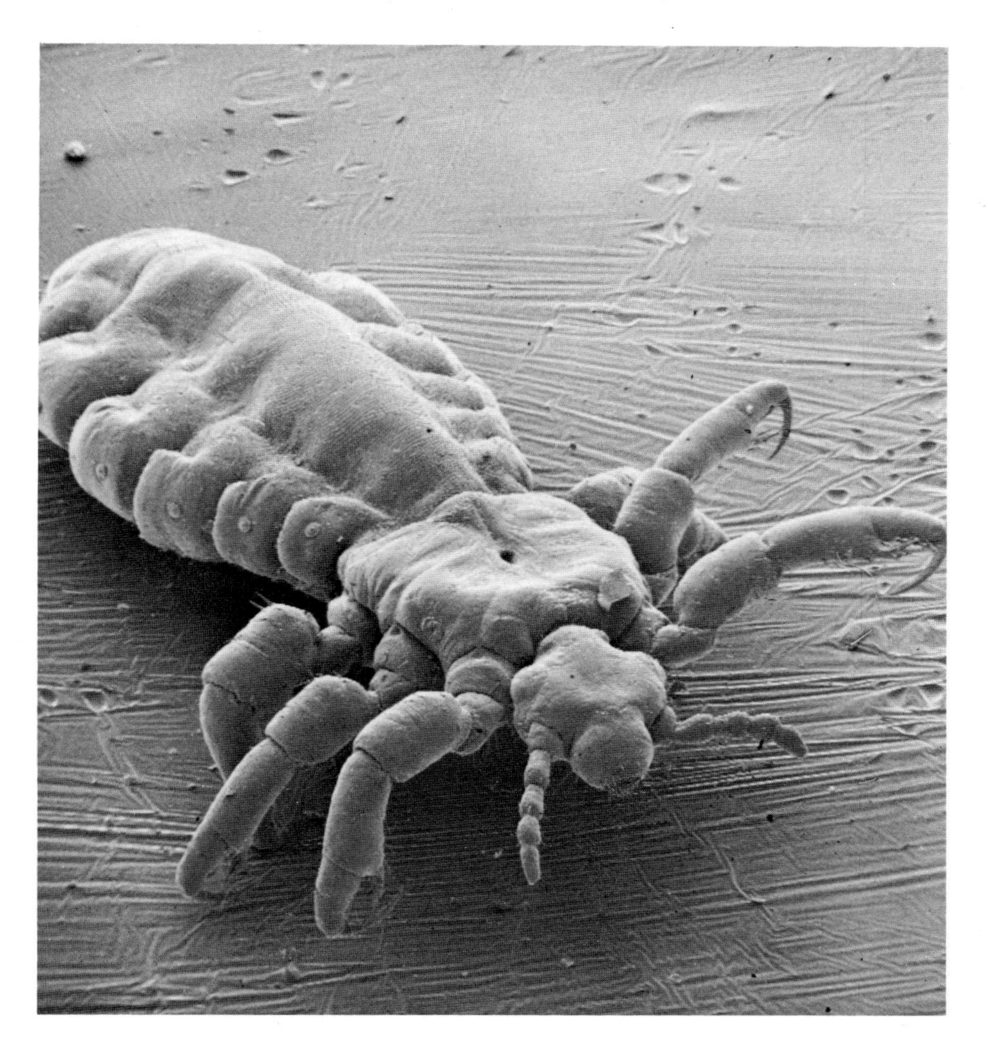

HEAD LOUSE

Meet *Pediculus humanus capitis*, the head louse—a tiny and bothersome pest that lives its life firmly attached to a single strand of hair. In the United States, head louse infestation has often reached epidemic proportions, particularly among schoolchildren. Magnification: × 50.

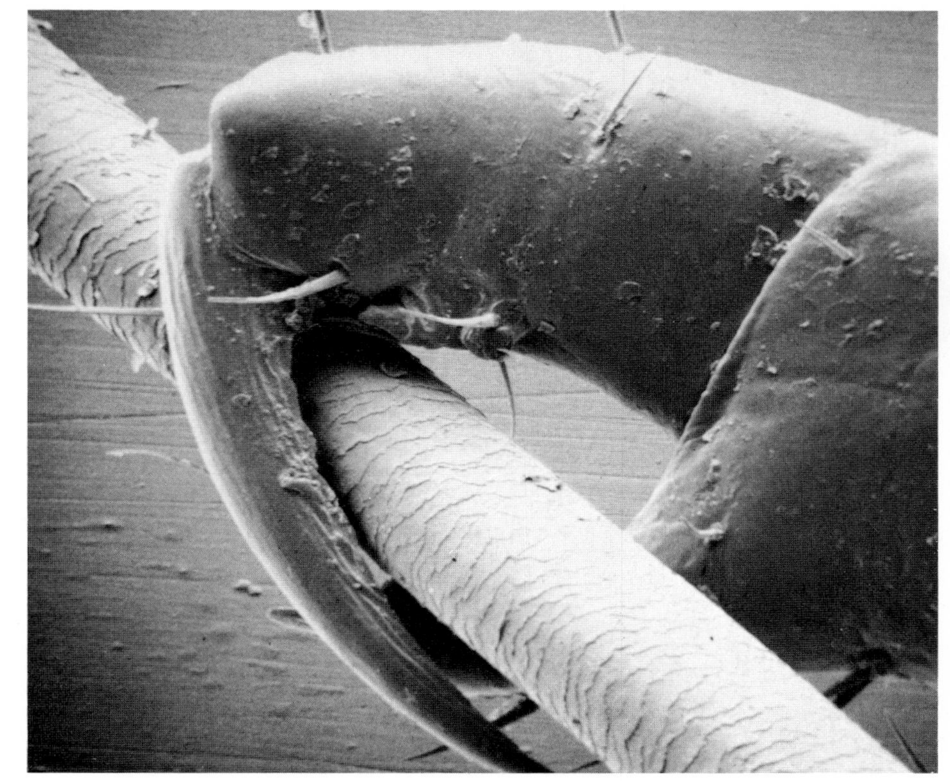

HEAD LOUSE CLAW

The head louse keeps a good grip on a strand of hair with powerful claws. Magnification: × 200.

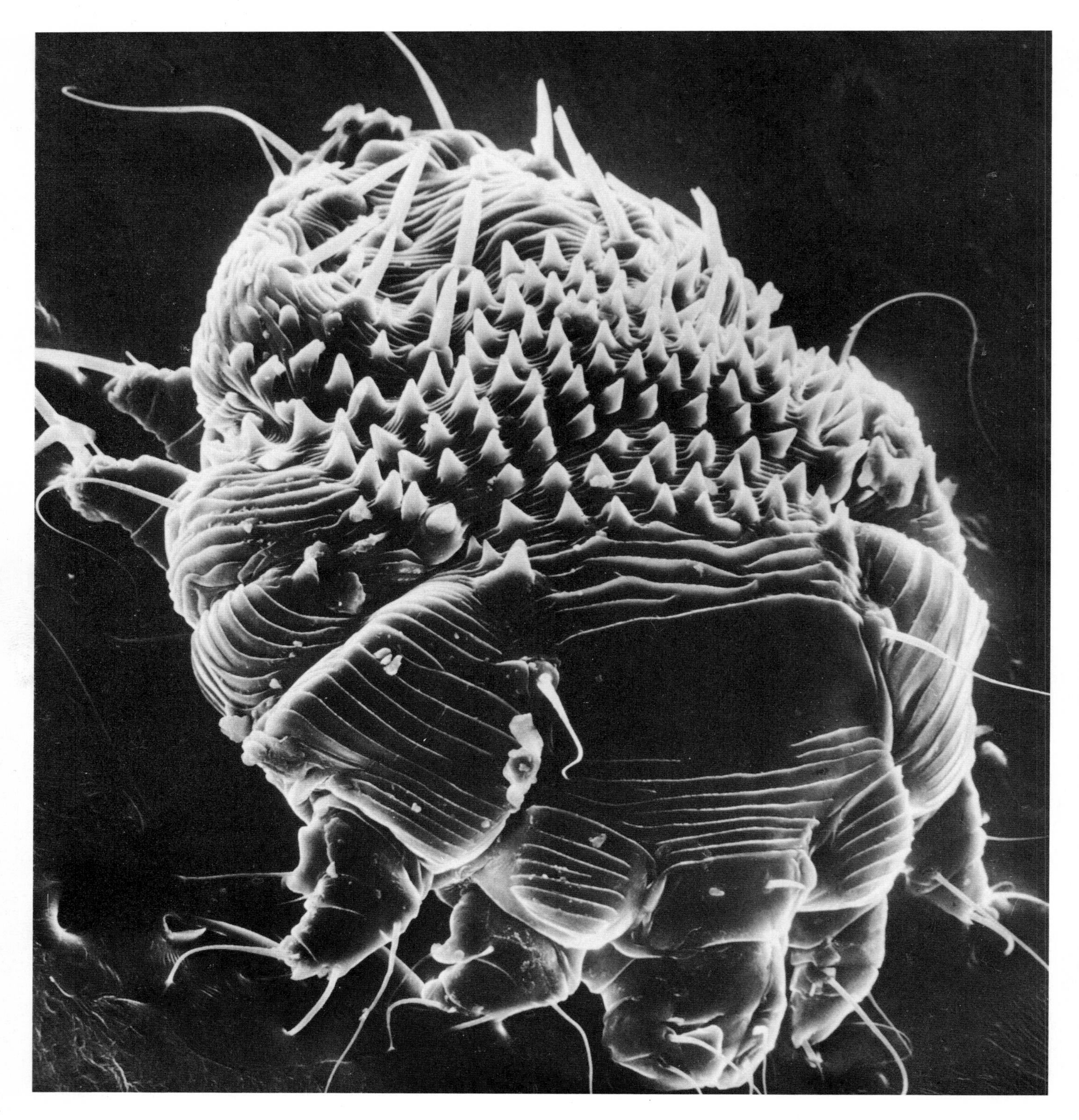

SCABIES

Sarcoptes scabiei, the scabies mite, is a microscopic parasite that makes a comfortable home below the surface of our skin. Magnification: × 300.

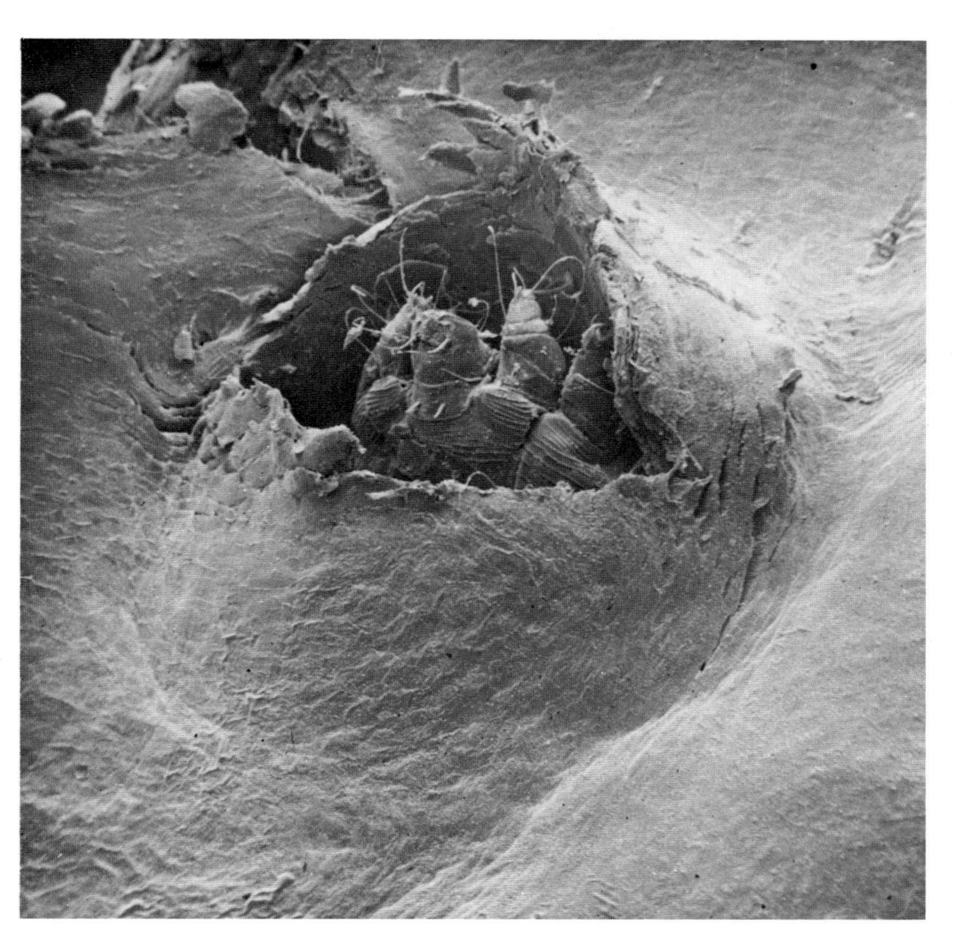

SCABIES AT HOME

The scabies mite burrows directly into our skin by chewing with its powerful jaws and cutting with its sharp front legs. Once dug in, the female mite lays several eggs daily, which hatch in three or four days. Magnification: × 350.

PUBIC LOUSE

The pubic louse—*Phthirus pubis*—lives on a steady diet of human blood and nothing else. As its name implies, it is usually found in the pubic hairs, but it can also live in the armpits or in a beard. It feeds up to a dozen times a day, using its mouth to dig directly into the skin. The presence of this creature on the body will eventually cause severe itching. Pubic lice are often passed through sexual intercourse. Hence their French name, *papillons d'amour,* or "butterflies of love." Magnification: × 70.

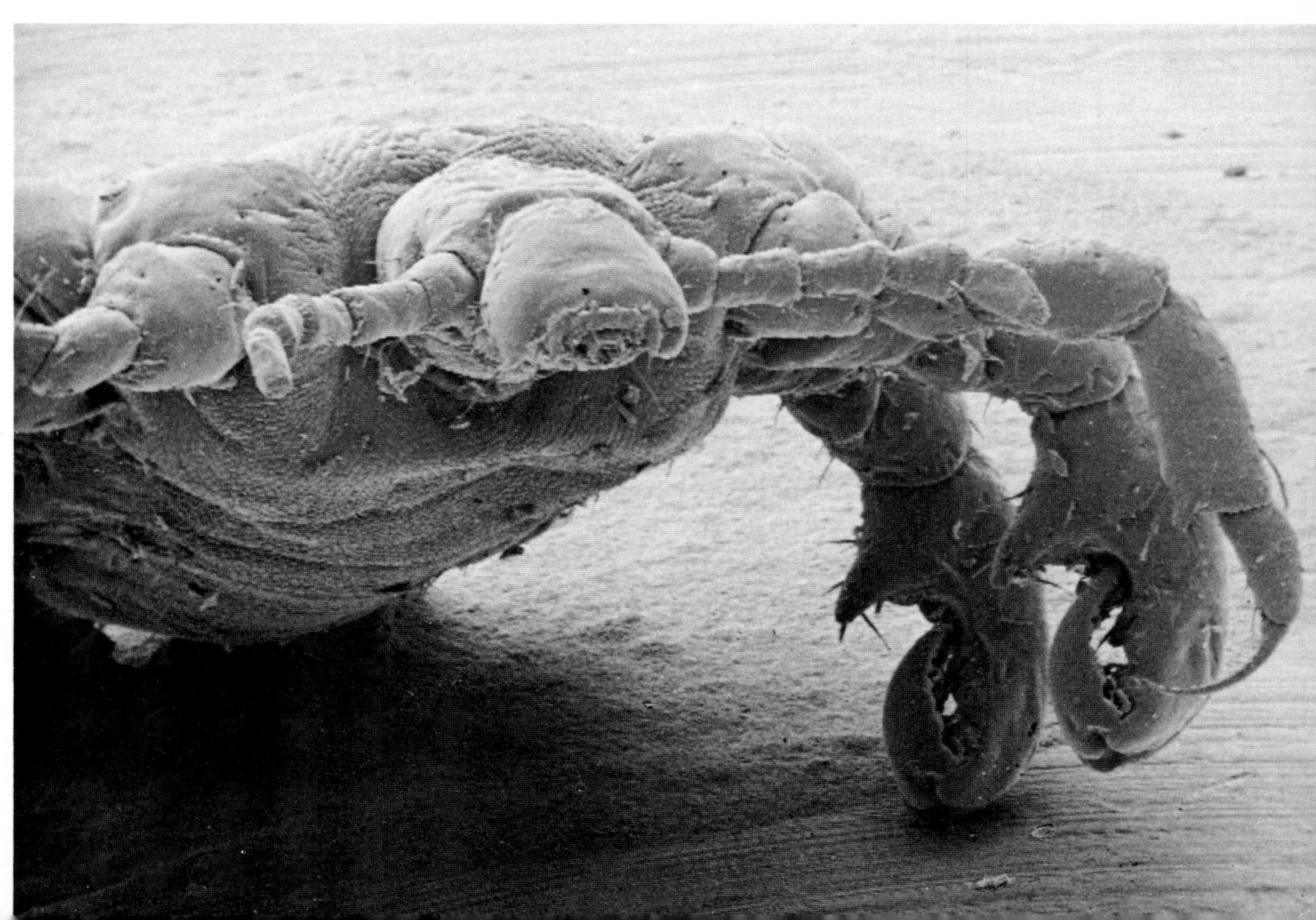

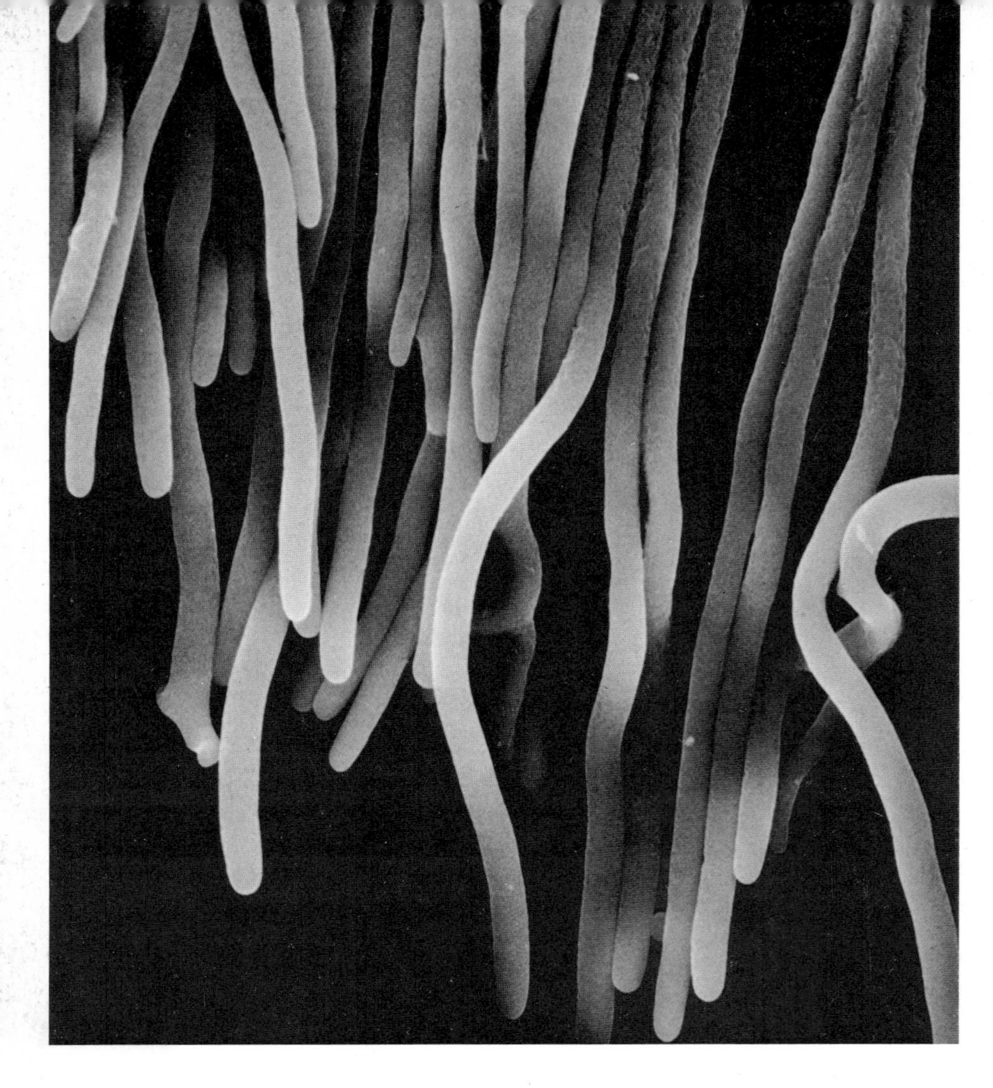

FUNGUS AMONG US

Several types of fungi have adapted to living on the surface of our skin. This variety, *G. candidum,* is a fungal parasite that thrives in warm, moist regions of the body. Magnification: × 750.

HAIRSCAPES

Human Hair and Hair with Fungus. On almost any strand of our hair, tiny fungi can be found. Our intimate fellow travelers, fungi have lived with us through evolution to establish a permanent niche in the habitat our bodies provide.

In numerous forms, their population on our hair and skin numbers in the tens of thousands. A sudden proliferation of fungi can totally engulf a strand of hair.

This variety is a keratinophilic fungus—it uses a keratin protein in our hair as a food source. It is called *Trichophyton mentagrophytes,* and occurs quite commonly in tropical climates. It can be gotten rid of by thoroughly washing your hair. Magnifications: Human Hair, × 910; Human Hair with Fungus, × 602.

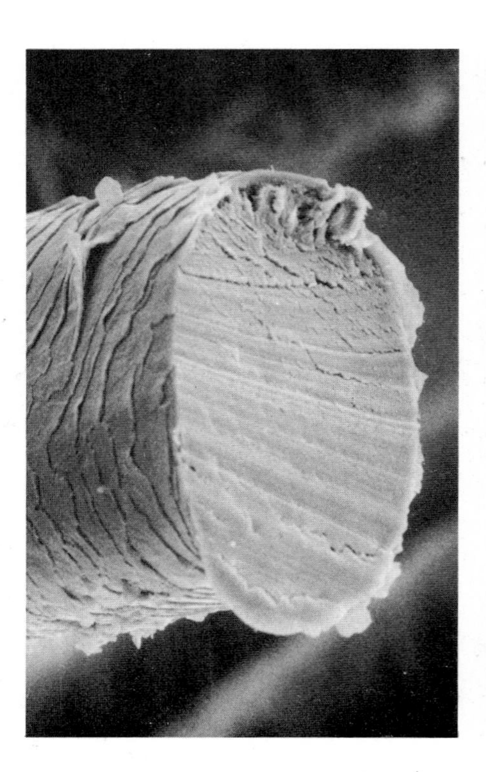

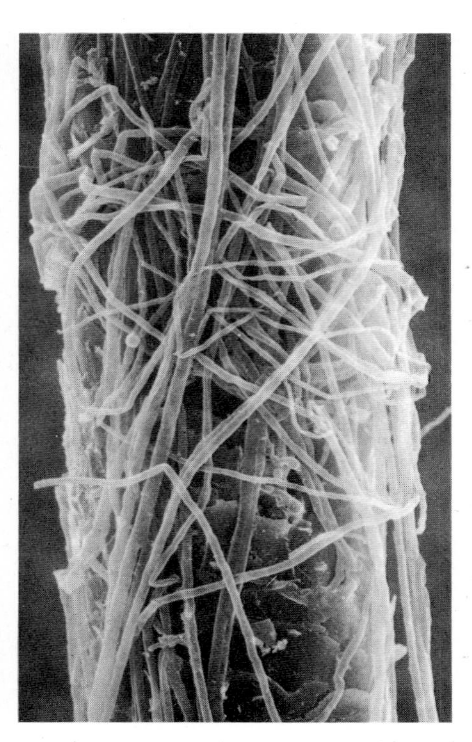

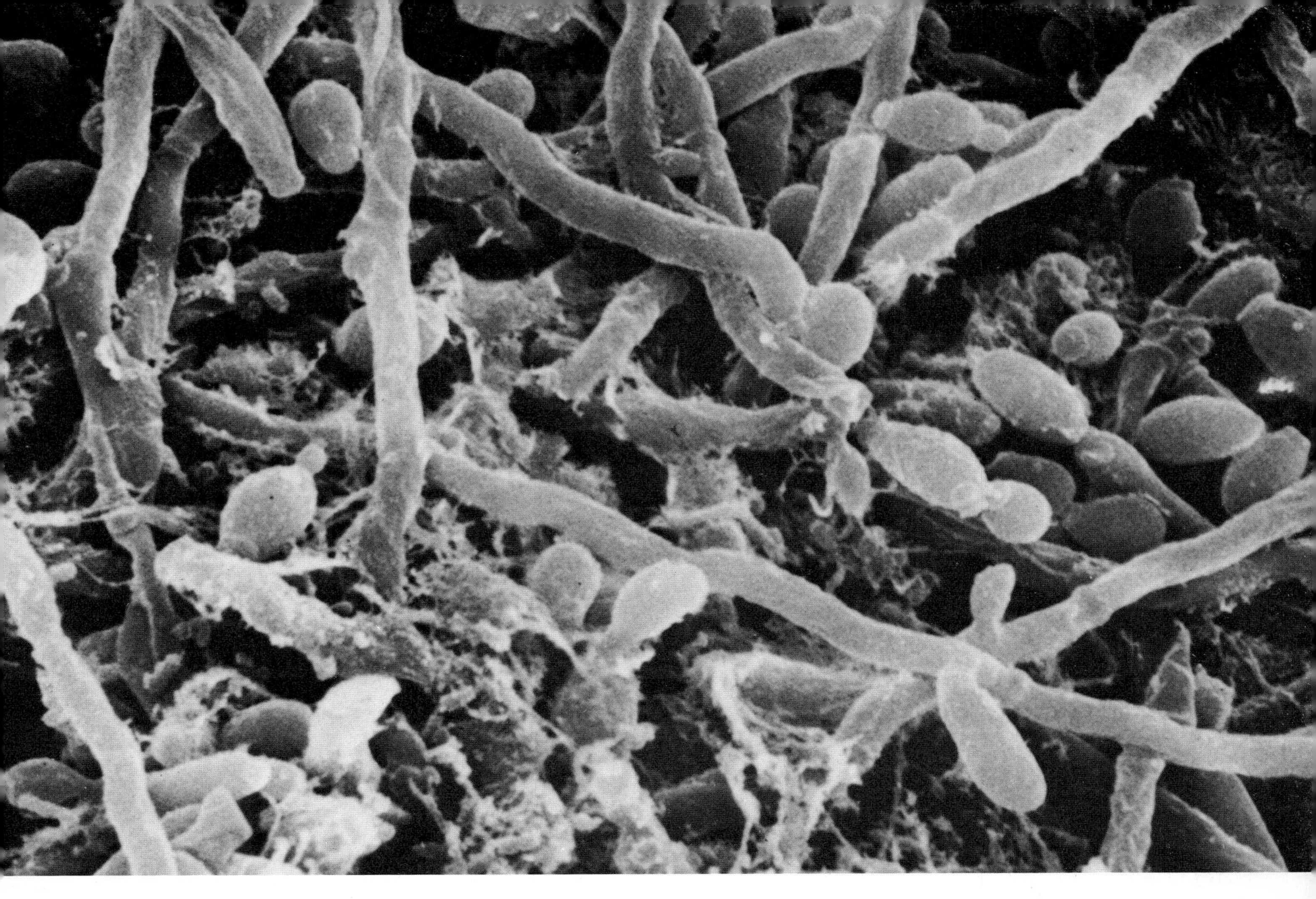

PLAQUE
Bacteria growing on the surface of a tooth, magnified 5000 times.

THE MITEY EYE
In the roots of everyone's eyelashes live tiny mites called *Demodex folliculorum*. Apparently they cause us no harm, but why they are there and exactly what they do has yet to be discovered.

Generation after generation of *Demodex* are born, live, and die without us being the wiser. One of their favorite foods is mascara. Magnification: $\times$ 500.

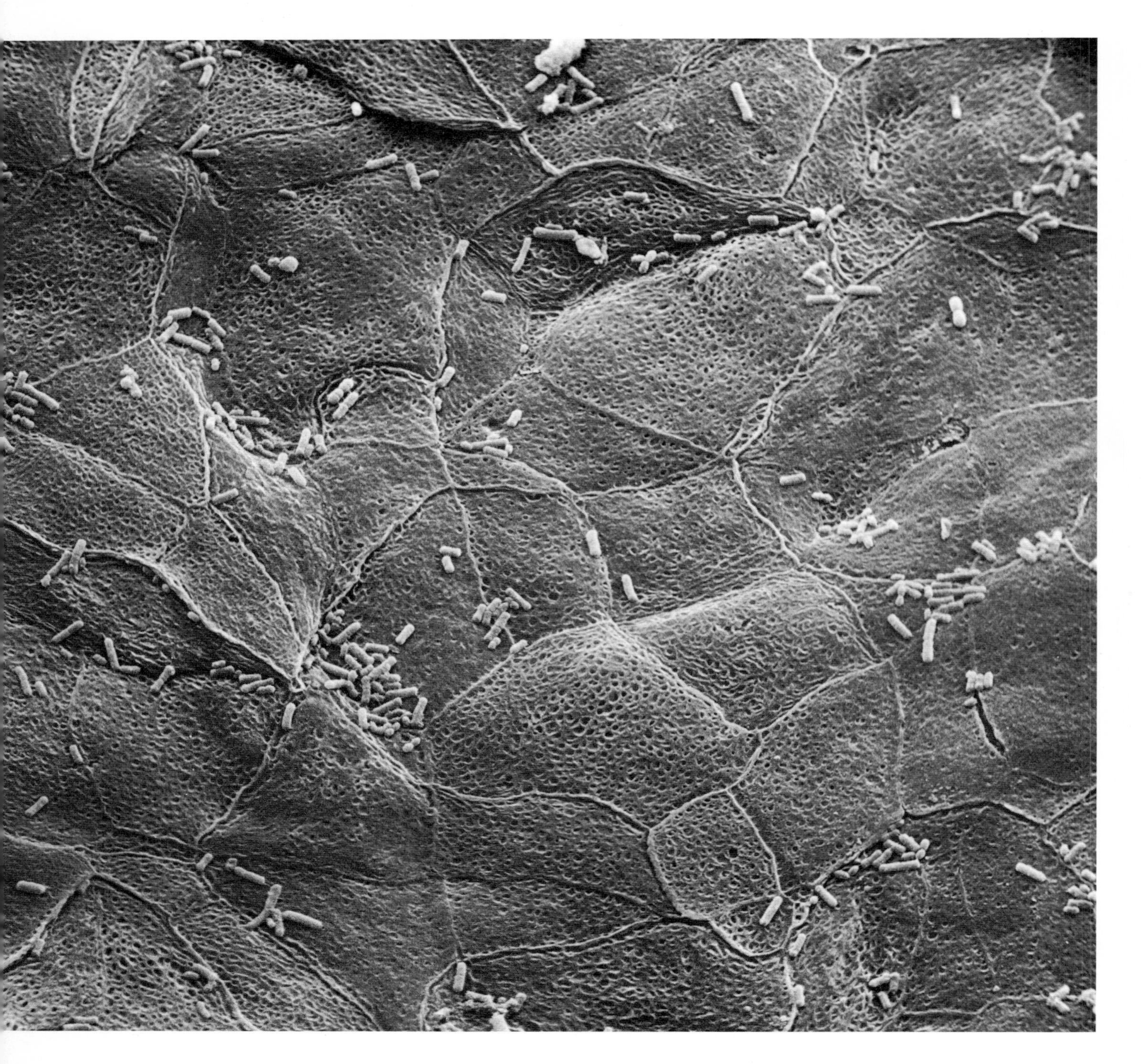

BACTERIA

Bacteria, the simplest form of free-living life, are constantly with us. They are most abundant on the warm, moist regions of our skin. Under the right conditions, a single bacterium can multiply to more than a million in about eight hours. No matter how often we wash, millions will remain with us. Magnification: × 1500.

REALMS OF TIME

Our eyes are exiled from other worlds by time as well as by size. In a world of motion there is infinite detail too slow or too fast for the unaided eye to see.

In 1872, an ingenious photographer named Eadweard Muybridge invented a way to record movements normally too quick to be seen. A wager about the stride of a running horse brought Muybridge to the stock farm of a wealthy Californian named Leland Stanford. Stanford was a horse lover, and had bet $25,000 that all four hoofs of a trotting horse were sometimes simultaneously off the ground.

With a battery of twenty-four cameras that were activated by threads stretched out across a track, Muybridge captured the stride of a horse as it had never been seen before. He also proved his patron was right.

The movement of people as well as animals became for Muybridge a passionate subject of study. Much more than just a technical curiosity, Muybridge's pioneering work was the first photographic analysis of the dynamics of physical motion.

Today, special cameras can record rapid motion with a clarity that Eadweard Muybridge could only have dreamed about.

With the aid of a flashing strobe light, cameras can freeze a flurry of movement or a tiny instant of time on a single photograph.

The stroboscopic light was developed and made practical by Dr. Harold Edgerton in the early 1930s. He was a student of electrical engineering at the Massachusetts Institute of Technology. Unable to see how electric motors behaved when they rotated at various speeds, he designed a light that could flash so quickly and brightly that motion seemed to stop. When coupled with a camera, a whole new age of high speed photography was born. Fractions of millionths of seconds can now be frozen in time. A once invisible world of motion has come within our grasp.

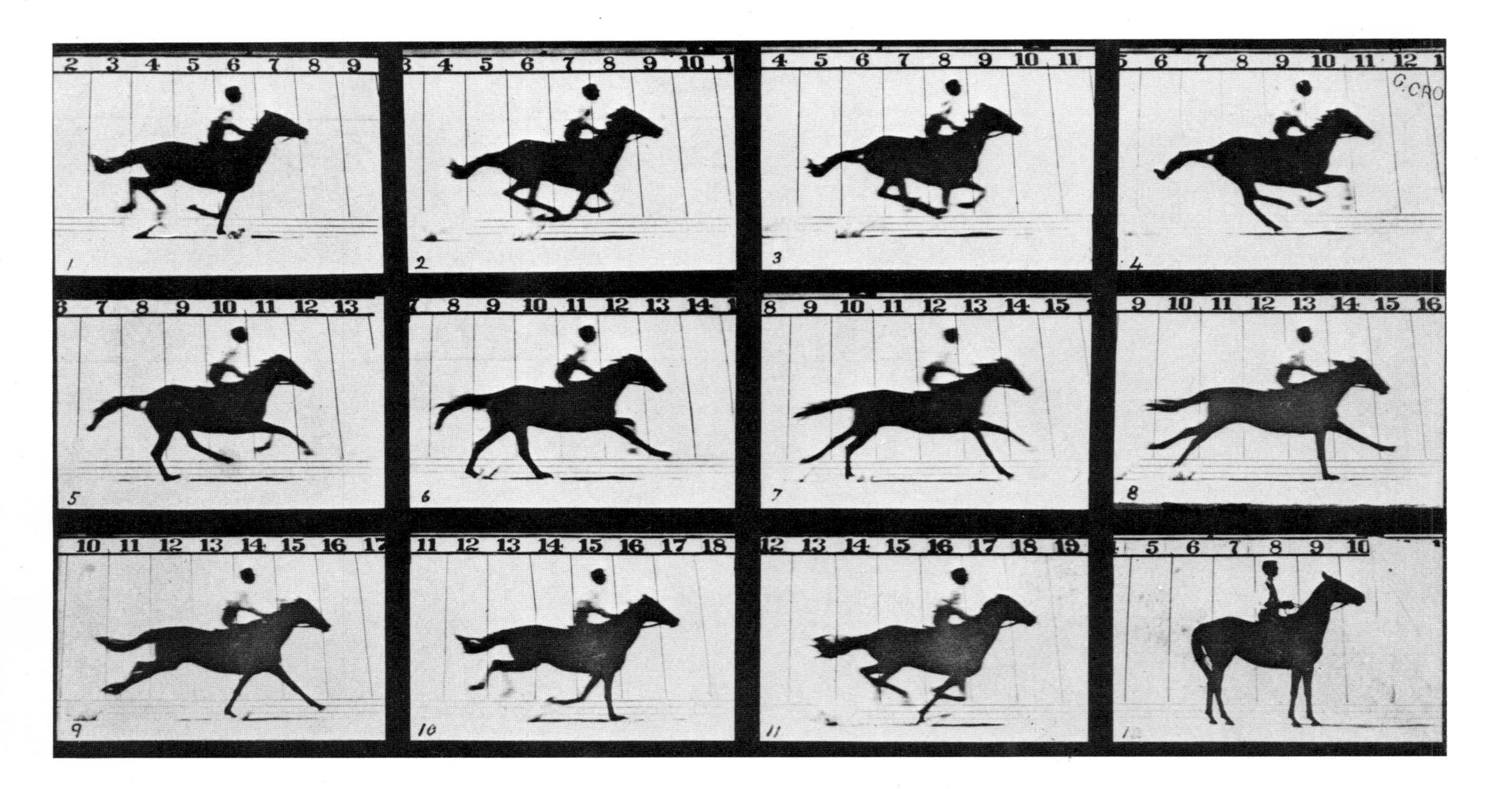

THE TROTTING HORSE

This classic series of photographs by Eadweard Muybridge proves that all four legs of a trotting horse are sometimes simultaneously off the ground. These pictures transformed the way artists rendered horses and other animals in motion. For the first time ever, they had an accurate picture of otherwise invisible movements.

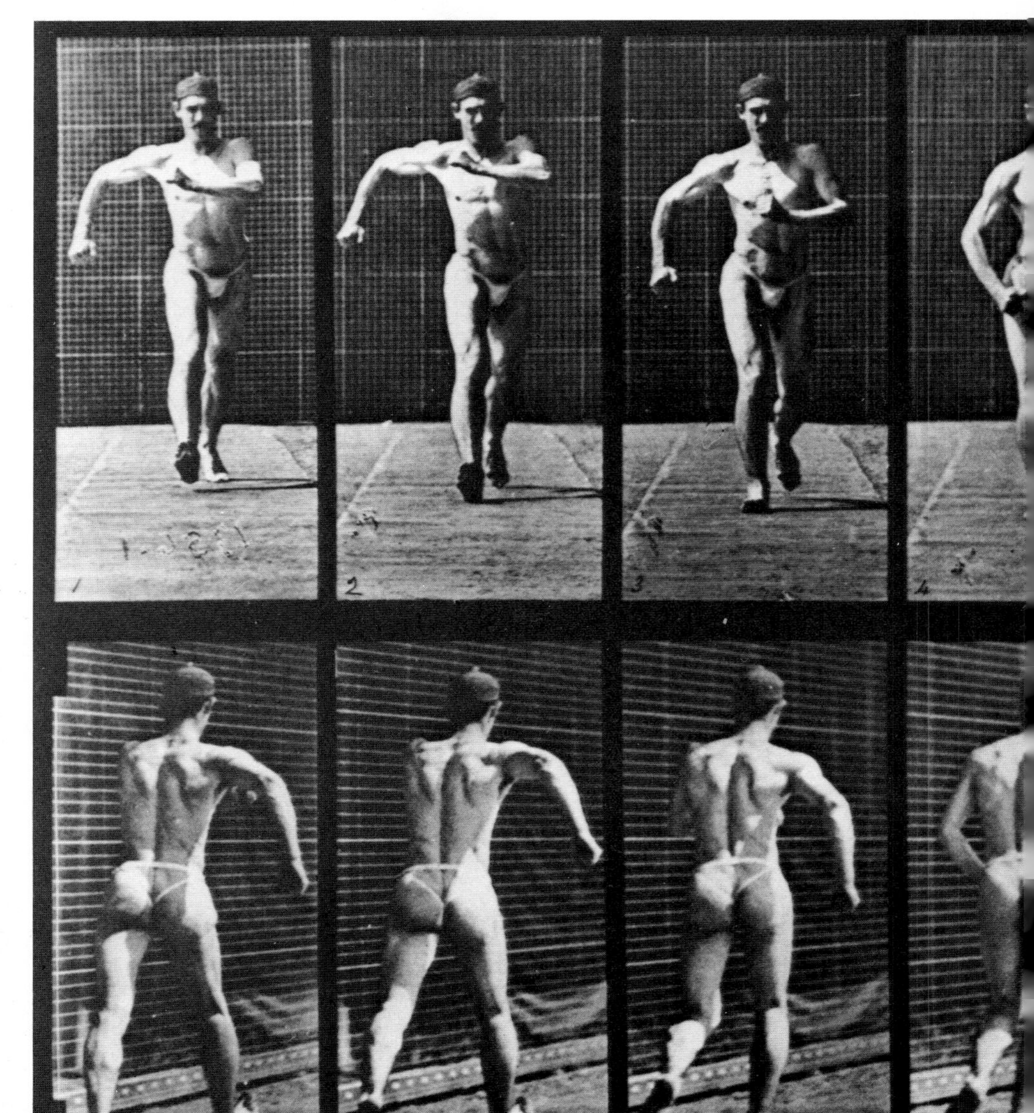

WALKING MAN

Muybridge's serial pictures of people in motion revealed the discrete aspects of simple movements that had never before been seen.

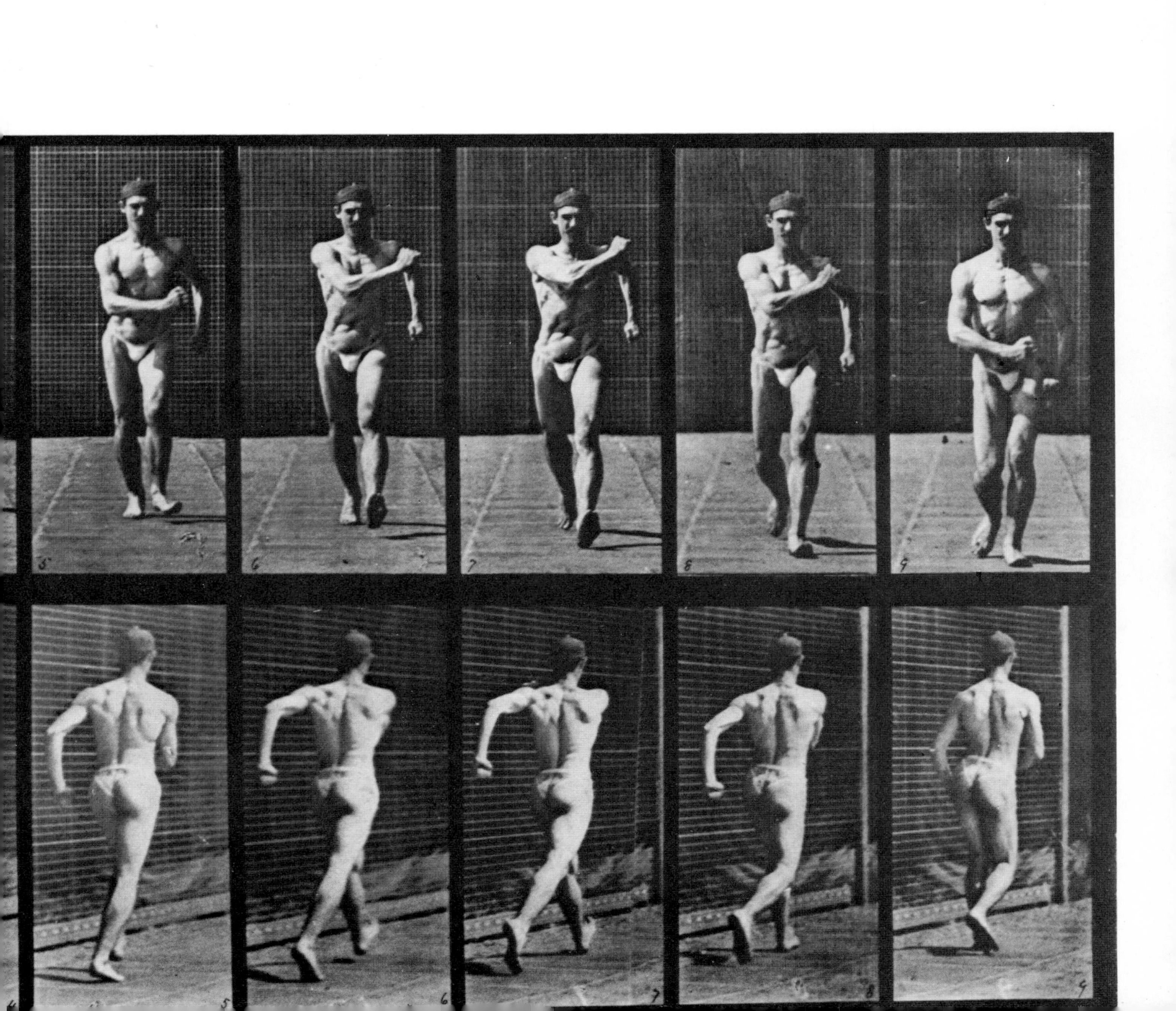

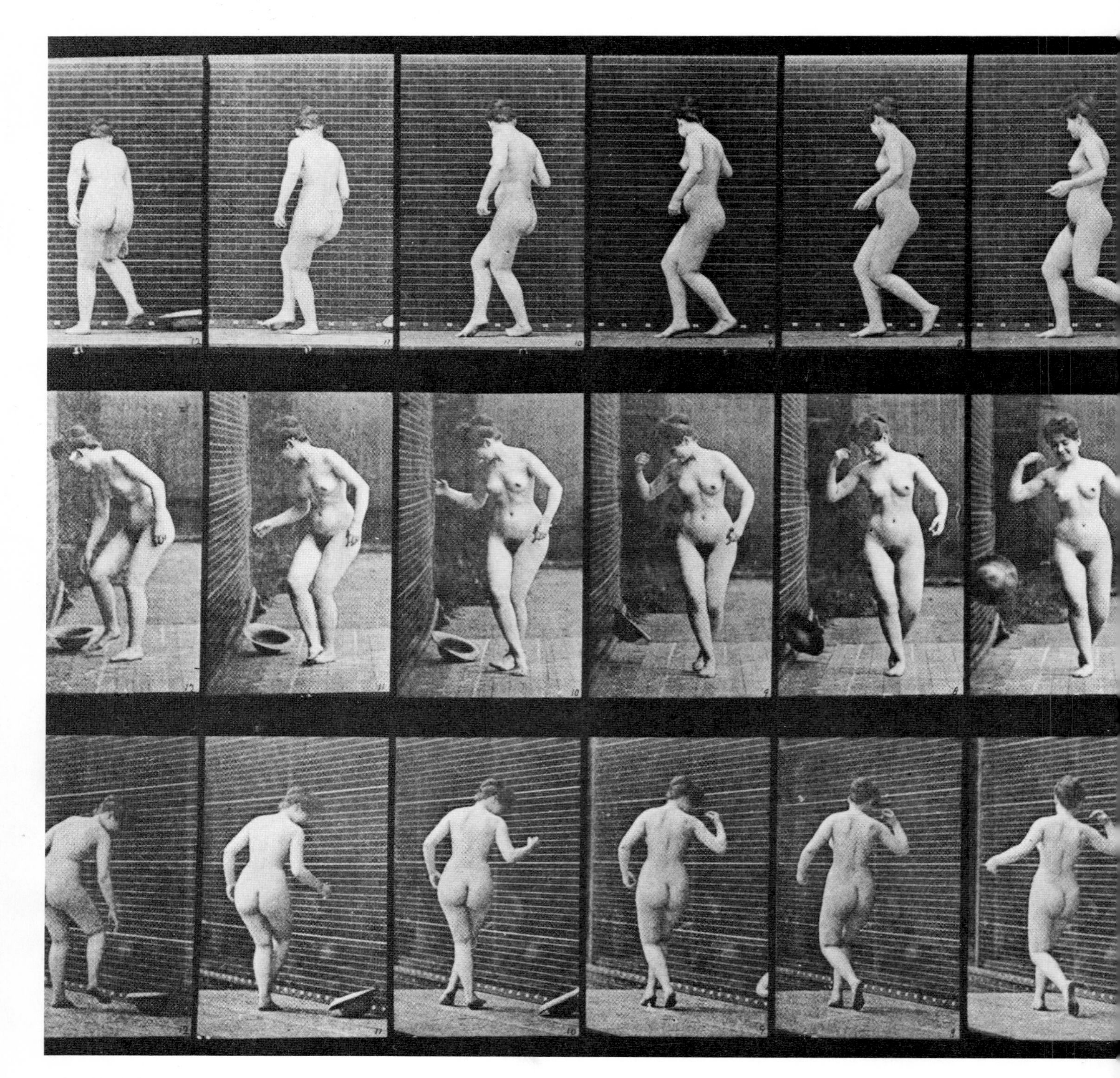

WOMAN KICKS HAT

Muybridge's photographs were often somewhat whimsical. His human subjects were nearly always nude. His pictures were sold to the general public, and in the late nineteenth century they were enthusiastically received.

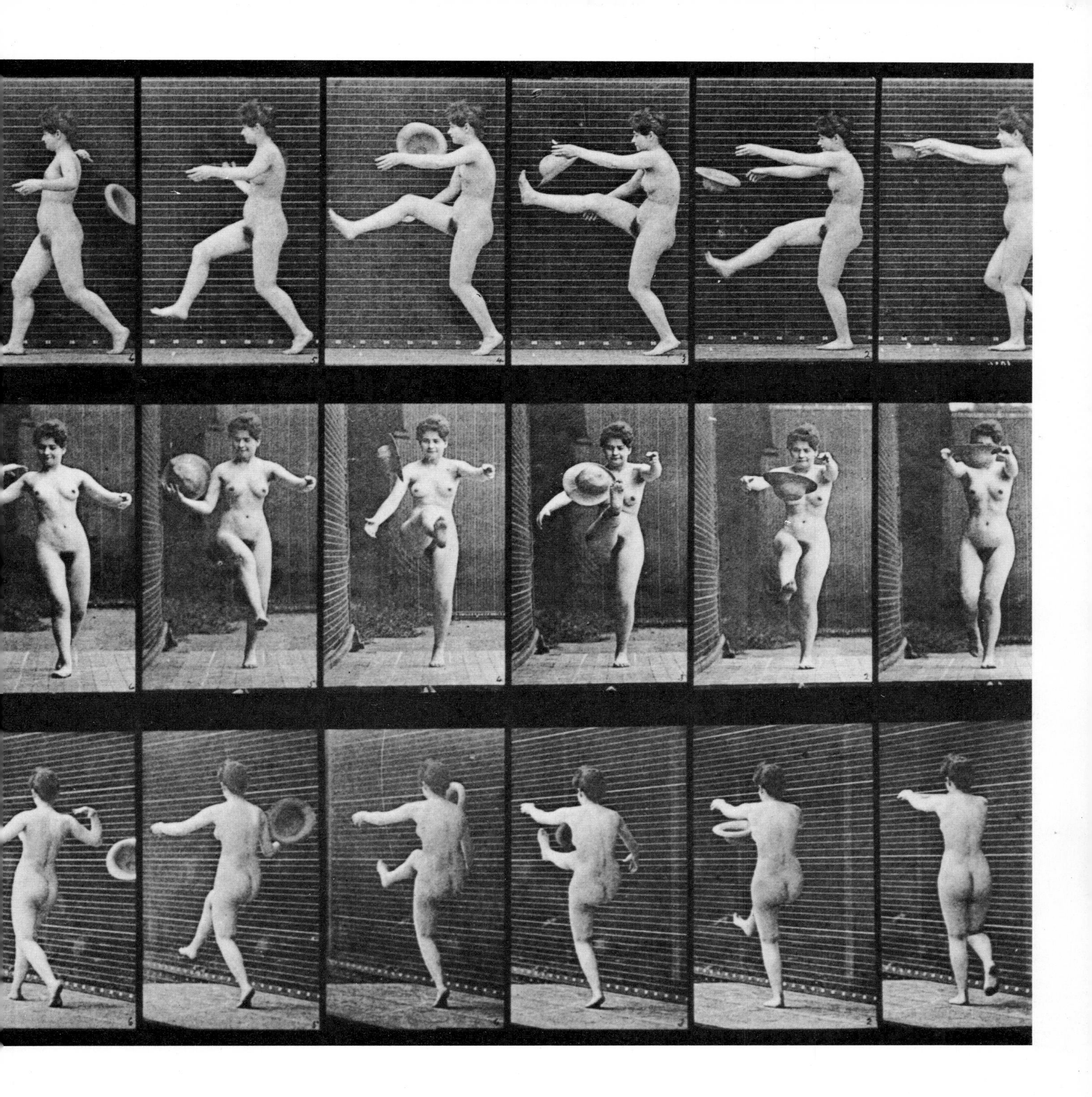

DRUM MAJORETTE ▷
Before a strobe light flashing sixty times a second, the majorette twirls the baton (at left) and grabs it as it falls (at right).

JUMP ROPE
This is what skipping rope looks like in front of a multiflash strobe light, blinking 60 times per second.

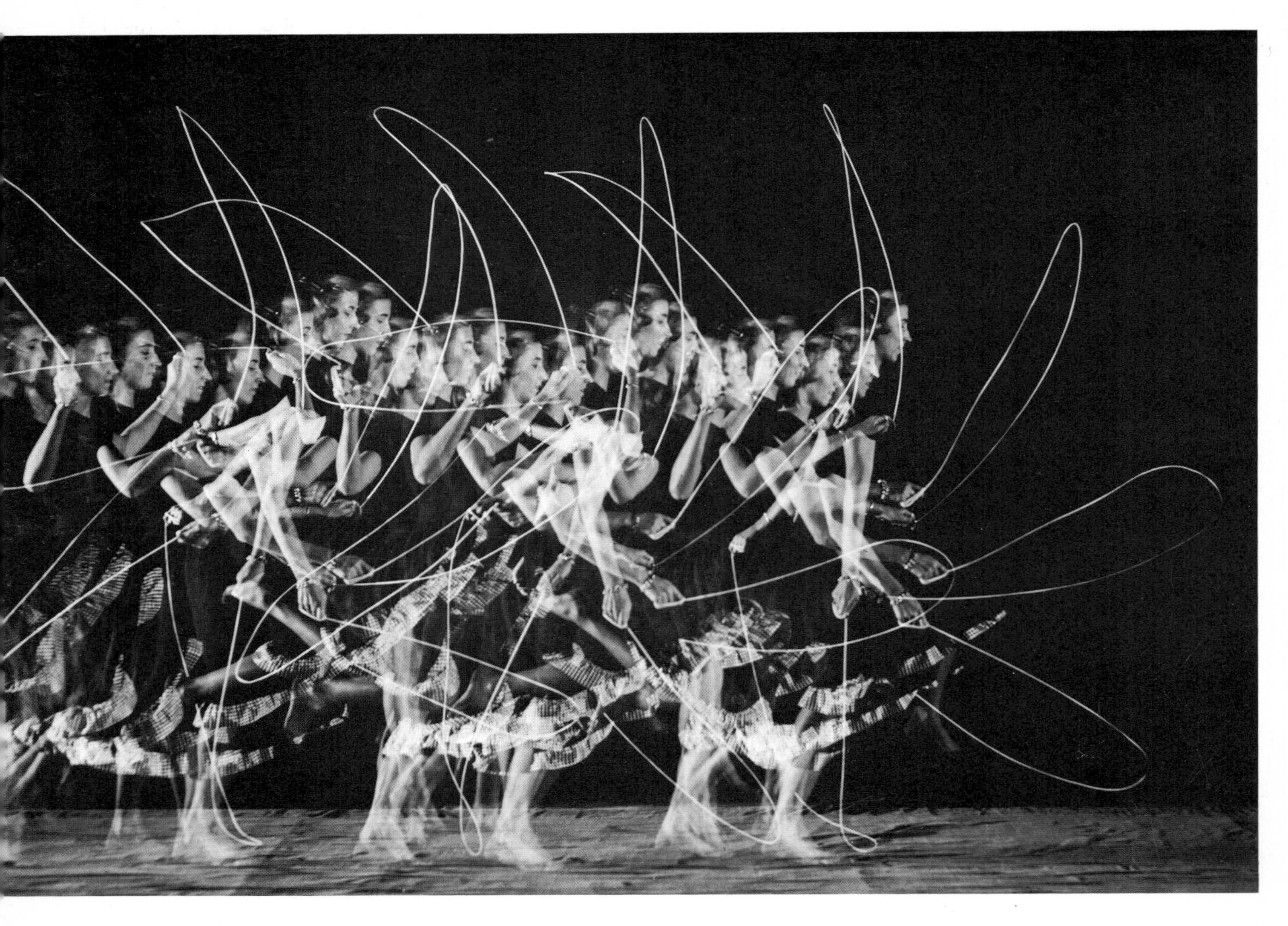

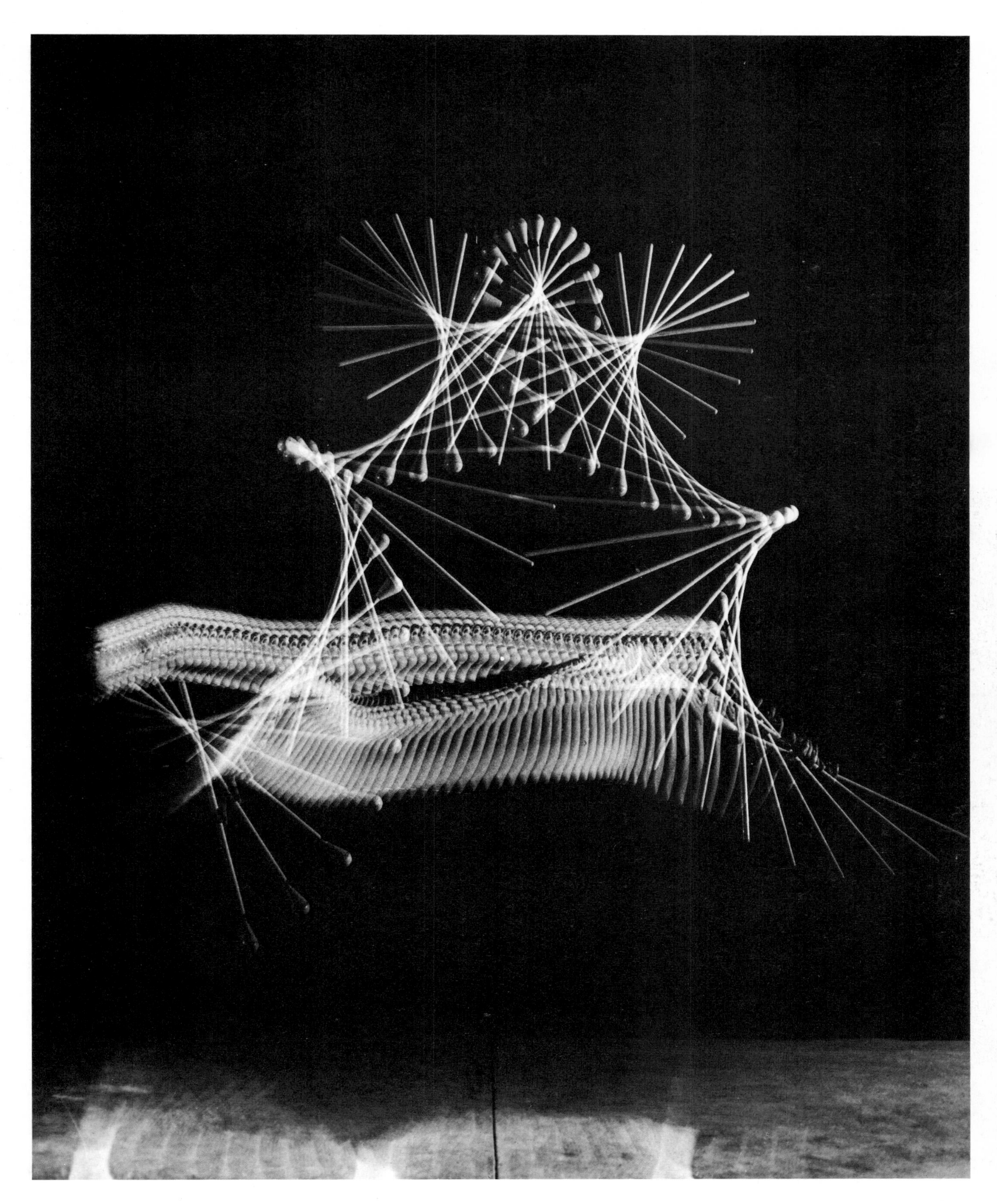

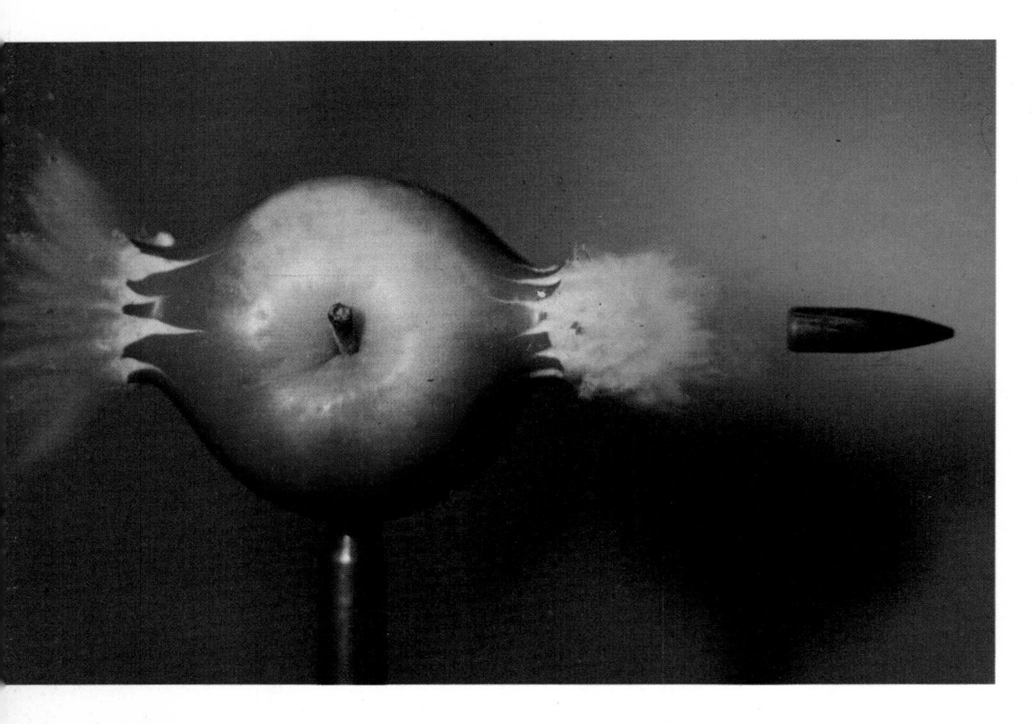

MAKING APPLESAUCE
An apple is shot with a bullet traveling more than 2000 miles an hour. The bullet was "stopped" using a microflash stroboscope at an exposure of one third of a millionth of a second.

CUTTING THE CARD
The eye of the camera is literally faster than a speeding bullet. Less than a millionth of a second is frozen in time using strobe light photography.

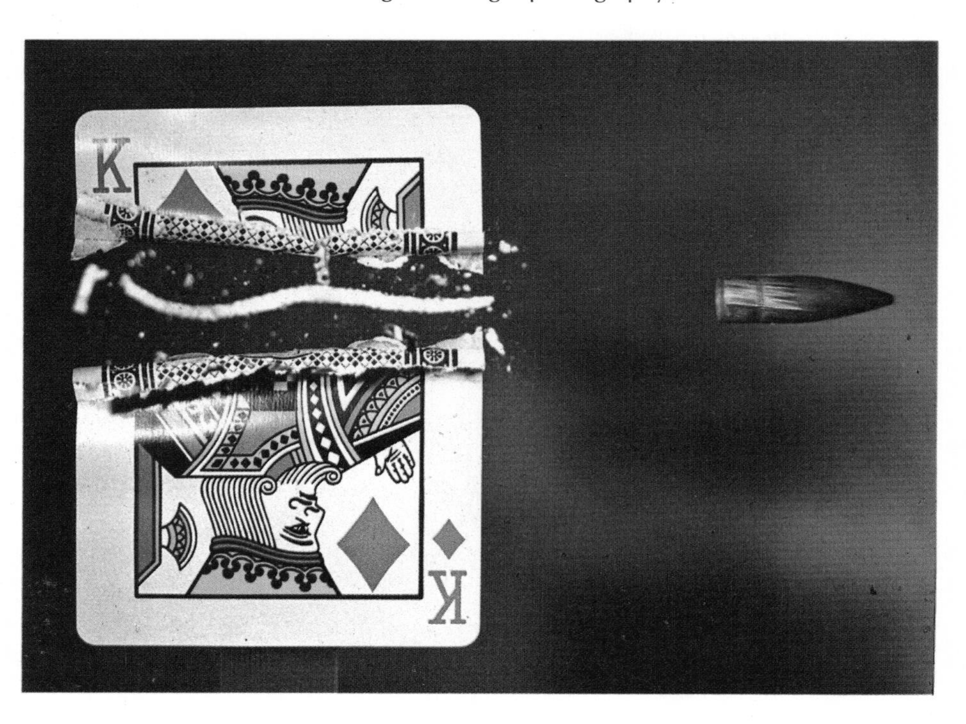

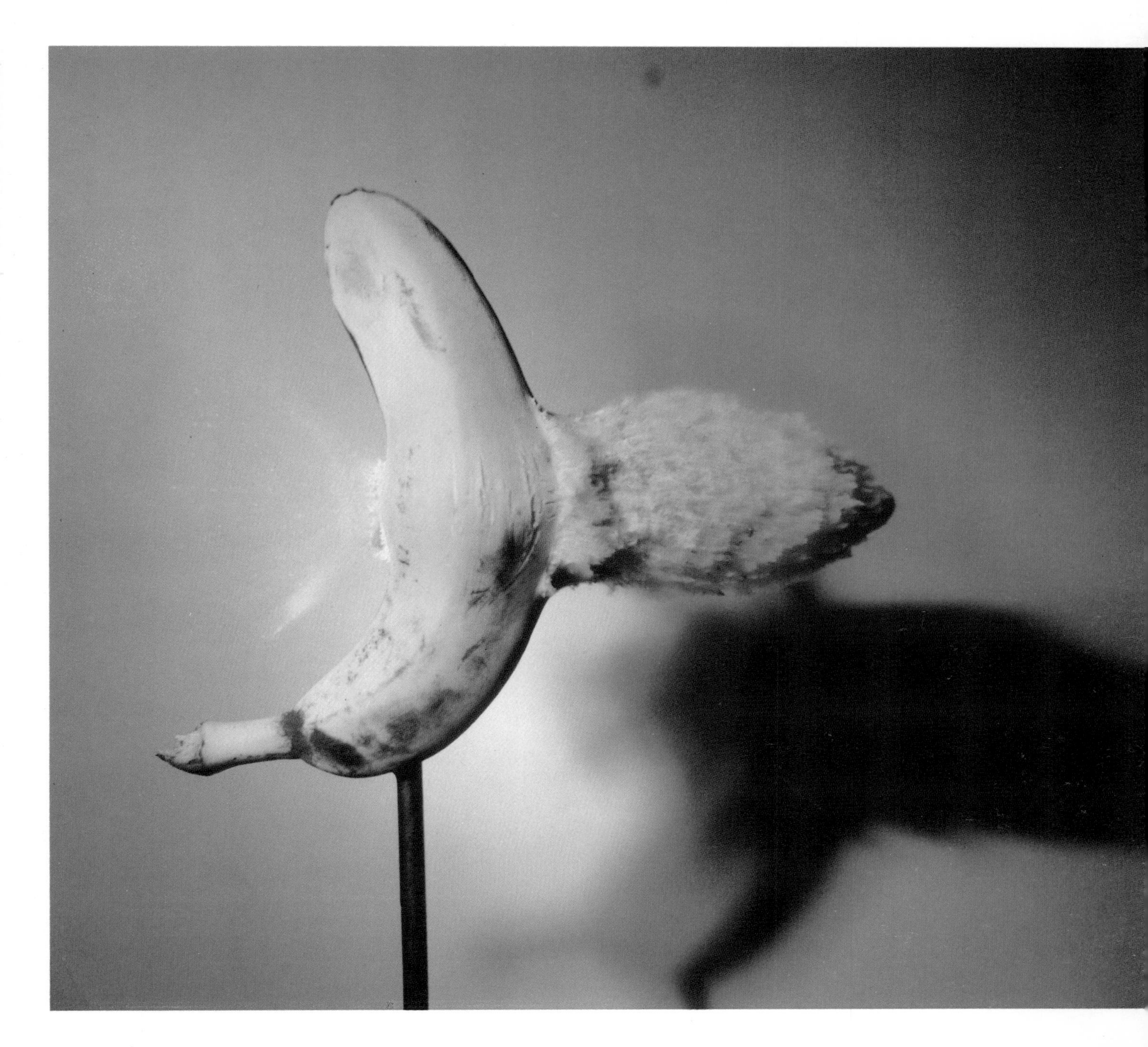

BANANA SPLIT

A speeding bullet—passing through a banana—is stopped in flight. The exposure is one millionth of a second.

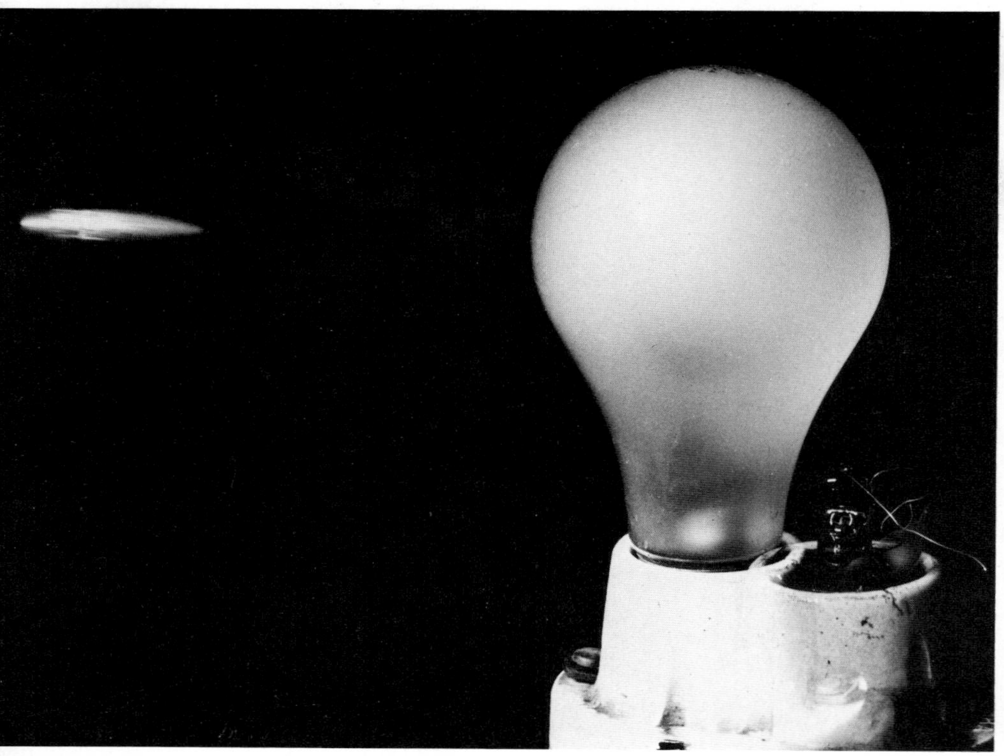

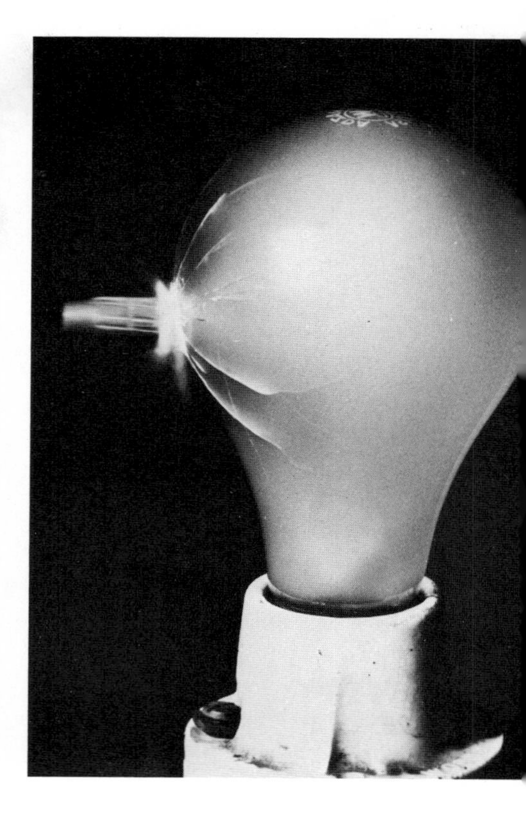

LIGHTS OUT

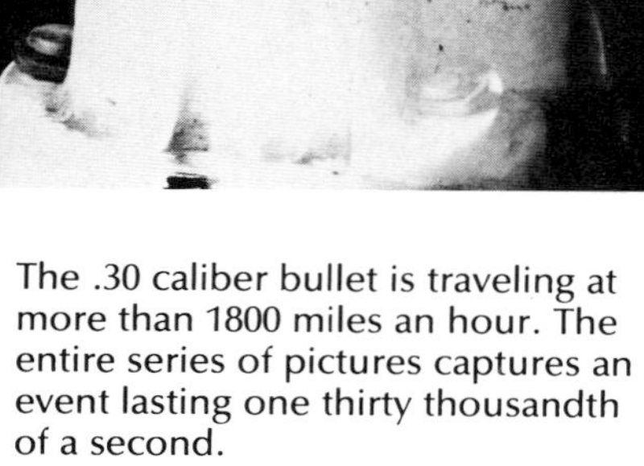

The .30 caliber bullet is traveling at more than 1800 miles an hour. The entire series of pictures captures an event lasting one thirty thousandth of a second.

In the second picture, impact has occurred, and the cracks in the bulb are moving faster than the bullet itself.

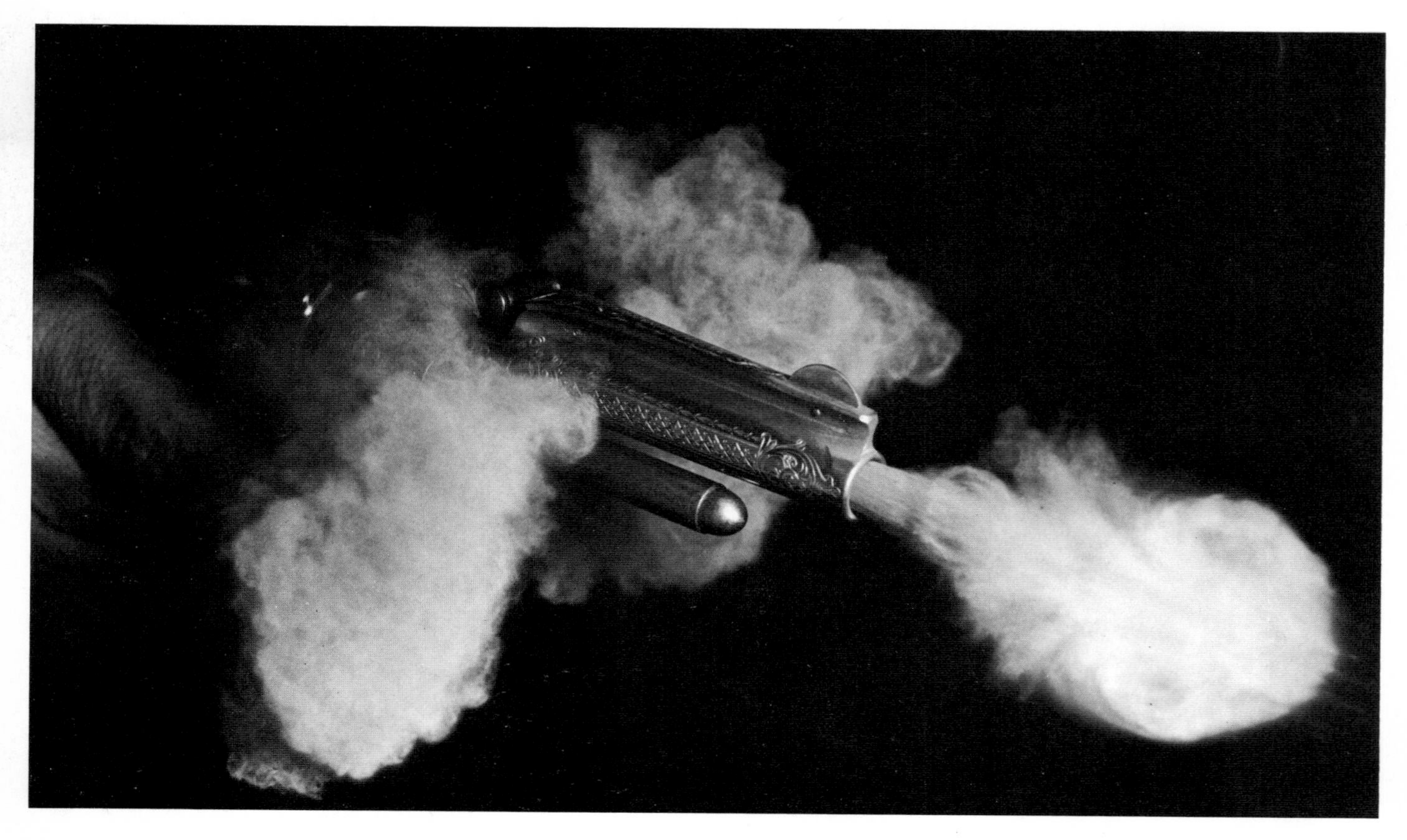

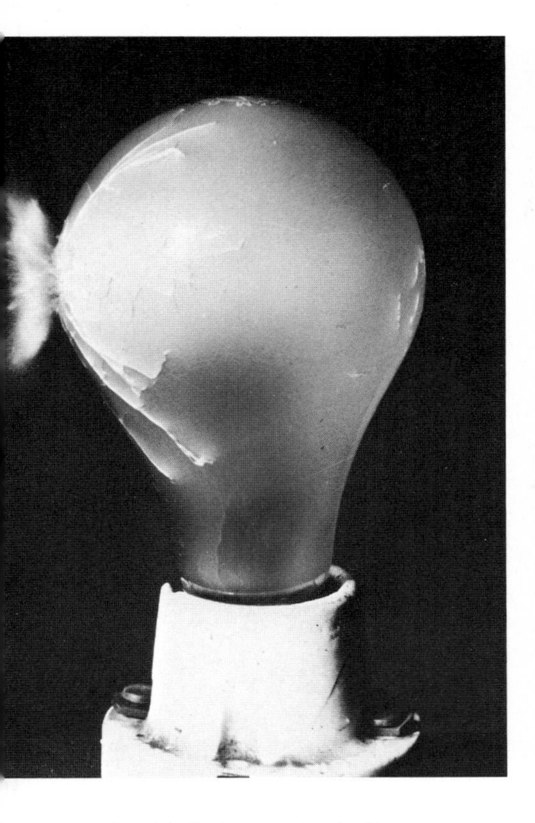

In the third picture, the bullet enters the bulb. A compression wave, moving inside the bulb at 15,000 feet a second, cracks the other side of the bulb before the bullet reaches it.

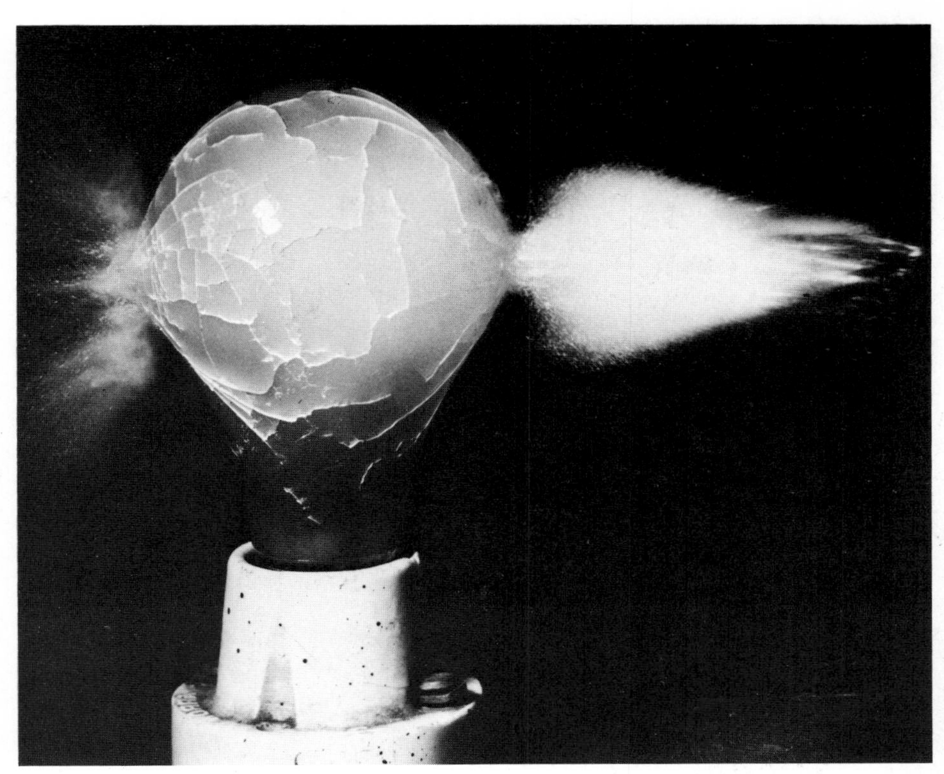

In the final photograph, glass fragments and gas form an arrow behind the bullet.

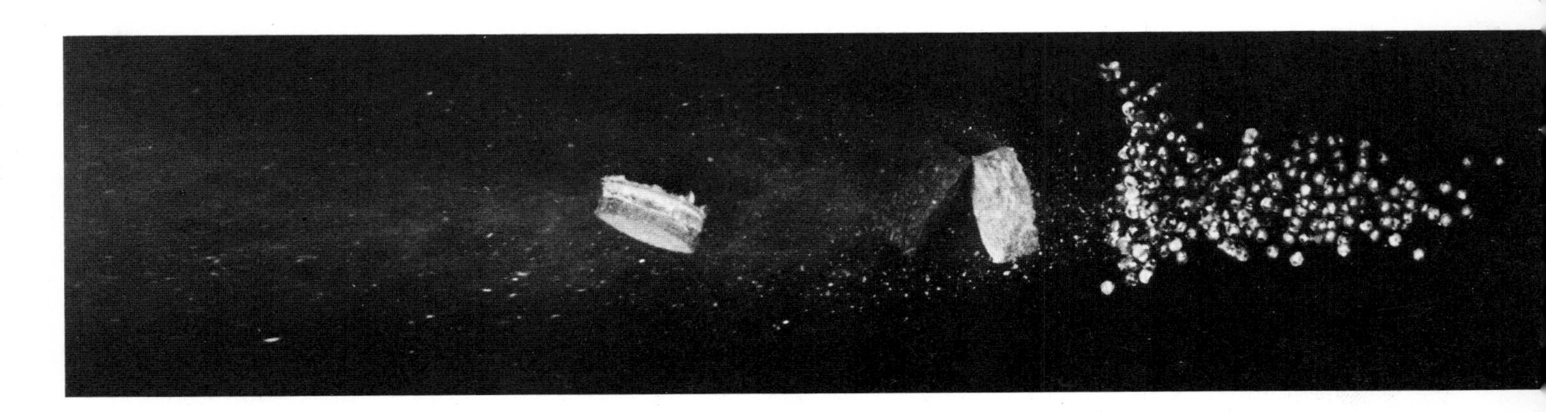

BOOM!
The blast of a shotgun shell is frozen in flight by a slit camera. Film in the camera moves horizontally at nearly five hundred miles an hour as the wad and pellets pass before it.

◁ **BANG!**
The bullet has just been fired. It cannot be seen yet because it is still surrounded by a cloud of normally invisible gas ejected by the gun. The exposure is one millionth of a second.

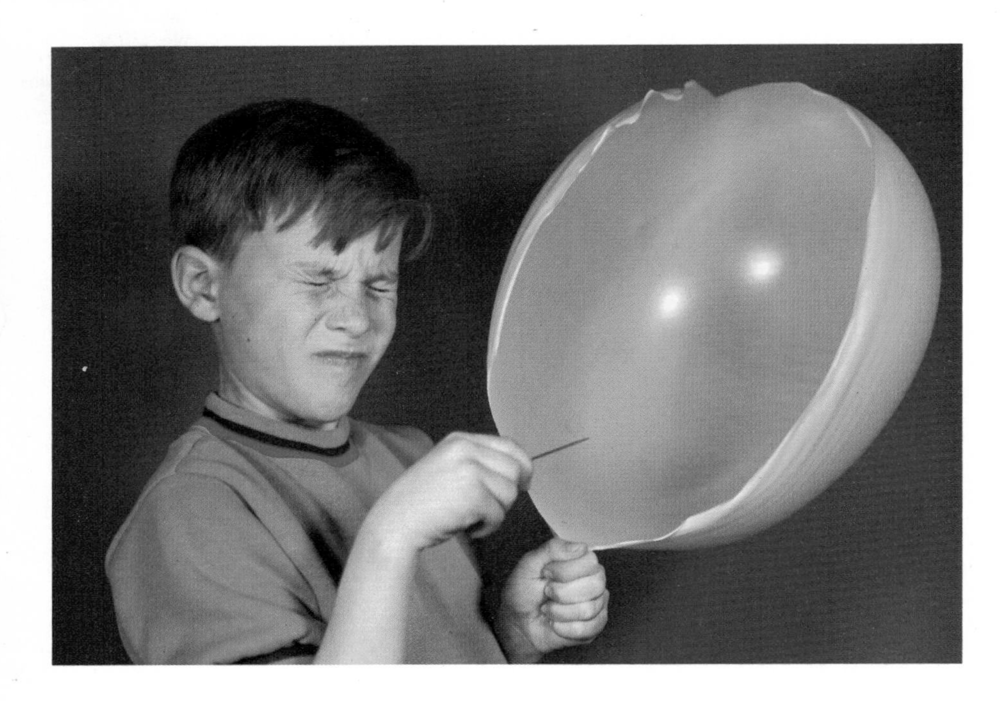

POP!

A sudden brilliant flash from a strobe light, lasting twenty-five millionths of a second, captures the moment a balloon is popped.

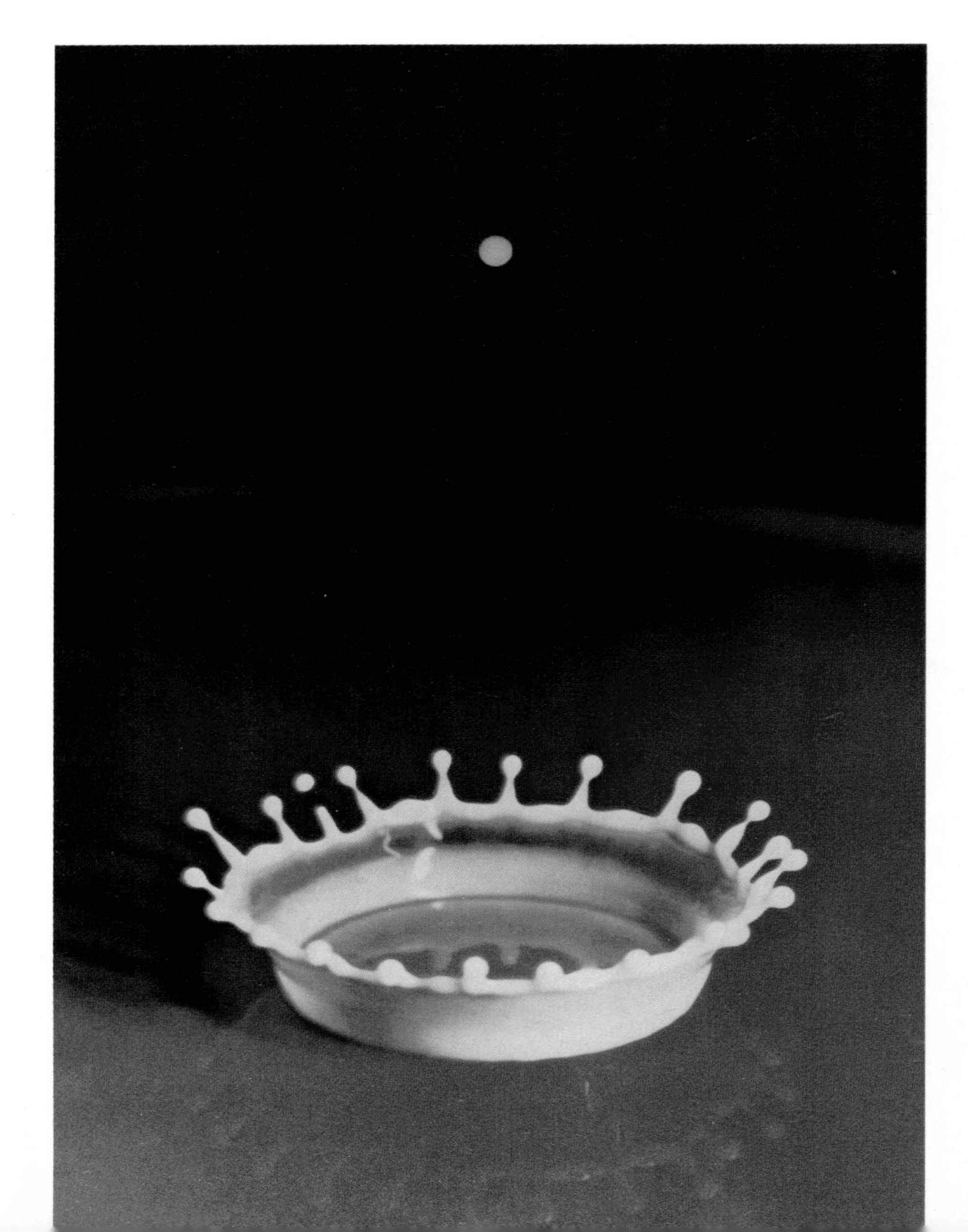

MILK DROP

The milk drop has just landed, shattering the surface tension that held it together. The crown that has formed is momentarily held together by its own surface tension, and within a minute fraction of a second it will fly free and collapse. The exposure is one millionth of a second.

PLOP!

A water drop makes a splash. This sequence of photographs captures the event—which takes place in one hundred millionths of a second.

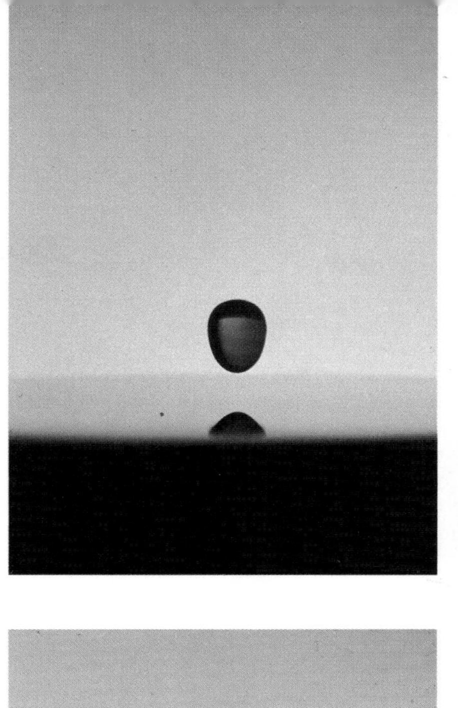

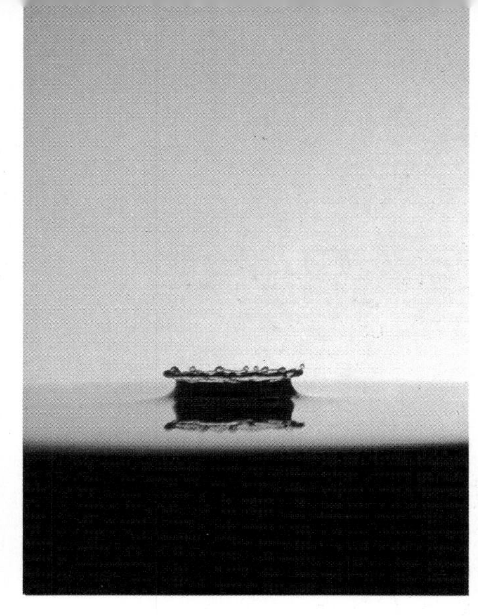

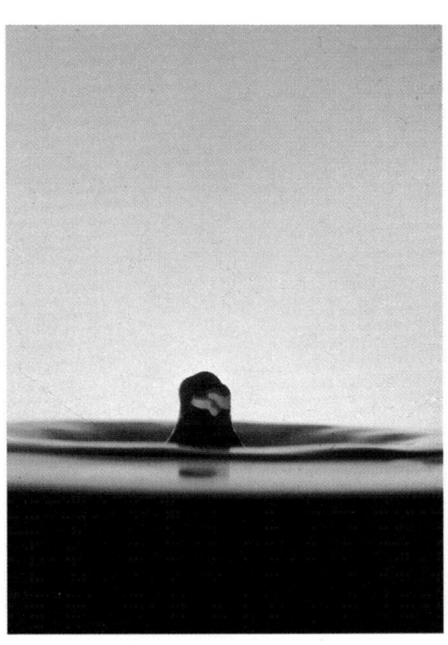

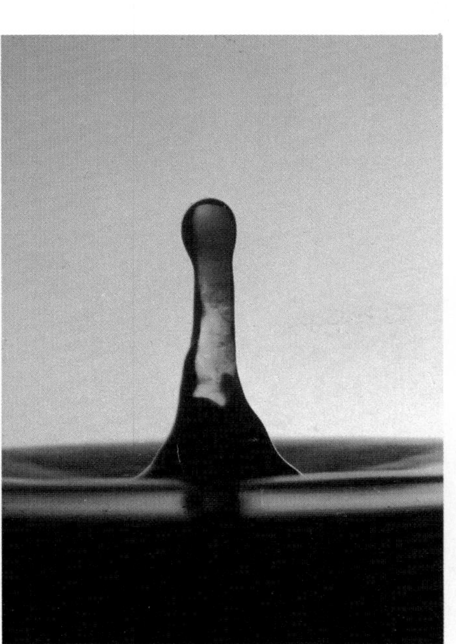

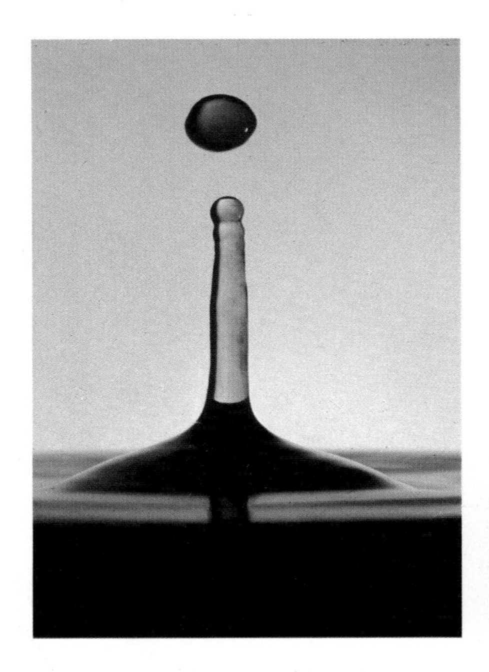

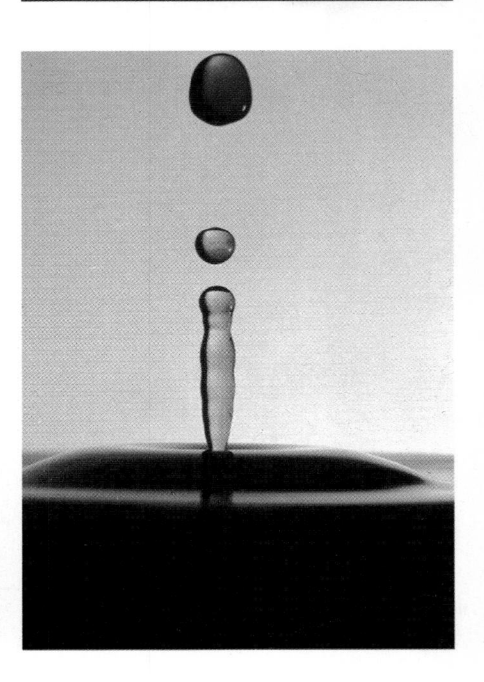

JUST FOLLOW THE BOUNCING BALL

This picture was made with a strobe light that flashes repeatedly for a millionth of a second. It records precisely the decreasing speed and height of the bouncing golf ball.

With each bounce, the ball loses energy and slows down. As the bounce becomes shorter and shorter, the images of the ball begin to overlap.

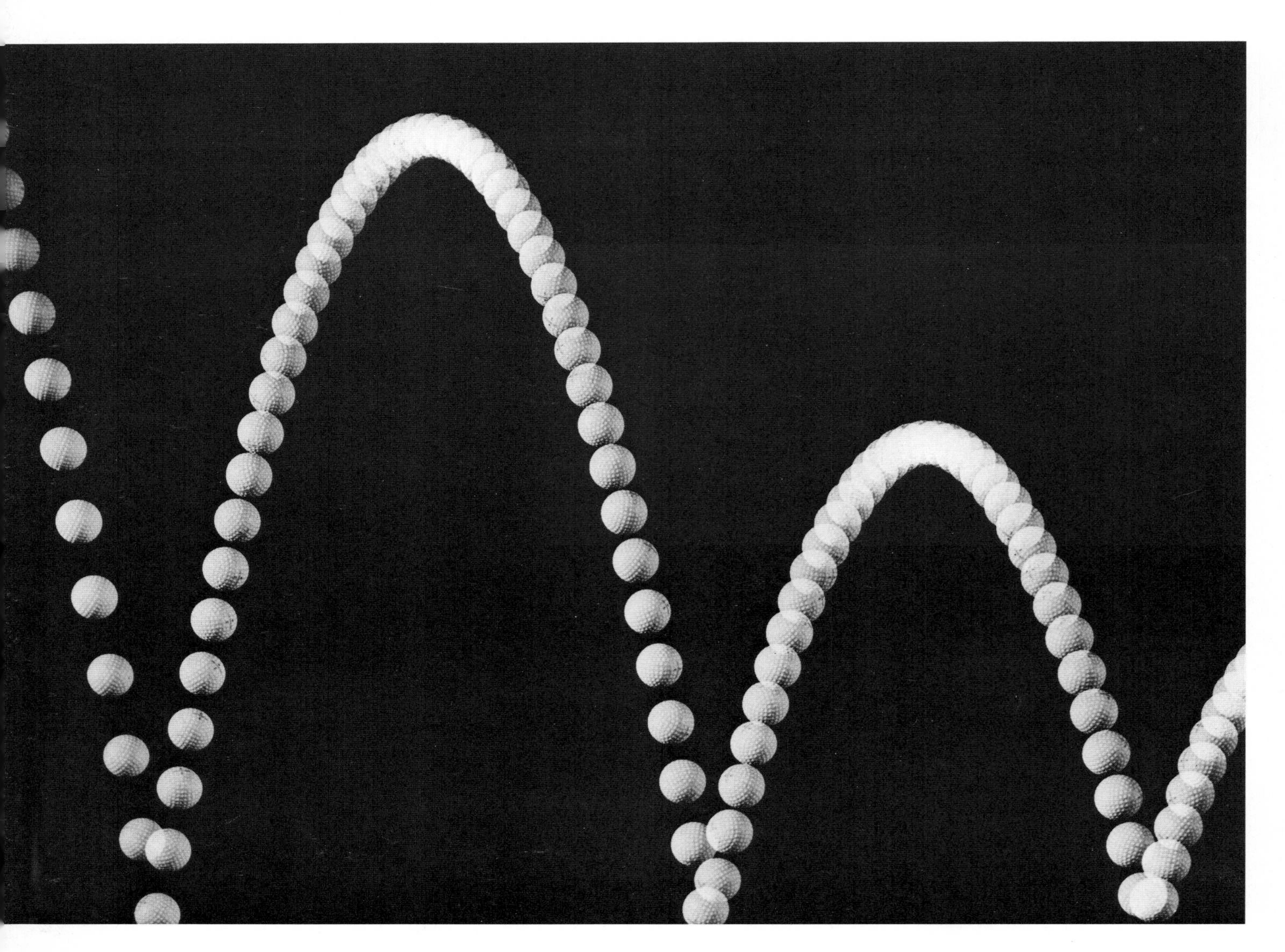

BEYOND LIGHT

The world hides numerous sights from our limited light-sensitive eyes. Light, visible light, is only a narrow slice of energy contained within an infinite spectrum of electromagnetic waves that constantly vibrate all around us.

Heat, sound, ultraviolet rays, gamma rays, x rays, even cosmic rays now can be used to create images that are just as real as those we see. Cameras are revealing the world in dimensions that were once completely unimagined and absolutely invisible.

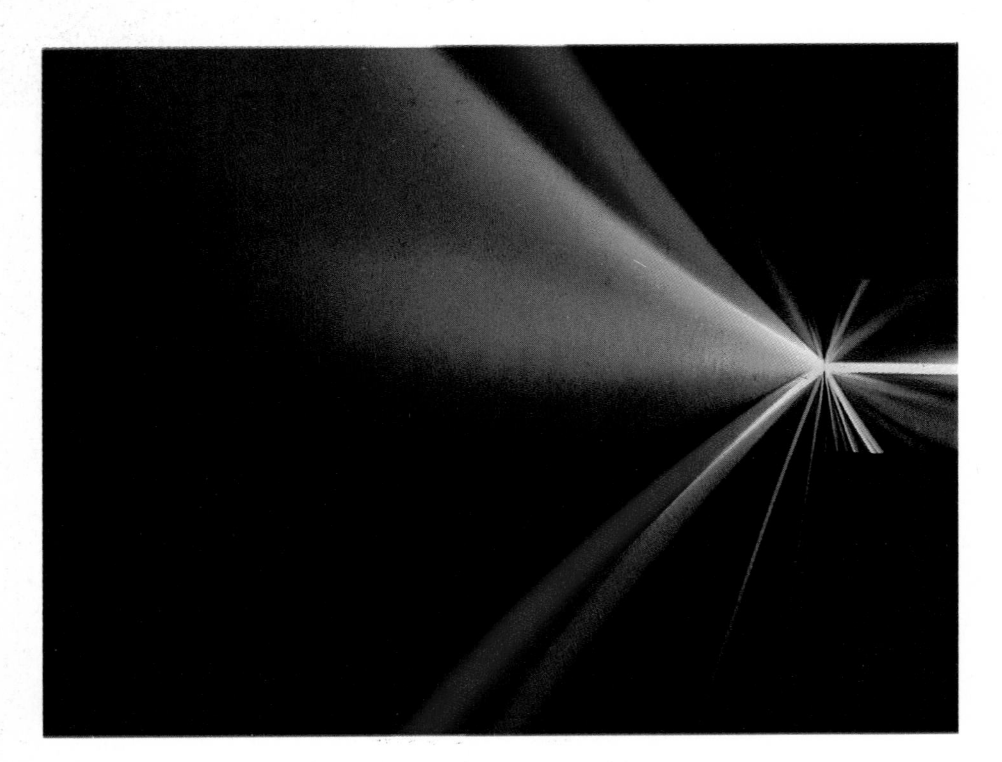

SOAP BUBBLE ▷

In the fragile film of a soap bubble lies a normally unseen world—a miniature liquid kaleidoscope too small for our eyes to see. The vibrant colors are caused by the random refraction of light.

VISIBLE LIGHT

When visible light is broken apart into its various wave lengths, the familiar rainbow of colors from red to violet appears. Colors, in fact, don't really exist. Colors are simply our brain's code for the wave lengths of light we can see. Beyond this band of energy our naked eyes go blind.

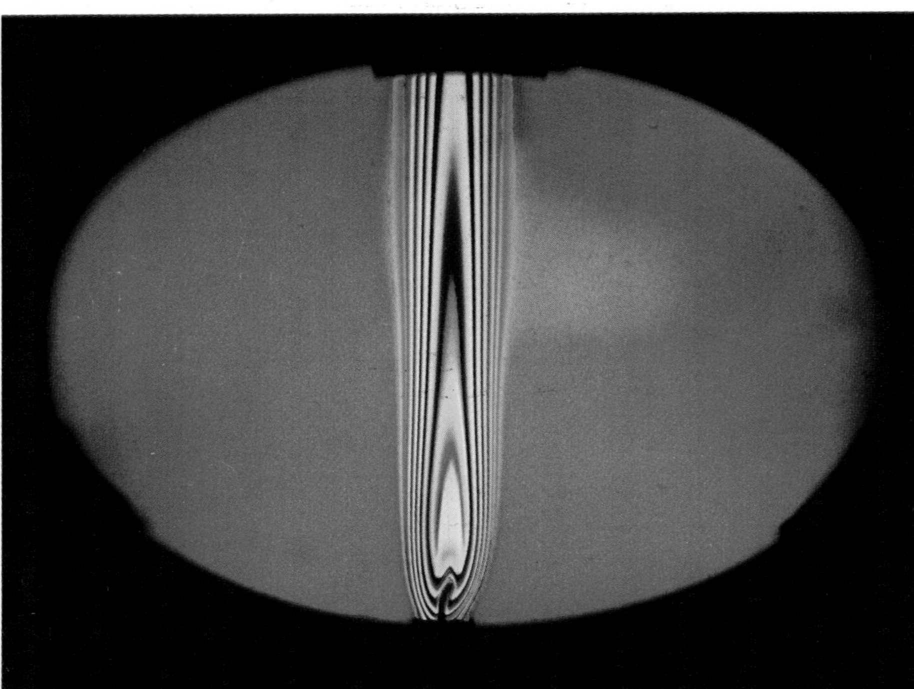

FLAME

The aura around the candle flame is a photographic effect caused by the many wave lengths of light either canceling out or intensifying each other. It is done with an instrument called an interferometer. The device slows down, ever so slightly, some of the flame's light as it travels toward the camera. Light behaves the same way when it creates a rainbow in the sky.

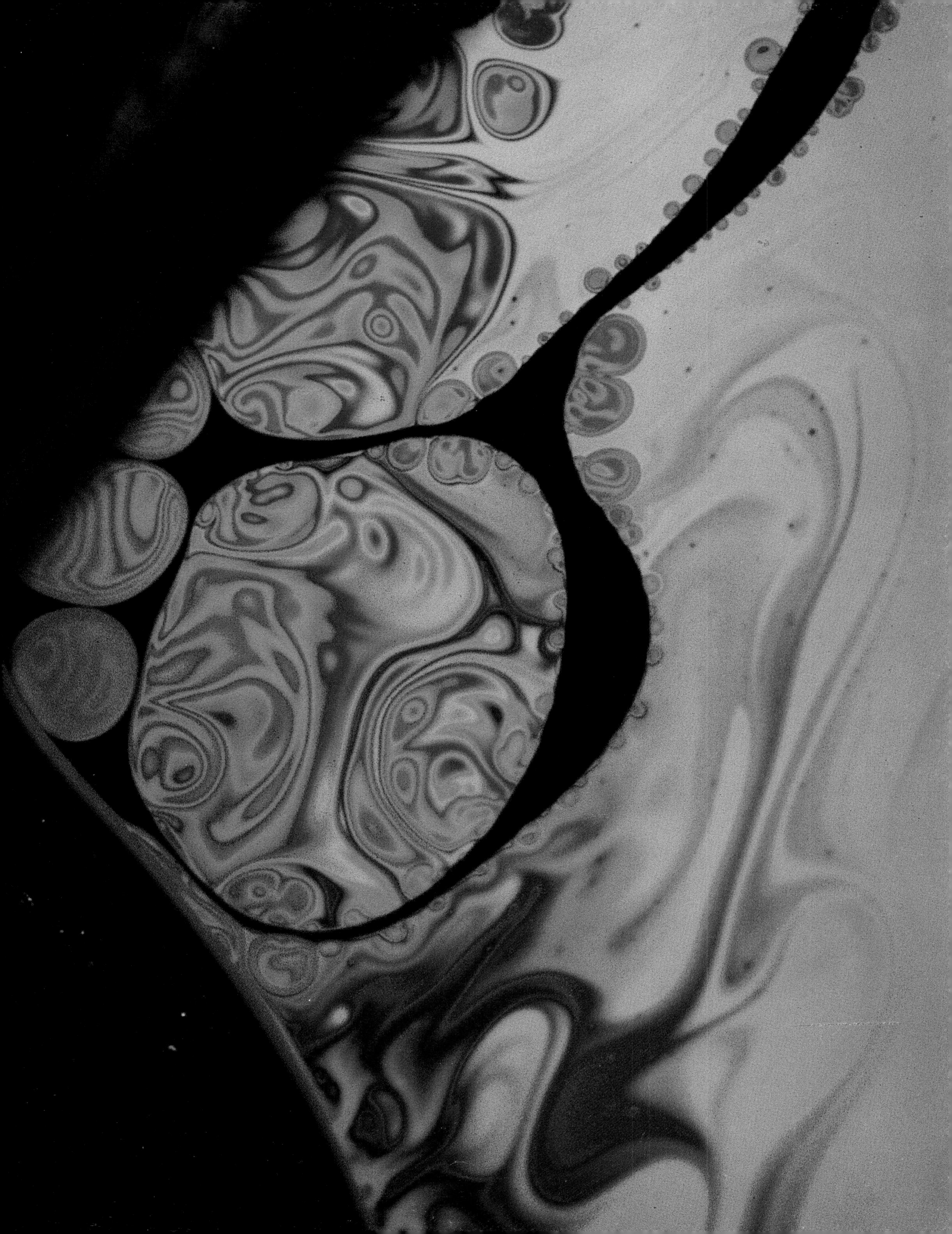

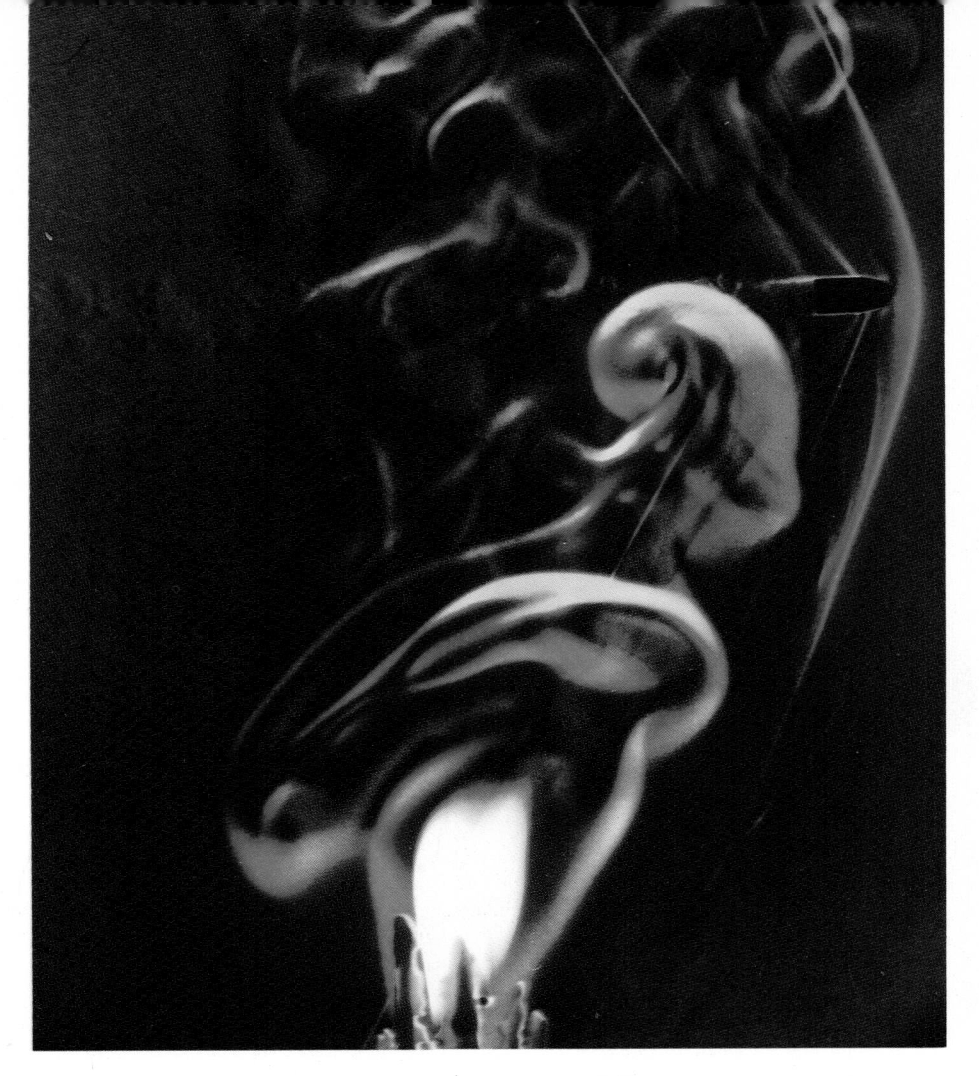

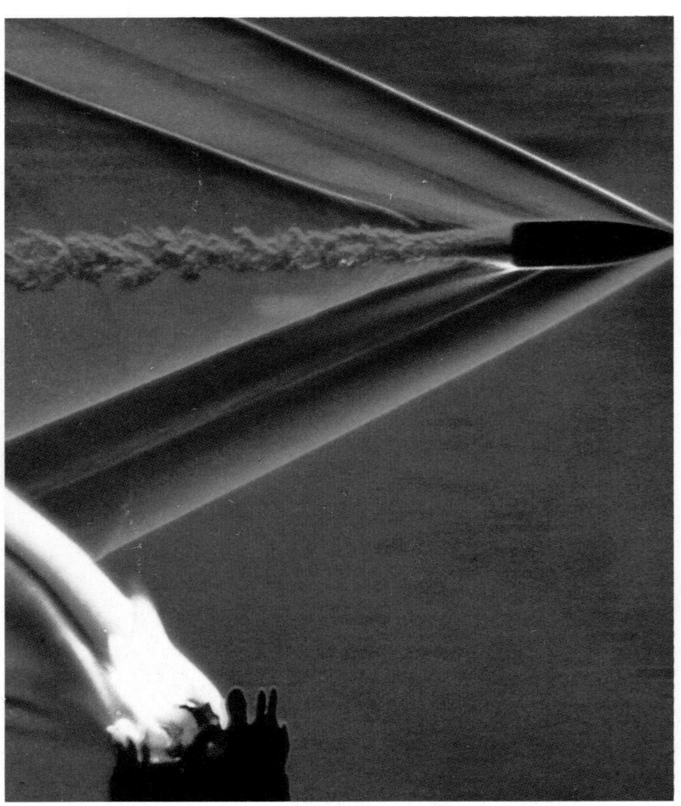

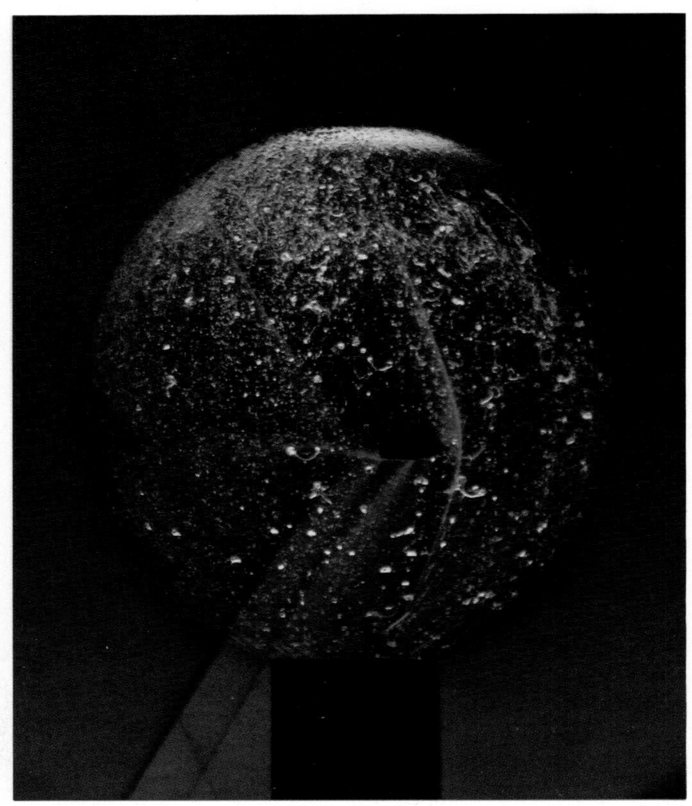

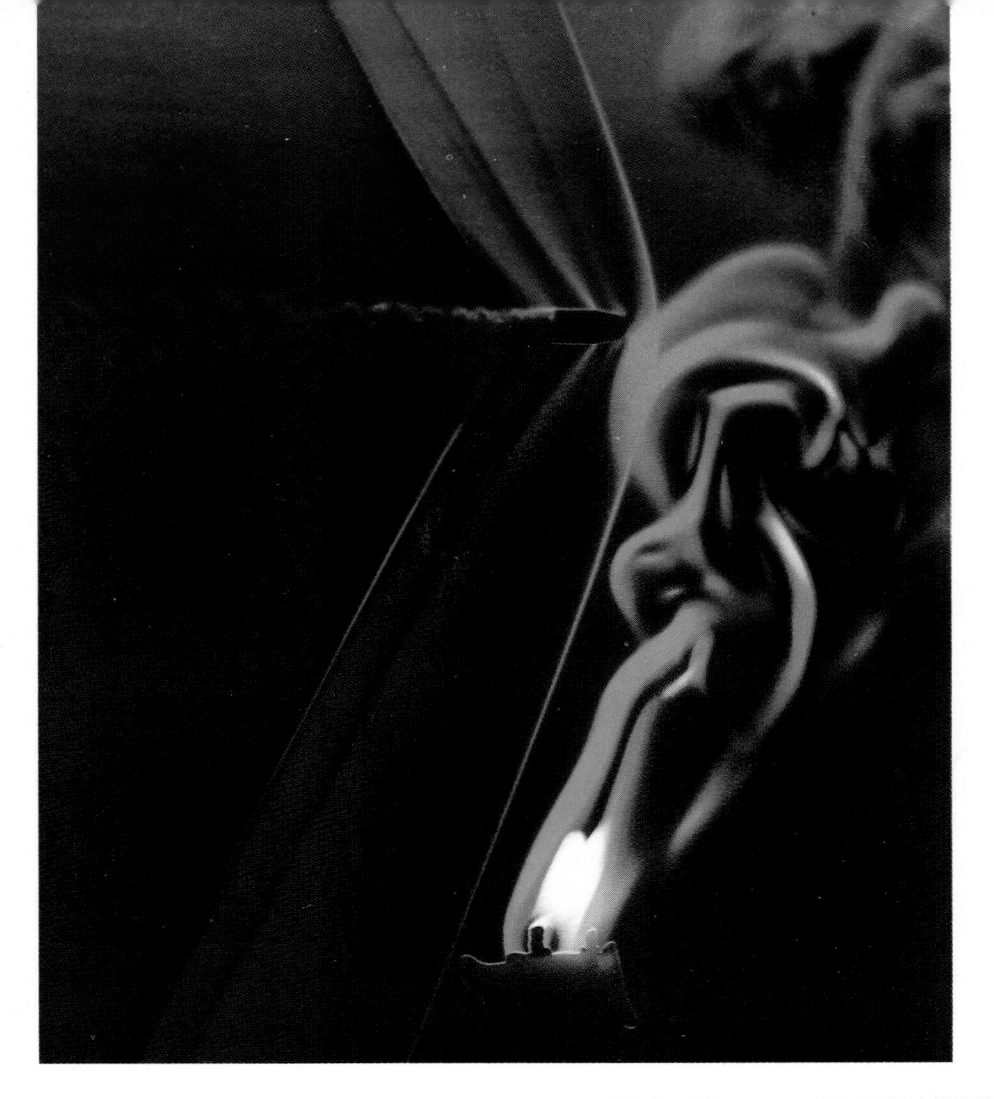

SEEING AIR

We think of air as invisible, but there are ways it can be seen. One method is by using schlieren photography, which slows and bends part of the light used to produce a photograph. By doing so, schlieren pictures reveal the varying densities of the air being photographed.

When the schlieren technique is combined with ultrahigh-speed stroboscopic photography, the results can be awesome.

Speeding bullets are stopped in flight . . . and the sonic boom the bullet creates is also frozen on film.

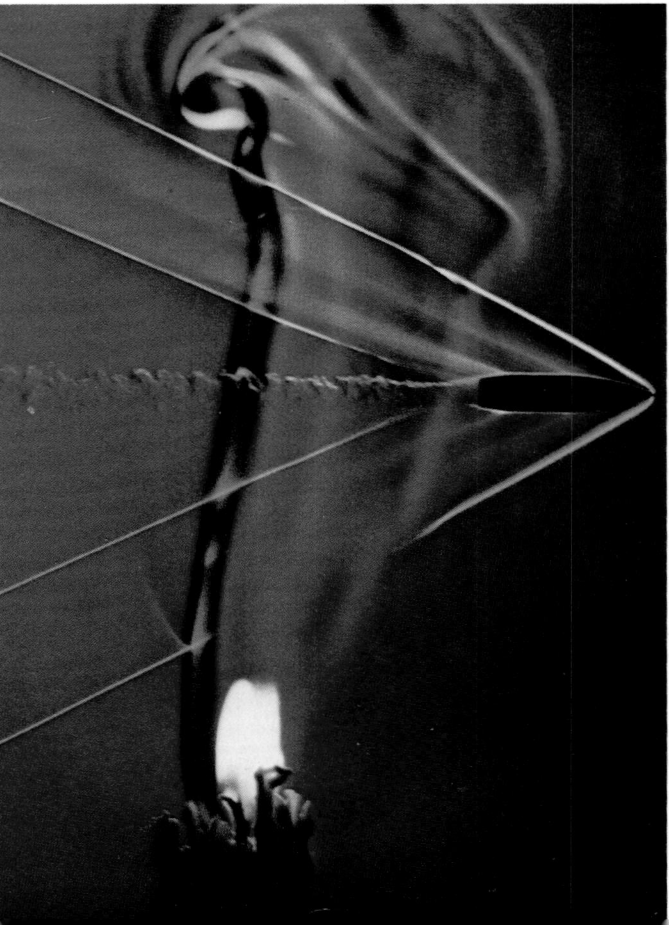

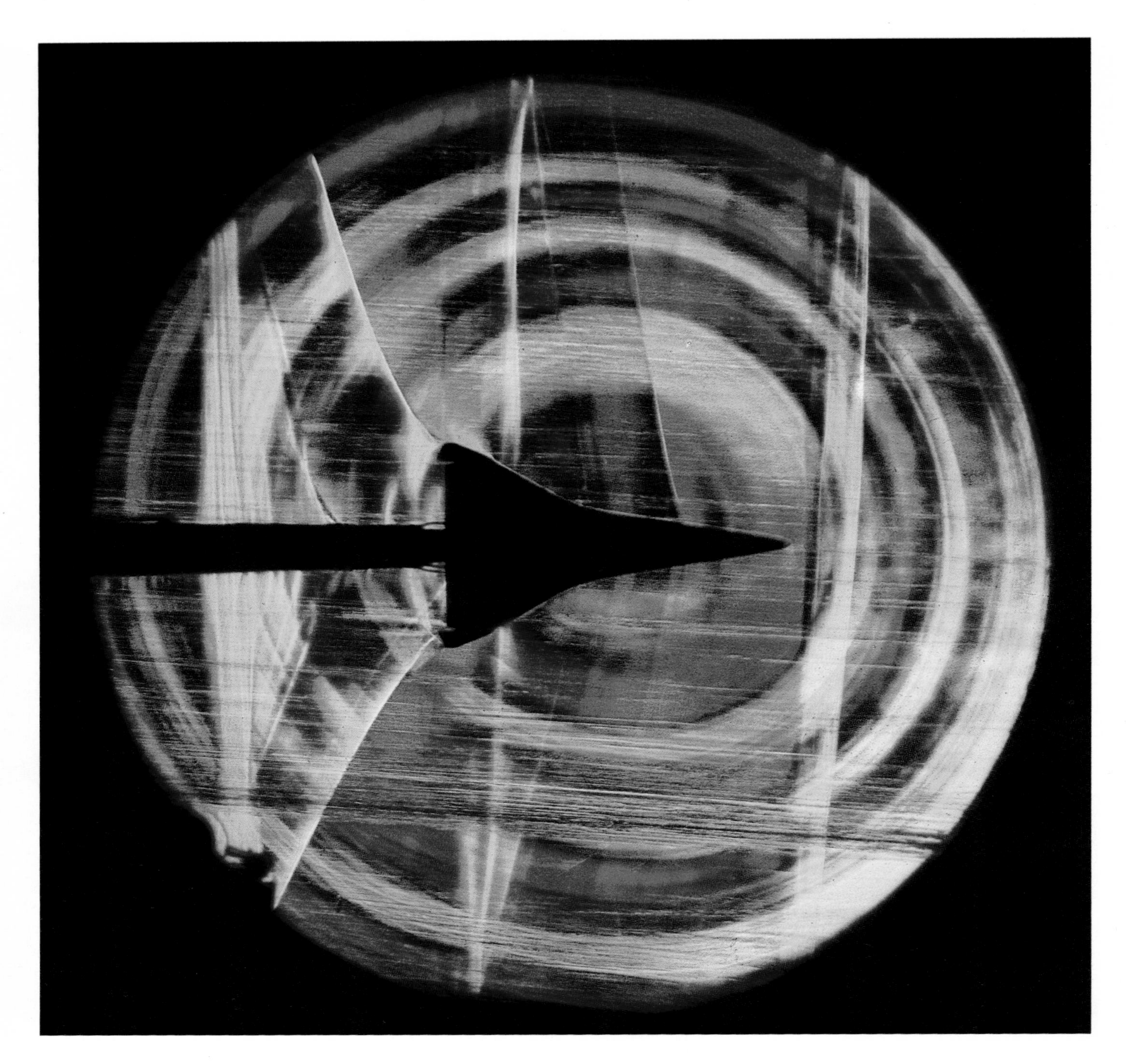

WIND TUNNEL

Schlieren photography is often used by scientists in wind tunnel studies. The aerodynamic qualities of everything from paper airplanes to space vehicles can be instantly seen by the otherwise invisible airflow patterns that surround them. The shock waves that buffet the model as it breaks the sound barrier provide information that will help perfect its design.

BREAKING POINT

Light can be directed to reveal normally invisible stresses and strains within a solid object. It is done by polarizing light. Light waves usually vibrate randomly in all directions. A polarizing lens—much like Polaroid sunglasses—filters through only the light waves traveling in the same direction.

When polarized light is shined on a plastic model of an object that is subjected to physical stress, its structural weak points become visible. The stresses and strains show as vivid color patterns.

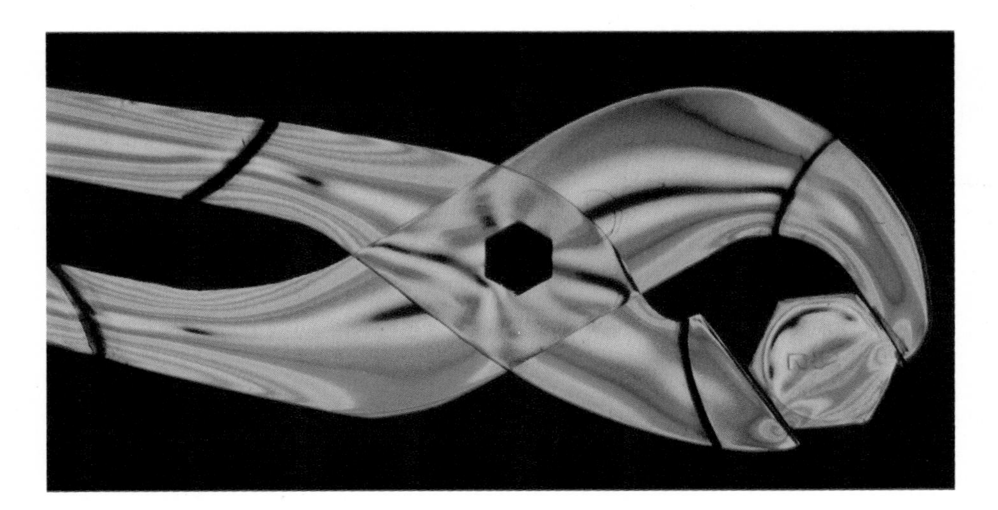

PUTTING ON THE SQUEEZE
Every time you squeeze a pair of pliers, this general pattern of strain will radiate through it.

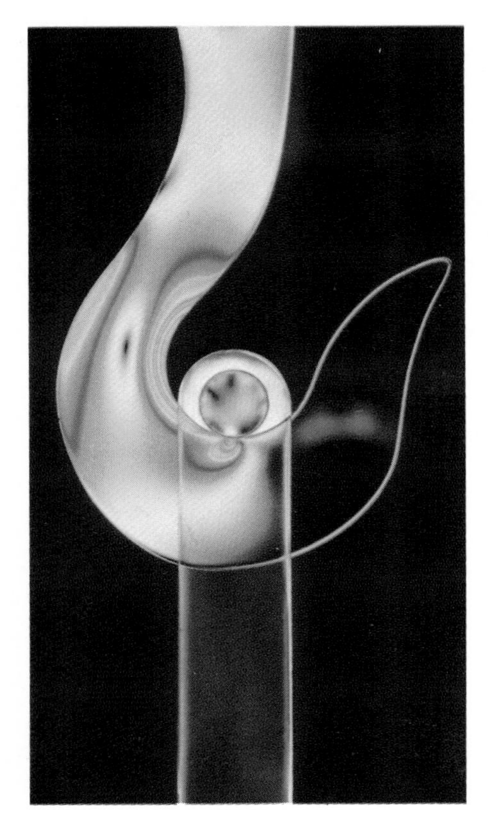

ON THE HOOK
Only a tiny section of the hook actually takes the strain of the weight.

THERMOVISIONS

If our eyes could see the part of the spectrum where red light turns to infrared, or heat, our view of the world would suddenly take on a new and expanded scope. Through the power of specialized cameras we can now see the world in terms of hot and cold as well as light and dark.

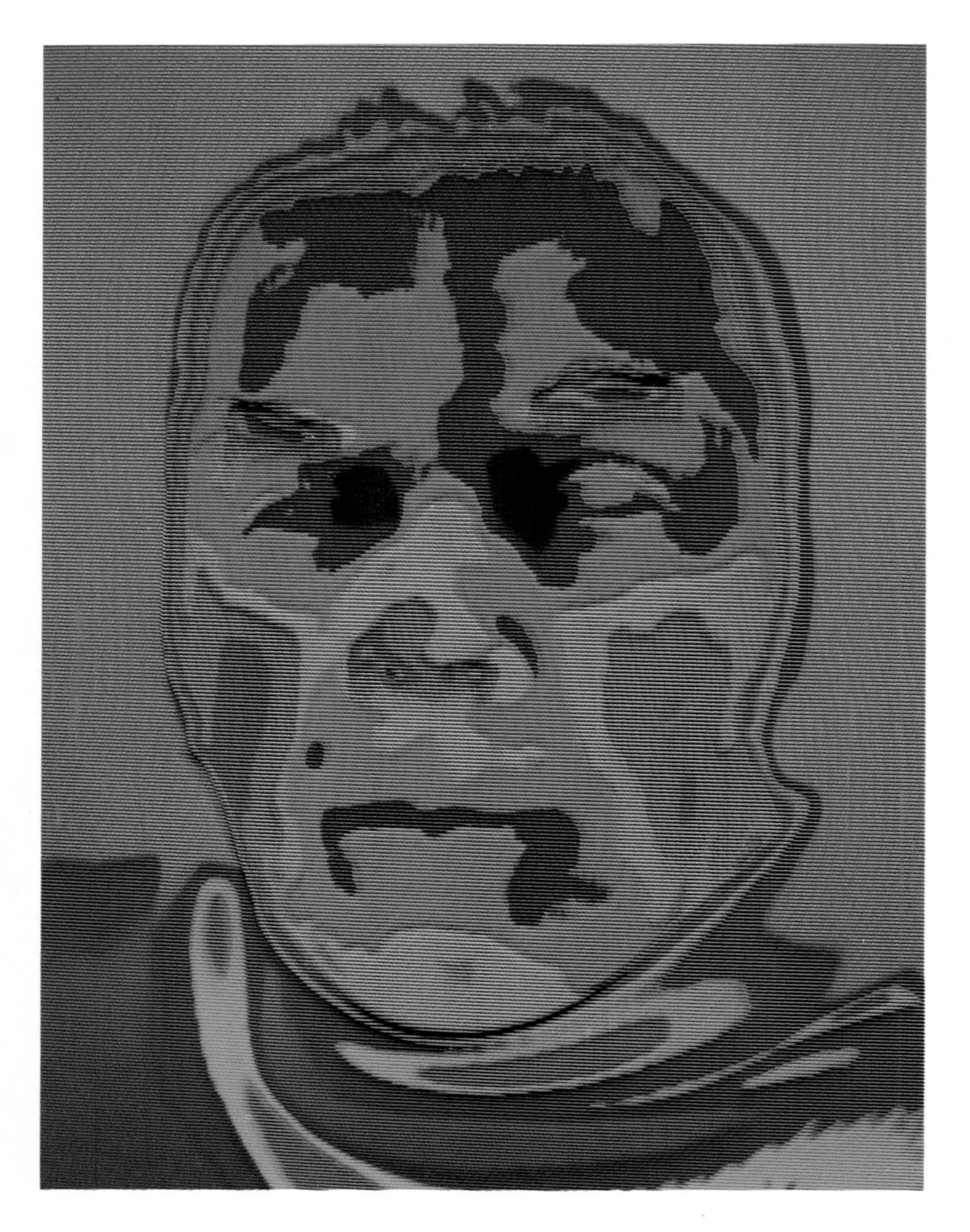

HOT HEAD

A yawn, a blush, a laugh, or a headache alters our infrared image. The color on this man's face reflects the subtle variations of his skin temperature. To the eyes of a thermal camera, we are an ever-changing kaleidoscope of color.

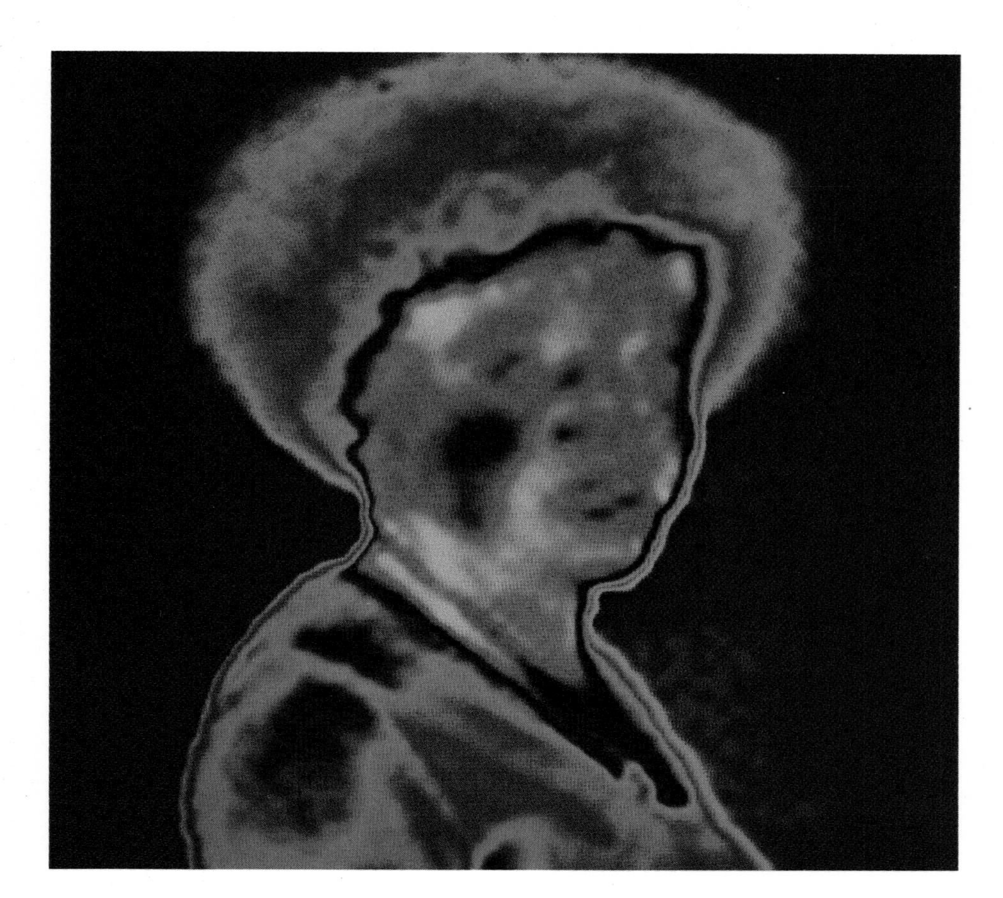

A PORTRAIT IN HEAT

Thermal cameras, a valuable new tool in medicine, can detect early warnings of tumors, infections, and constricted blood-flow. This portrait is a picture of health.

THERMO KID

In this thermal photograph of a child, red and yellow represent the warmest areas of the body; blue and green the coolest. There is one obvious observation that doesn't require medical training: The child's feet and bottom are cold.

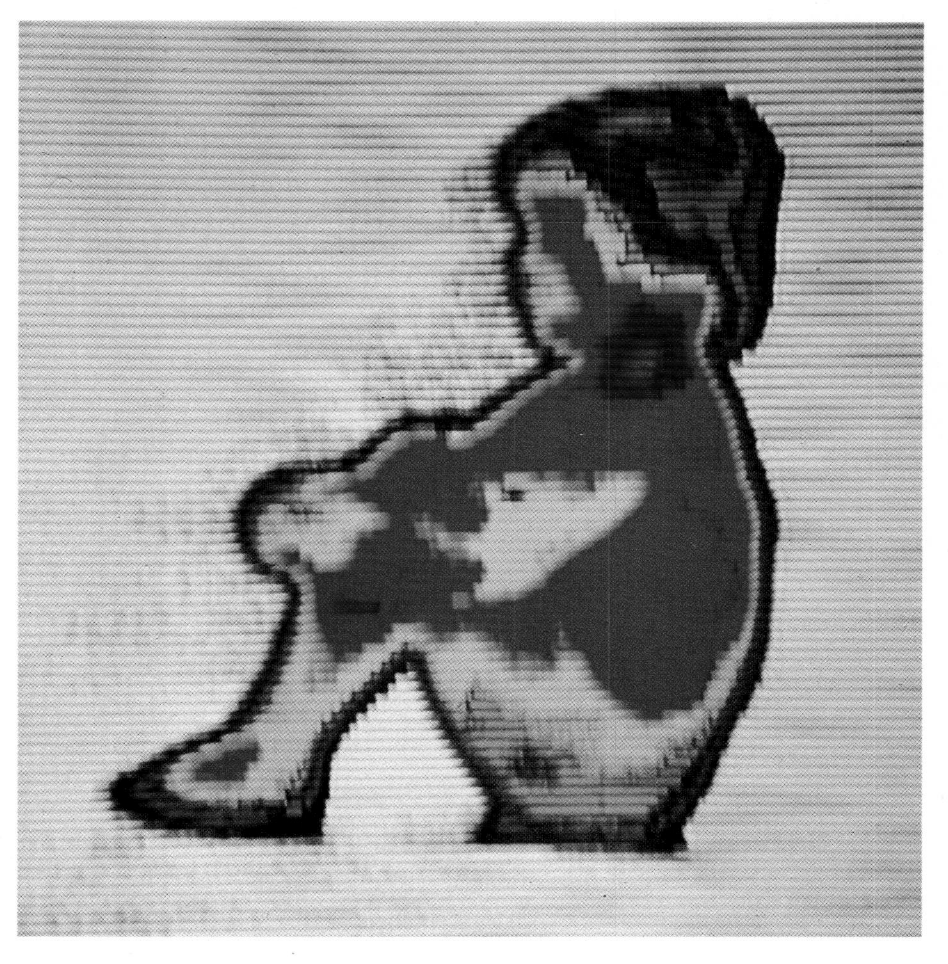

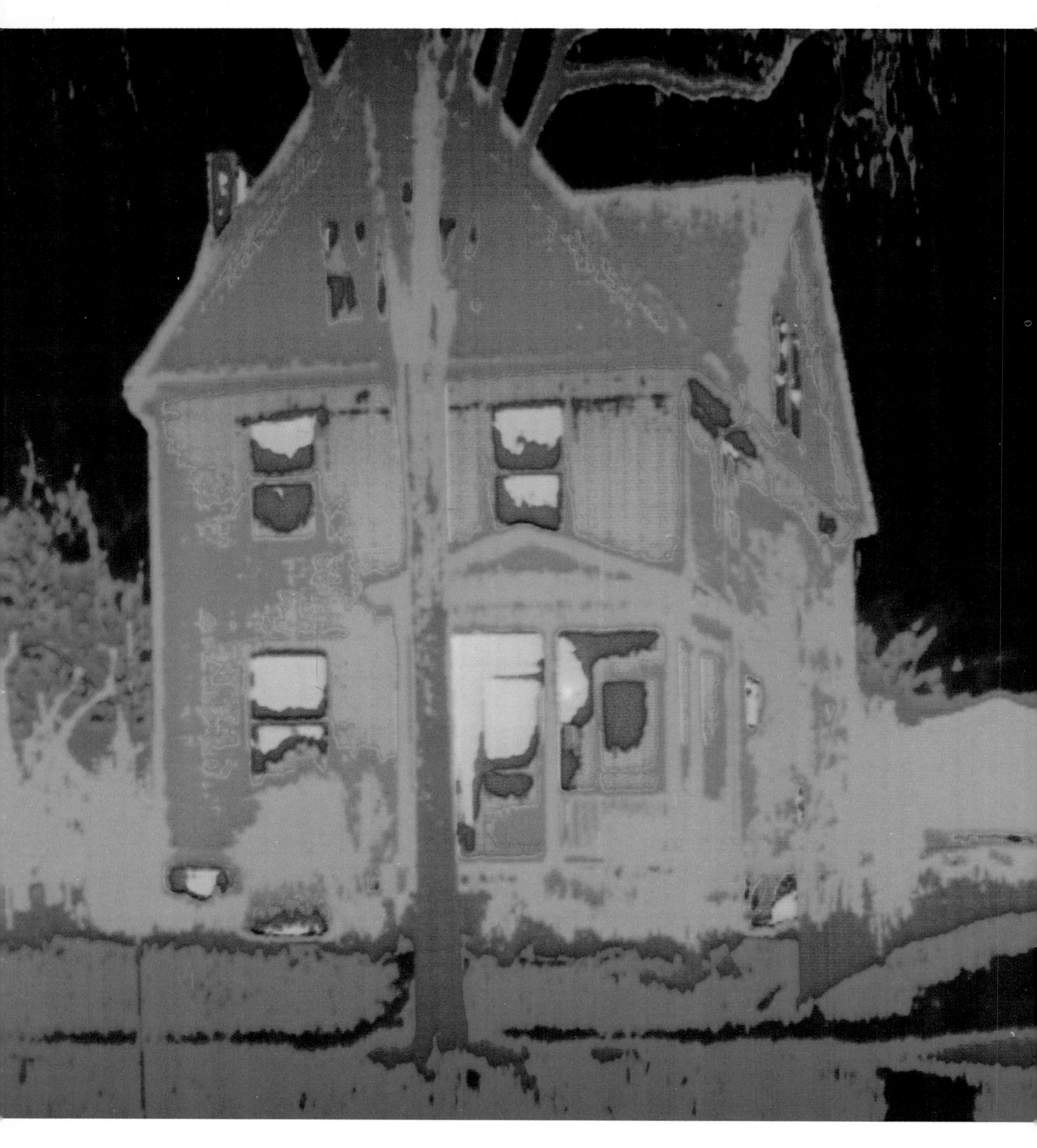

HOT HOUSE
To the eyes of a thermal camera, a poorly insulated house is instantly recognizable. Costly heat energy can be seen radiating through the windows, roof, and walls.

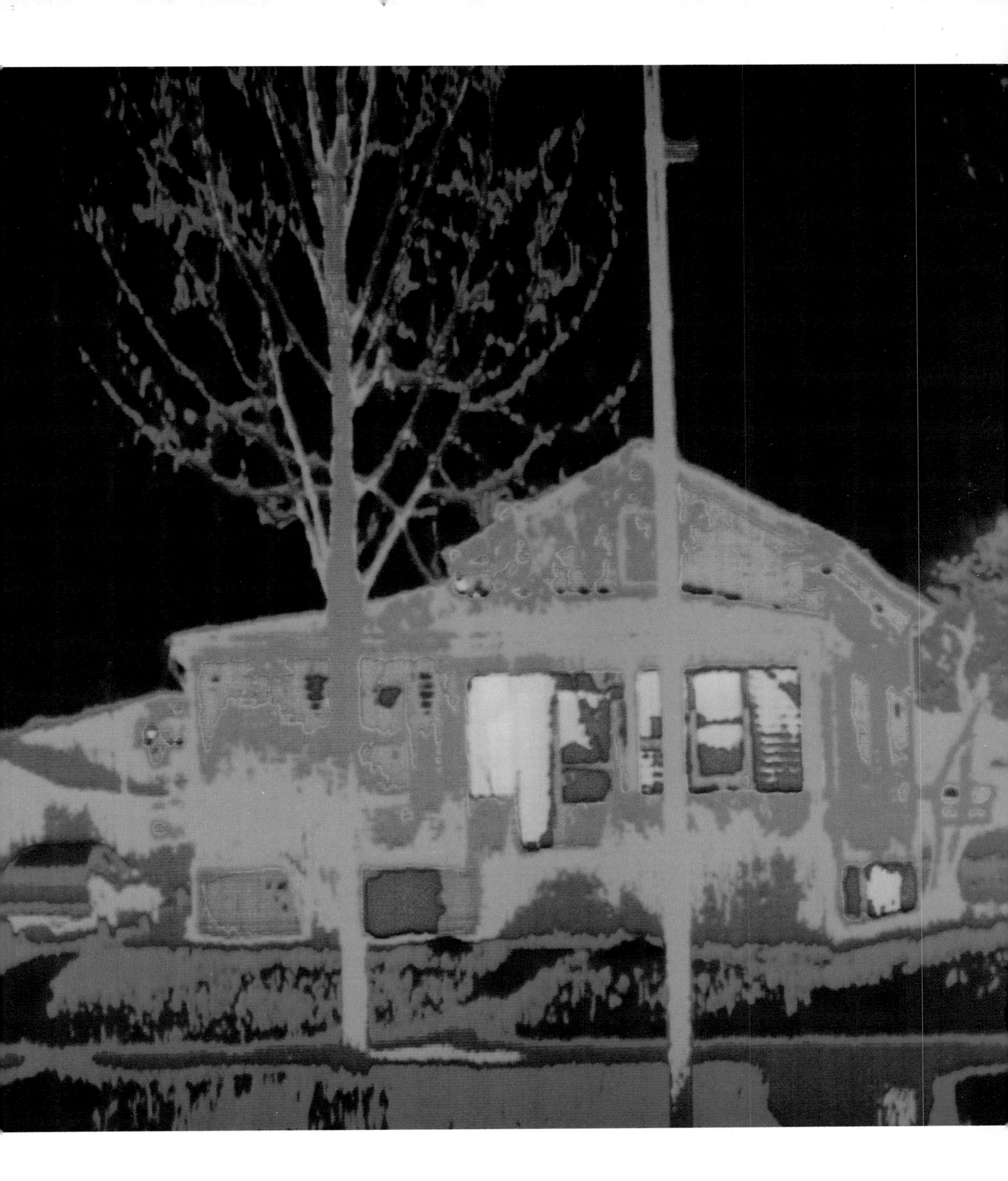

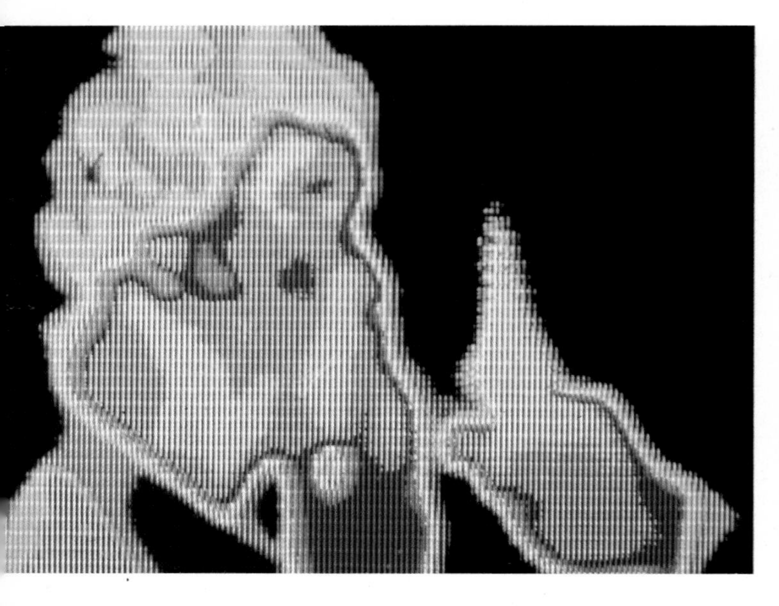

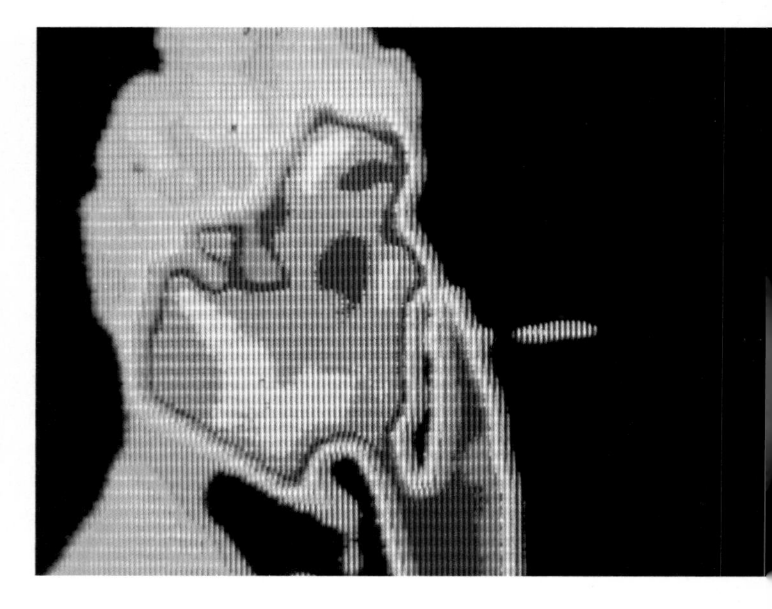

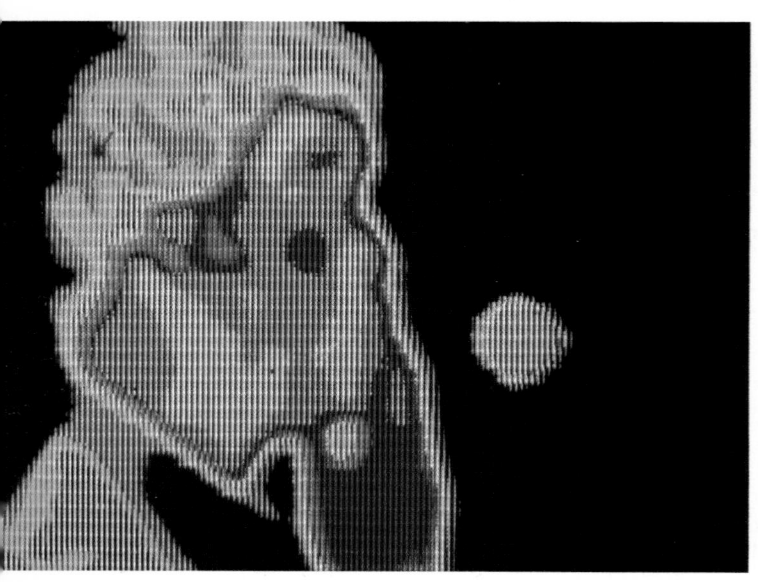

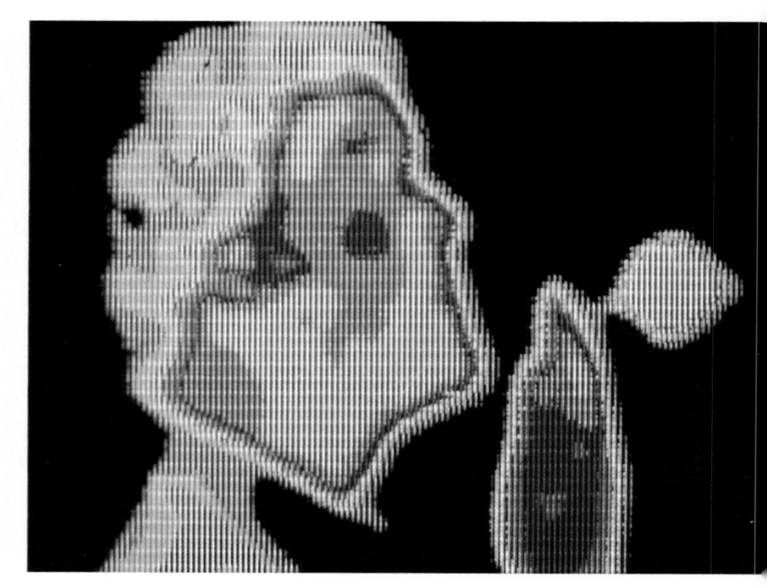

SMOKING

The simple act of lighting and puffing a cigarette reveals the effects of nicotine to a thermographic camera. Blood vessels quickly constrict and cool the surface of the skin.

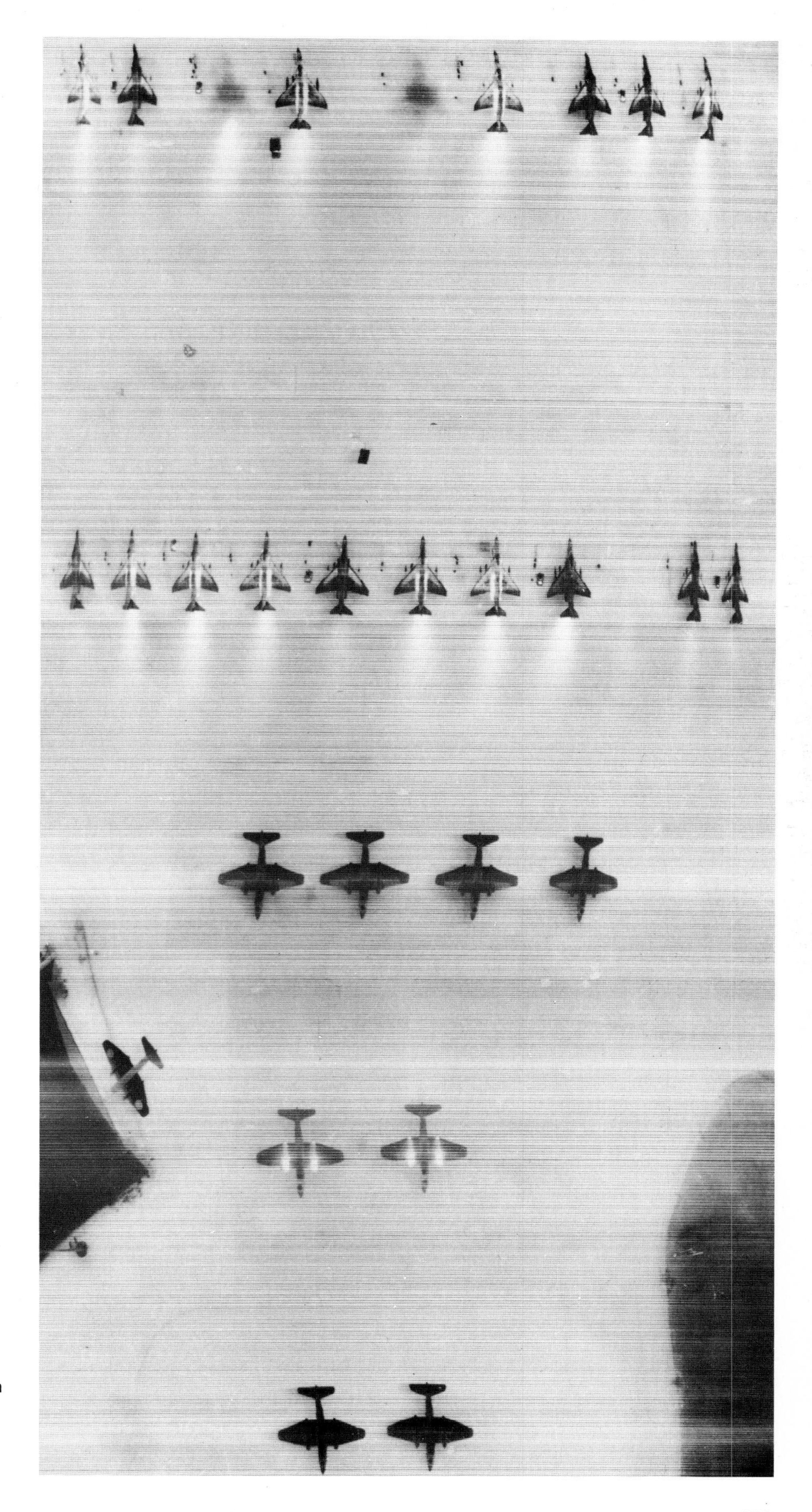

EYE IN THE SKY

To an infrared-sensitive camera, an airfield reveals much more than would be apparent in normal light. The full fuel tanks of jets glow much hotter than the cooler body of the plane. So do warm engines that are ready for takeoff. Jets that have already departed leave a visible shadow of heat.

SEEING INSIDE

If something is photographed with visible light, only the outer surface details are recorded by the camera. With another form of energy, invisible to the eye, solid matter can be penetrated to create an image of what is inside.

X rays have the power to do that. Their existence was discovered in 1895 by a German scientist named Wilhelm Roentgen. It was a revolutionary find. Even so, x rays were briefly considered by some to be a threat to feminine modesty. Fears, however, were quickly allayed at first sight of the x-ray image.

SHOT IN THE DARK
If our eyes were sensitive to x rays as well as visible light, the sight of a gun being fired might look something like this. This picture was created by superimposing an x-ray image upon a normal photograph.

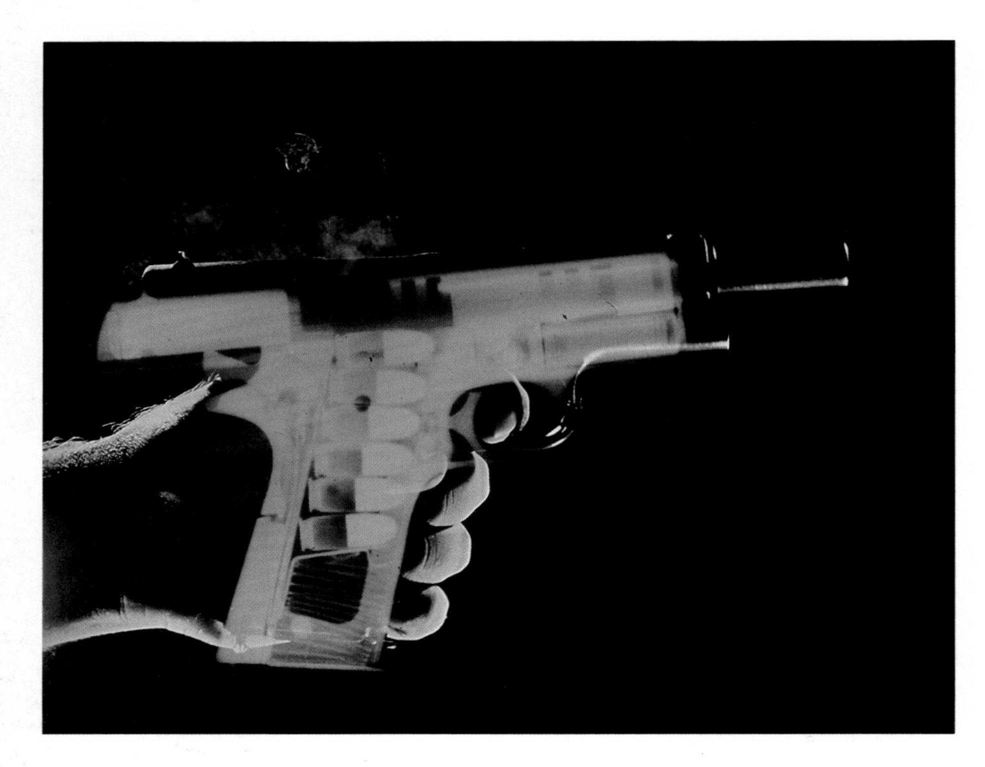

X-RAY MAN ▷
A computer enhancement technique called density slicing can transform a black-and-white x-ray photograph into a strikingly colorful image. Each subtle shade of the x-ray picture was given color electronically.

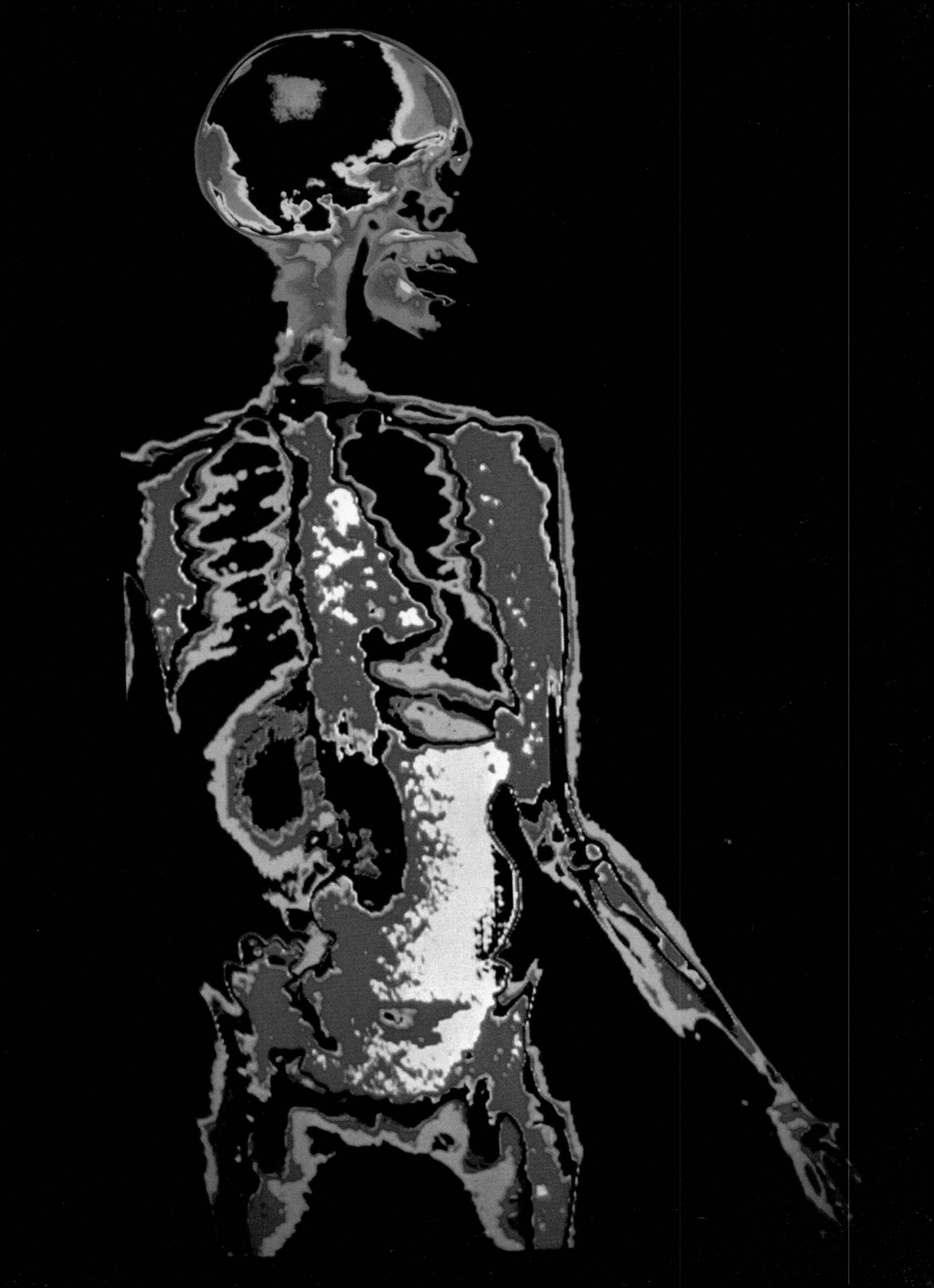

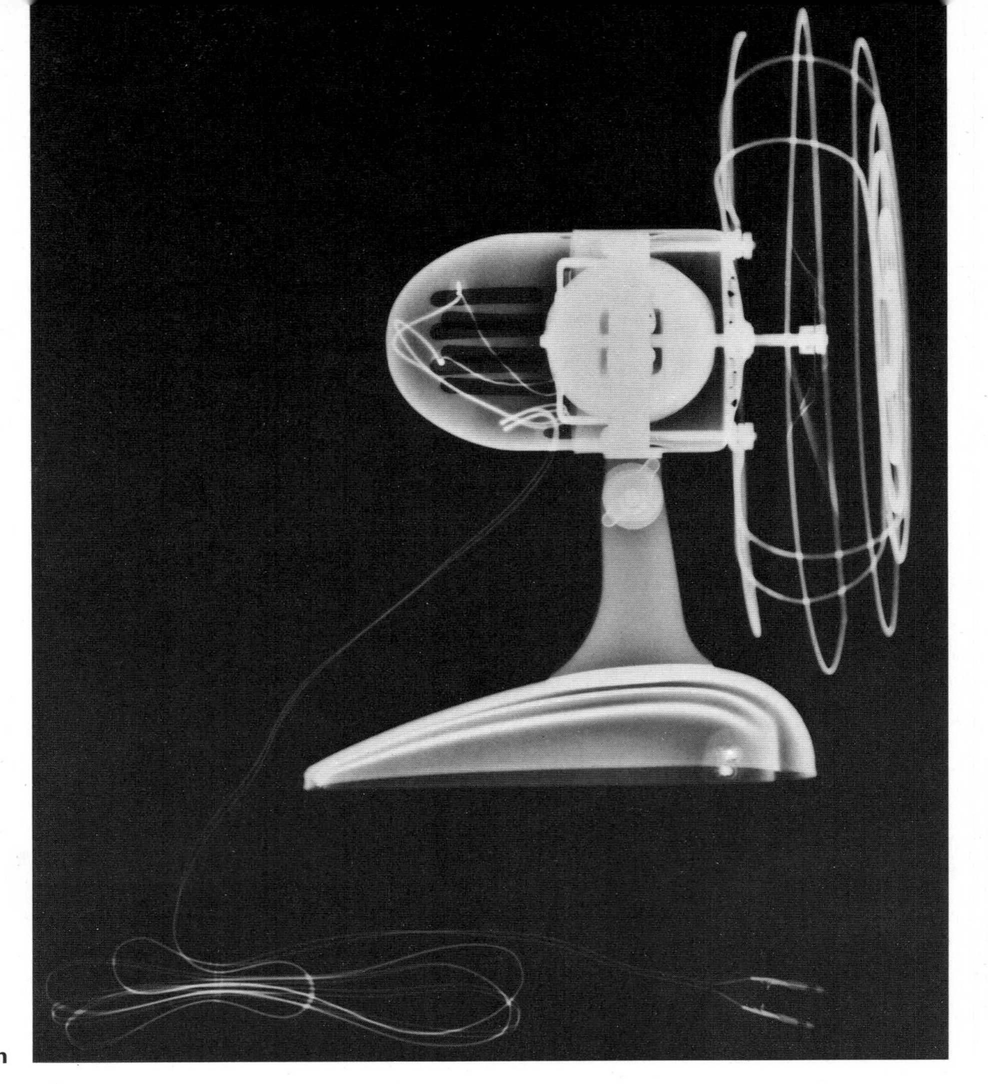

Electric Fan

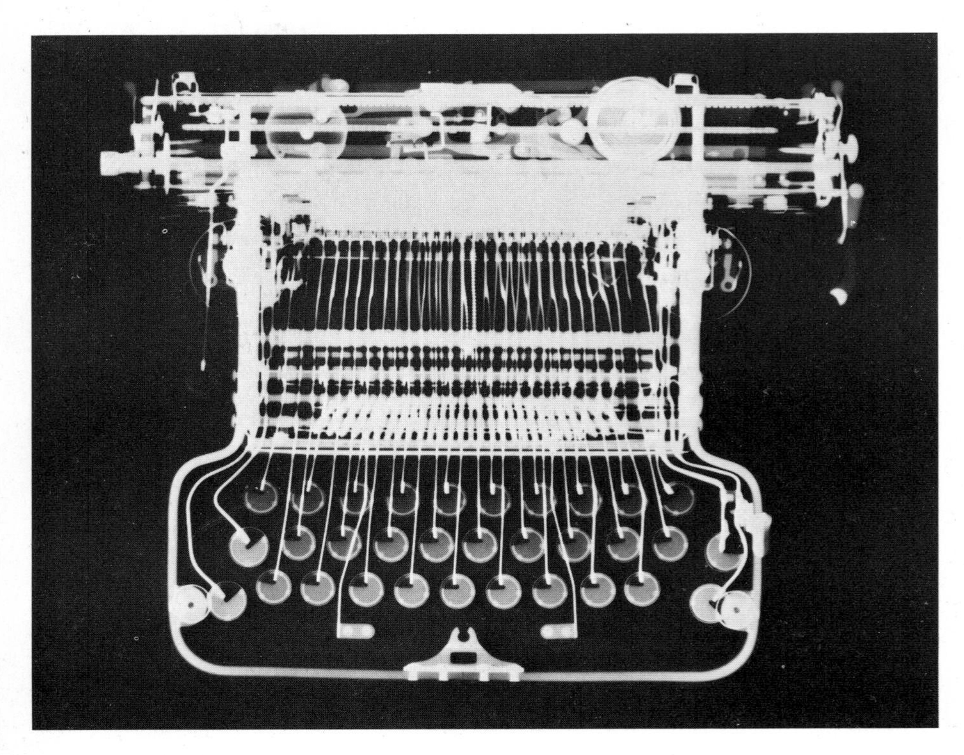

Typewriter

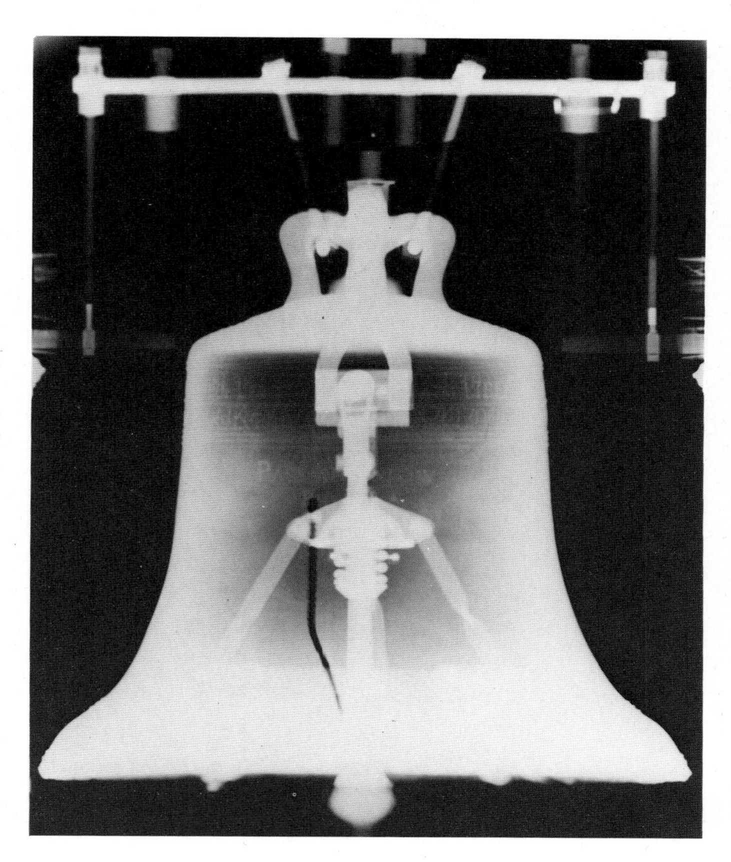

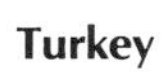

The Liberty Bell

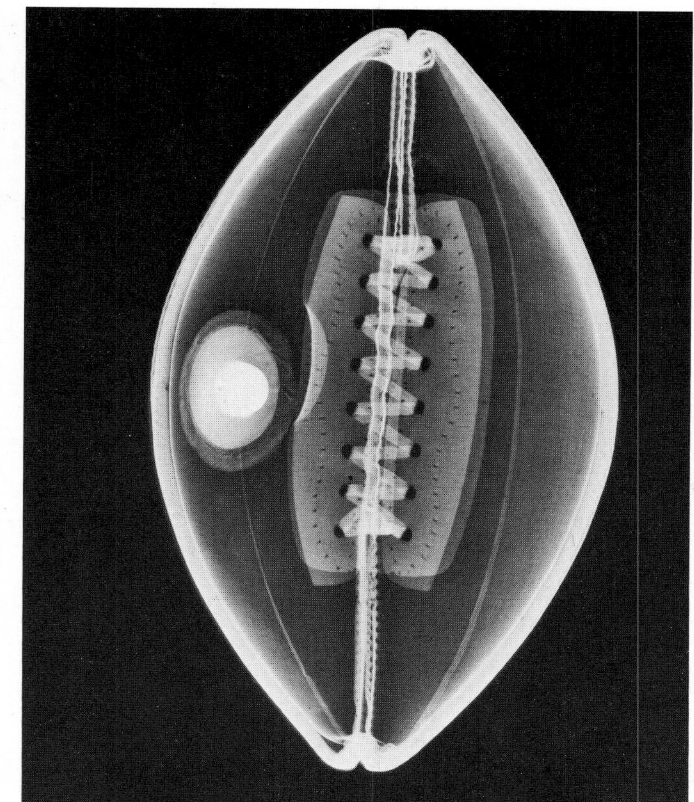

Football

Turkey

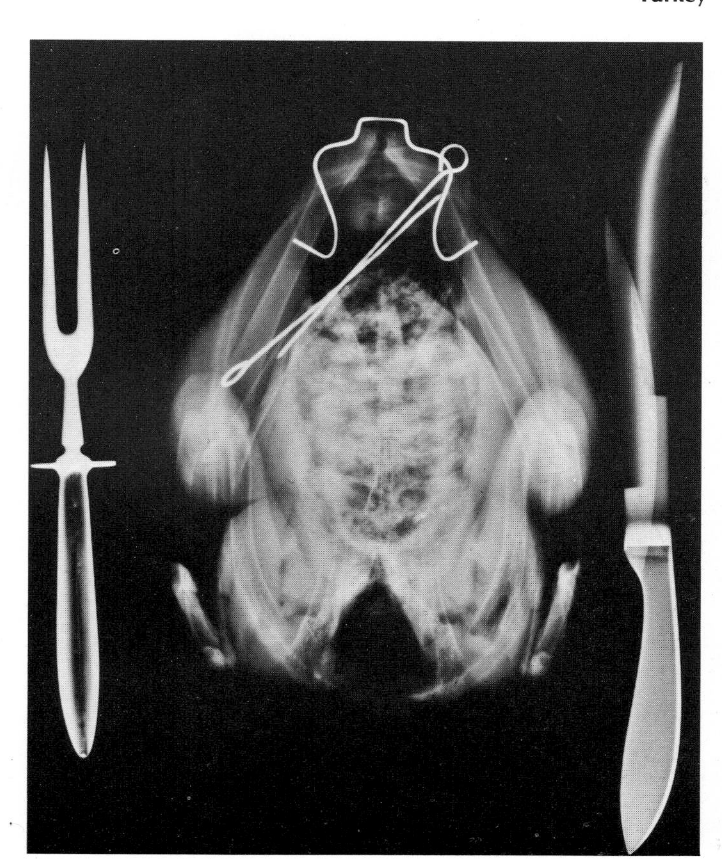

Box of Candy

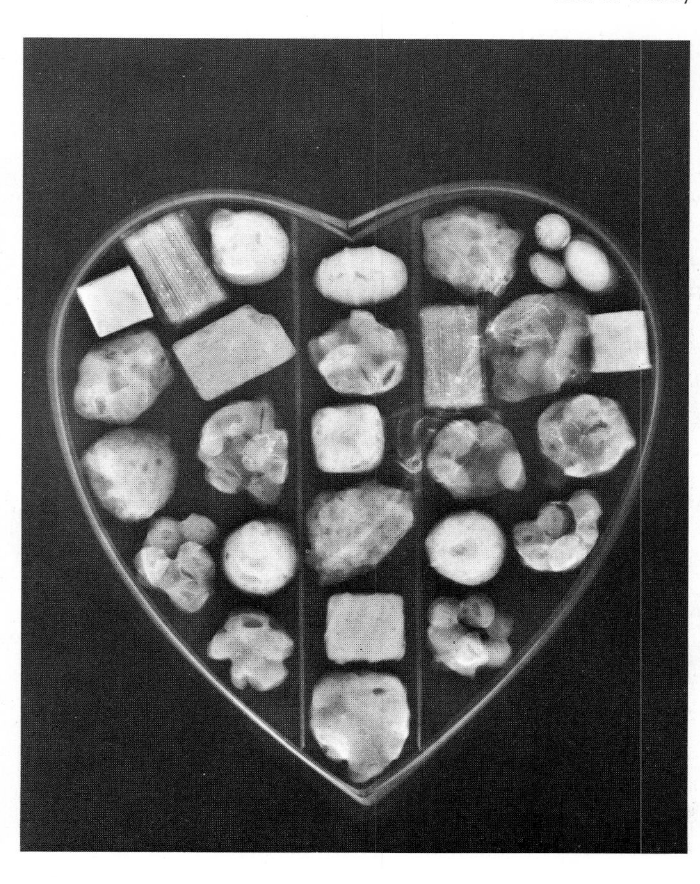

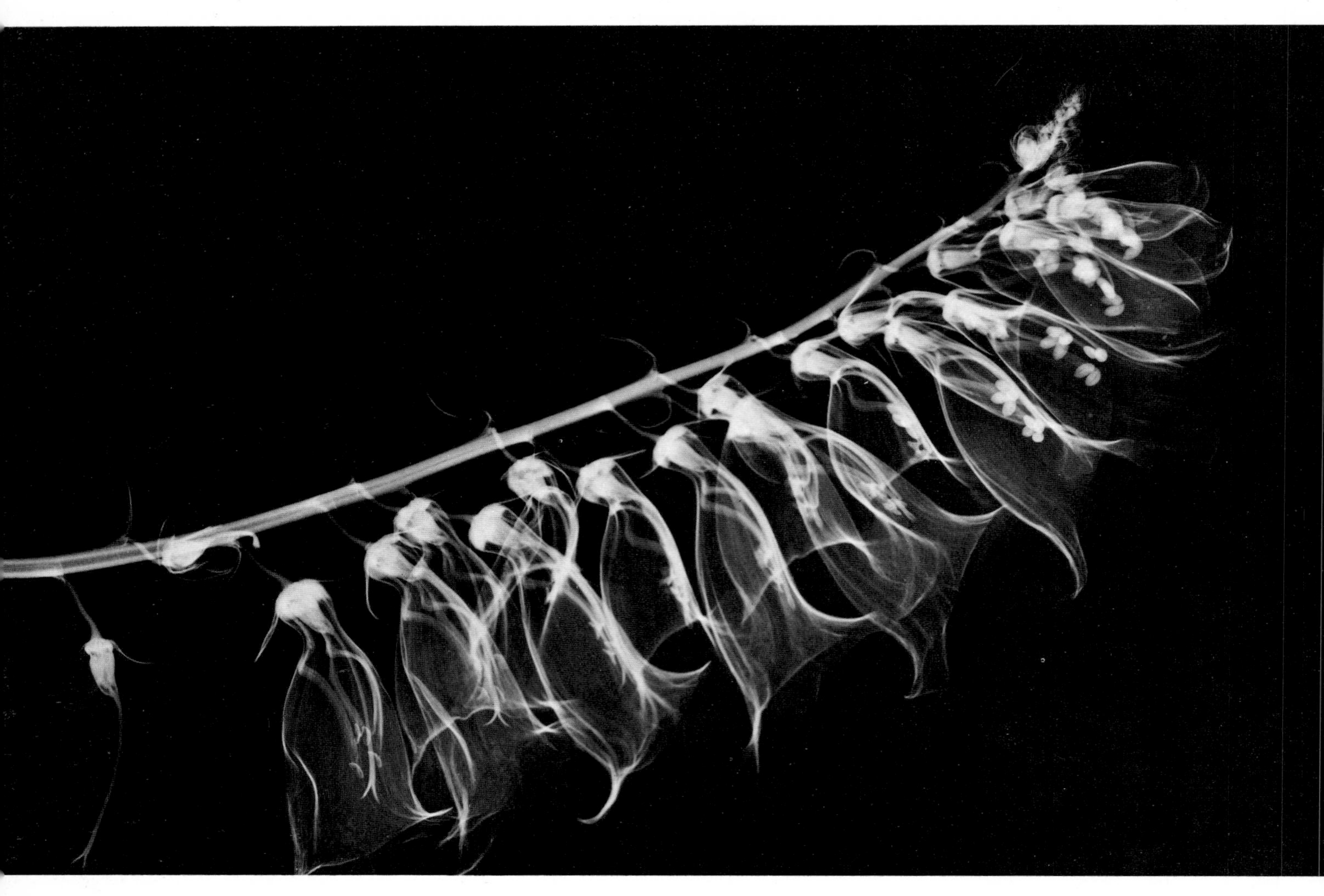

Foxglove Flowers

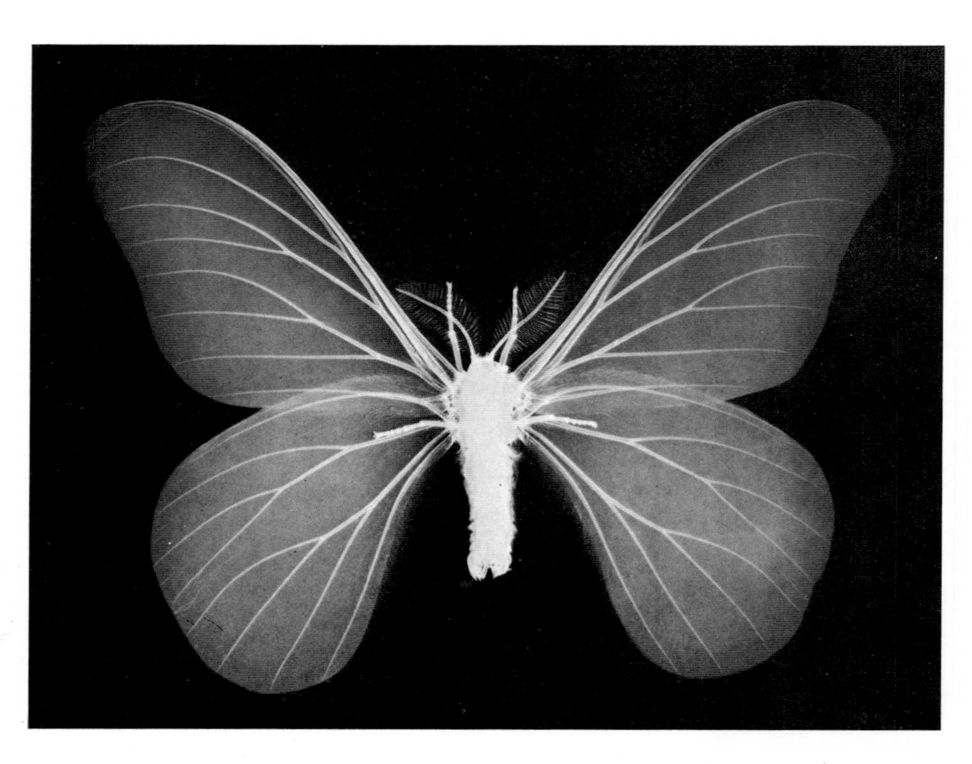

Moth

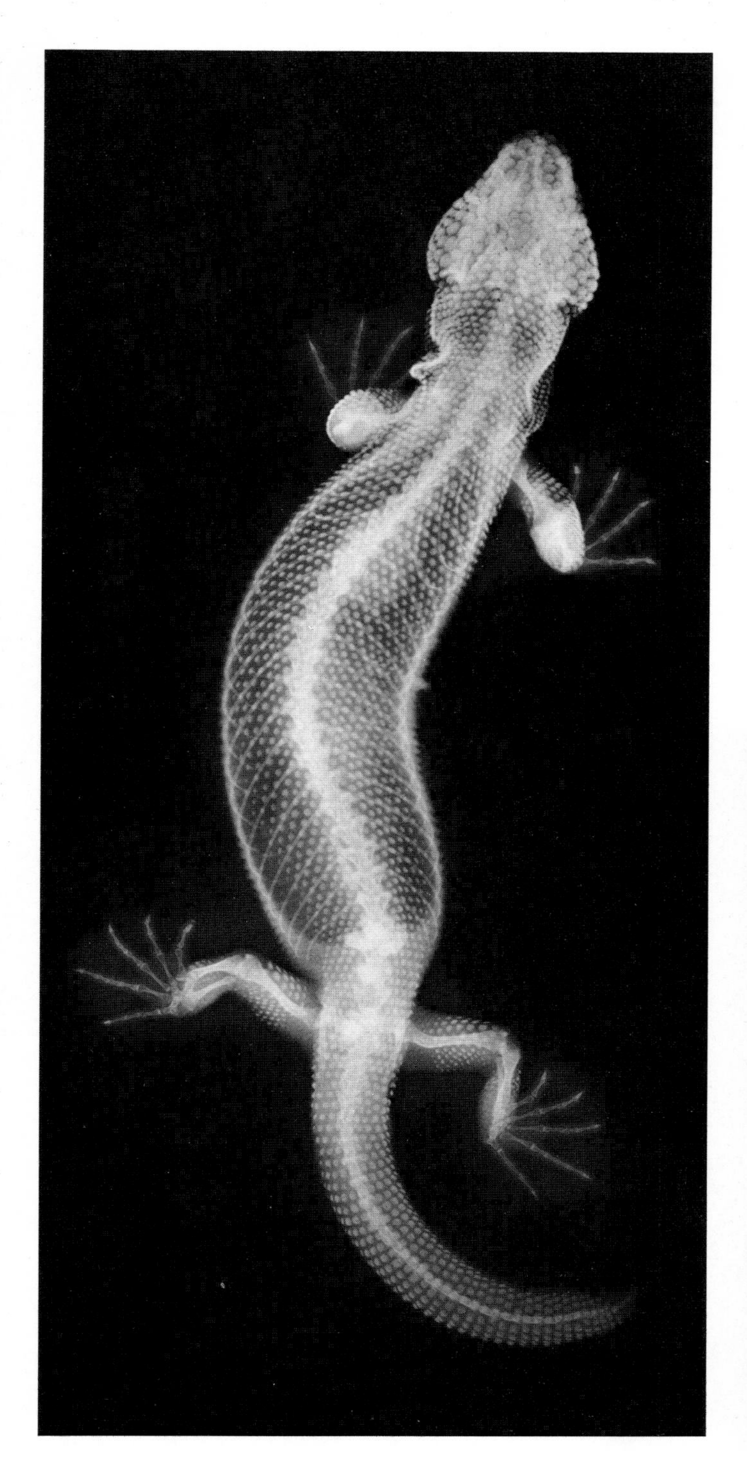

Gila Monster

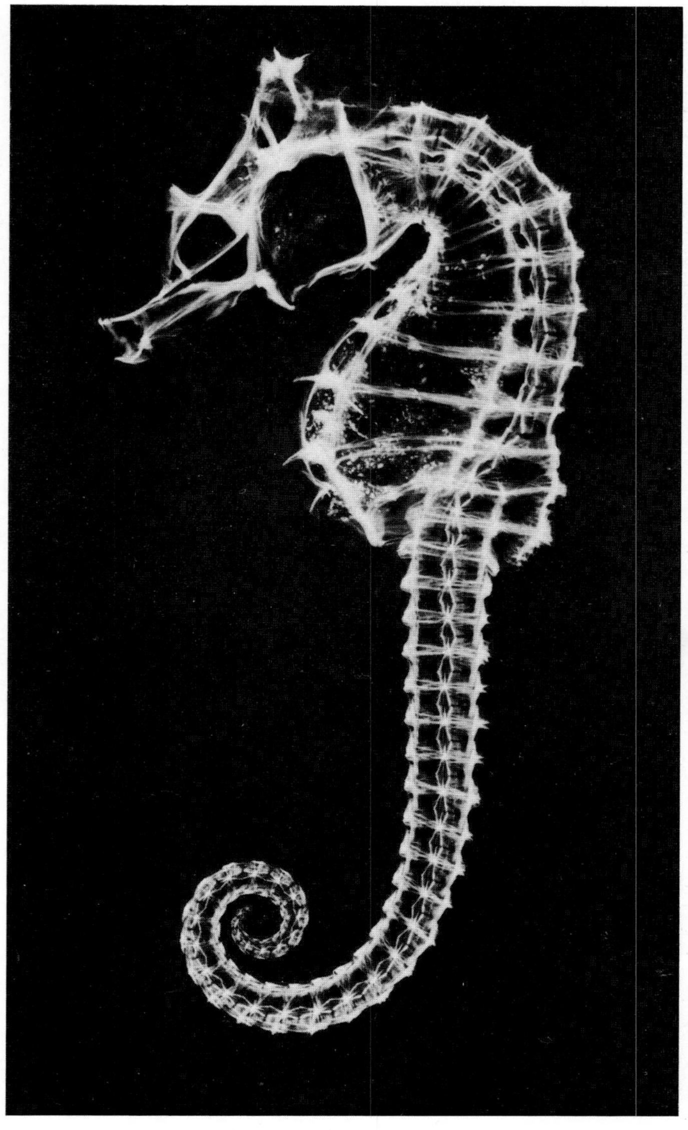

Sea Horse

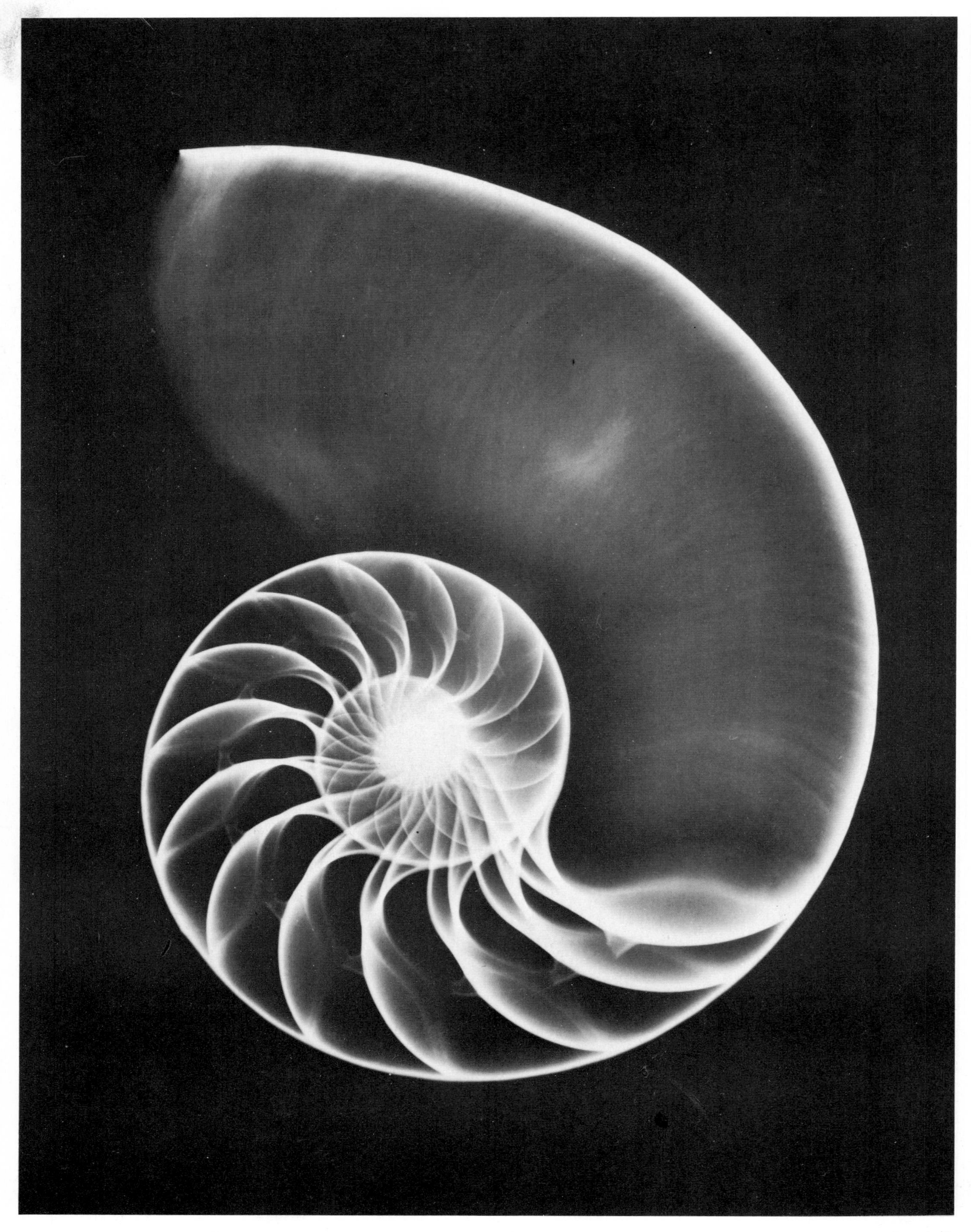

Nautilus Shell

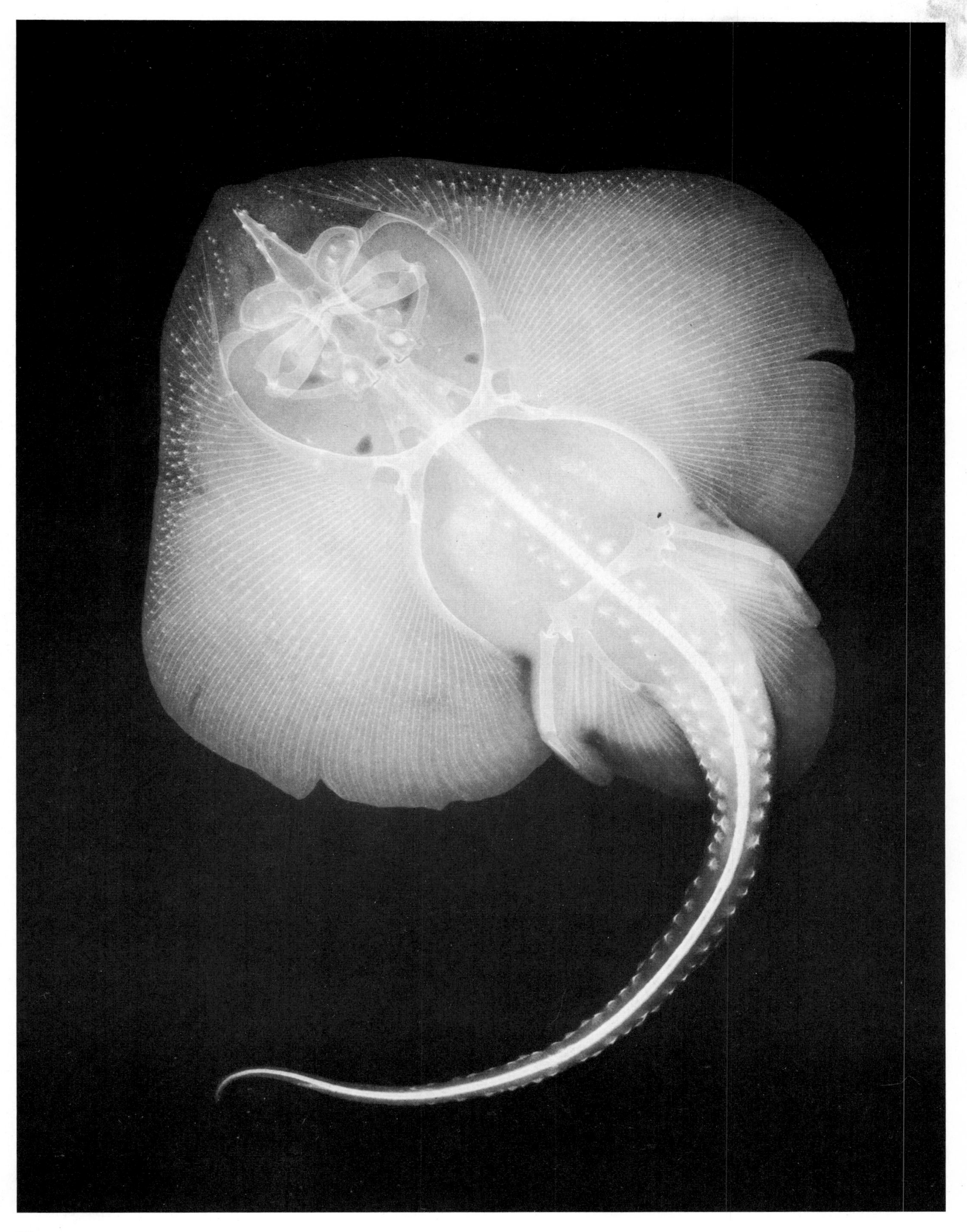

Stingray

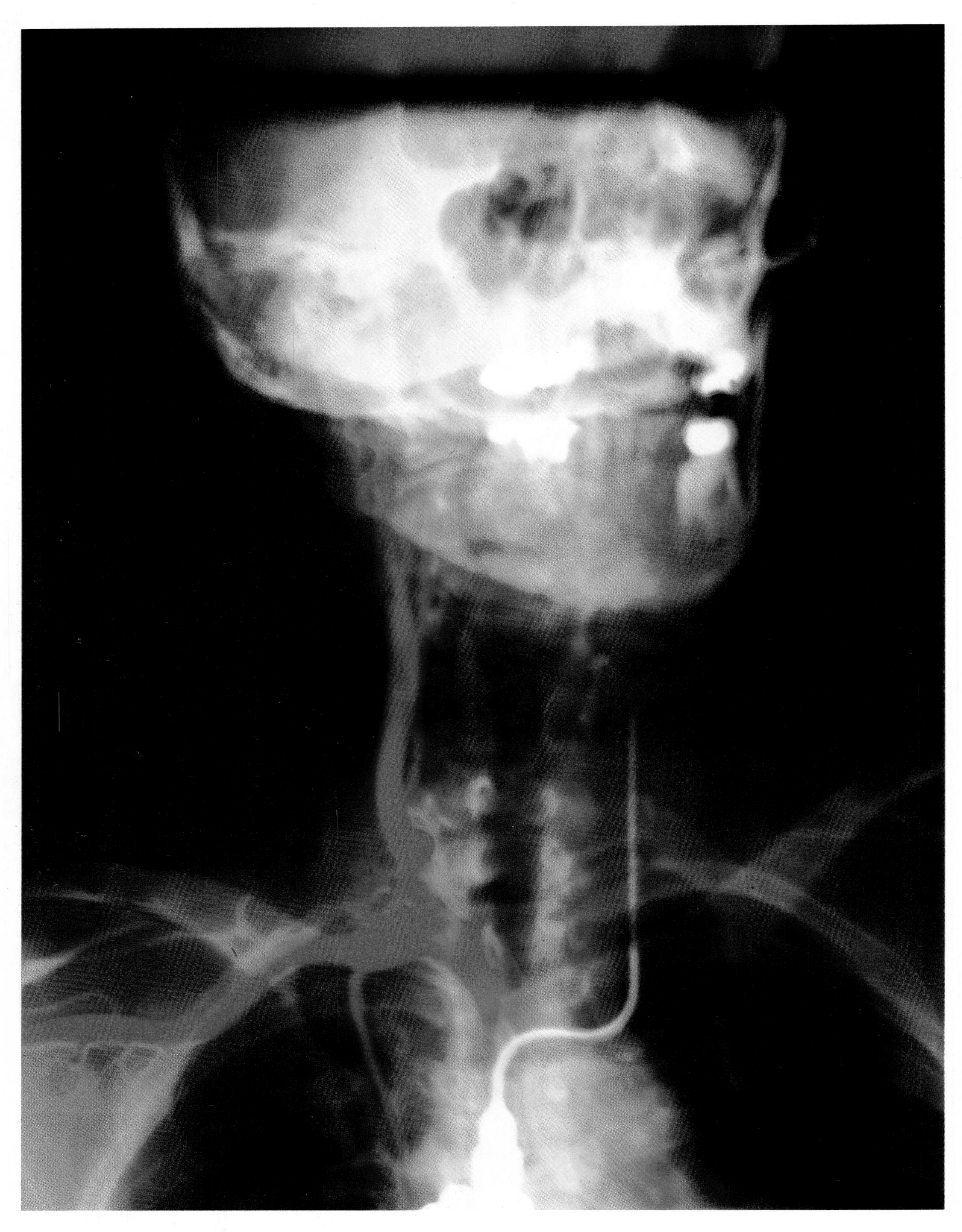

◁ **X-RAY ARTERY**

A dramatic and clearer view of our body's internal structure can be achieved through the color enhancement of x-ray photographs. The large red blood vessel is the carotid artery. It supplies blood and oxygen to the brain. Blocking or constriction of this artery can be an early warning of a stroke.

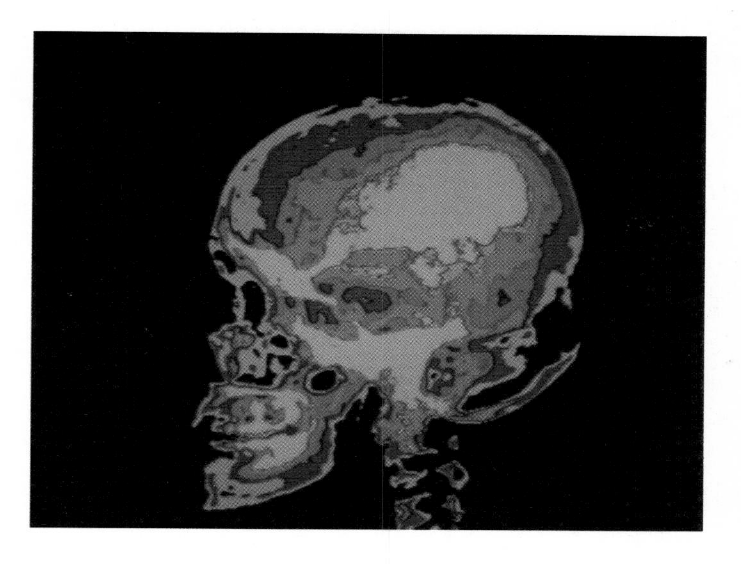

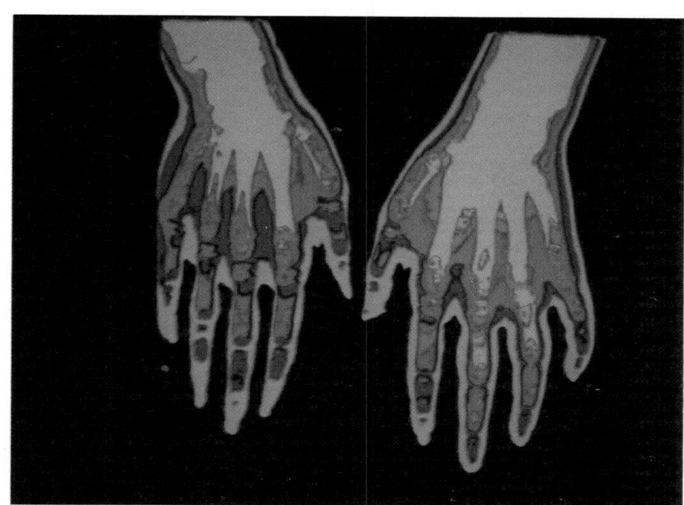

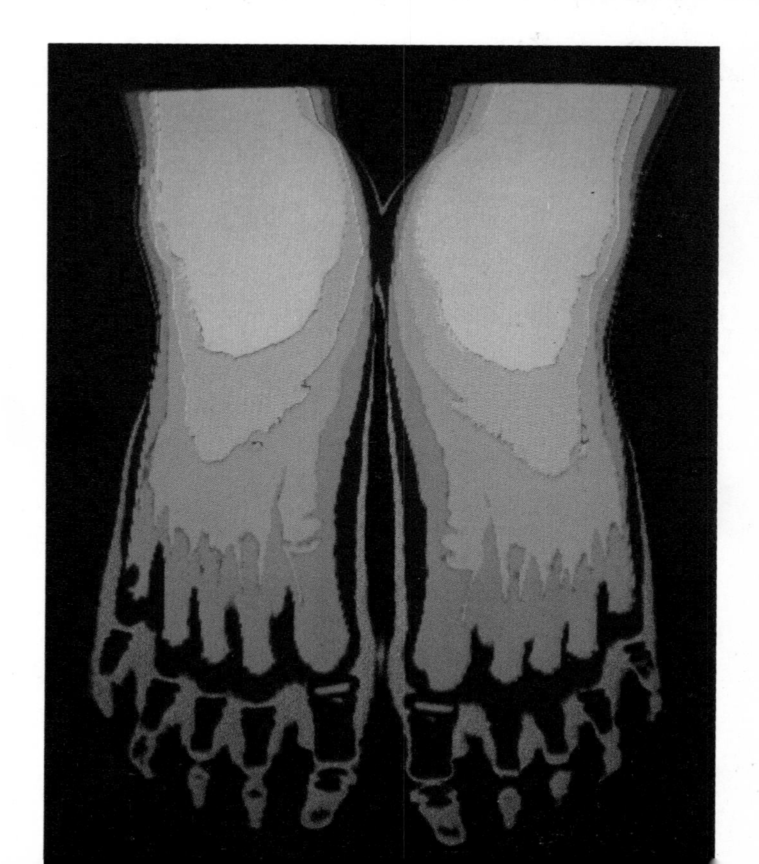

FEET, HANDS, AND HEAD

X-ray pictures can be so radically color-coded by a computer that our bodies become pop art.

LOOKING BACK

The modern x ray is expanding our understanding of the distant past. When Egyptian mummies are subjected to modern x-ray analysis, scientists gain new insight into the culture and lives of the ancient Egyptians. What time and wrappings have hidden, x rays can still reveal.

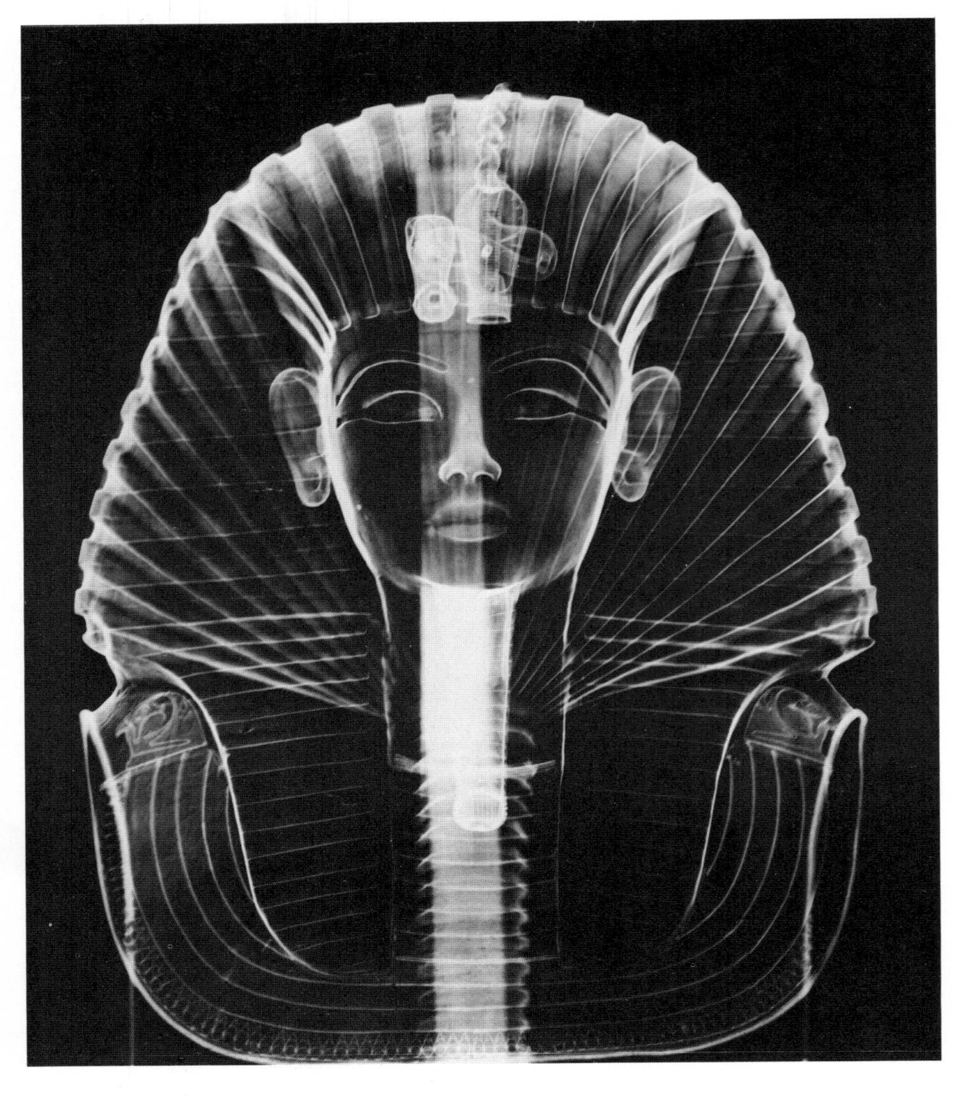

KING TUT'S MASK

Perhaps no pharaoh is better known than the young Tutankhamen. Penetrating gamma rays—which are even more powerful than x rays—show that his golden mask was constructed in several parts. His beard was added last, attached to the chin by a tapered peg.

The body of King Tut itself has undergone careful analysis in hopes of finding evidence as to the cause of the young pharaoh's death. X rays, however, show a young man in good health. Unless there is evidence still to be discovered, the reason for Tut's early death may remain a mystery forever.

MYSTERY MUMMY ▷

For an unidentified mummy, an apparently awful fate. Legs and head are intact, but the torso is mysteriously missing. Perhaps he was the victim of a hurried discount funeral.

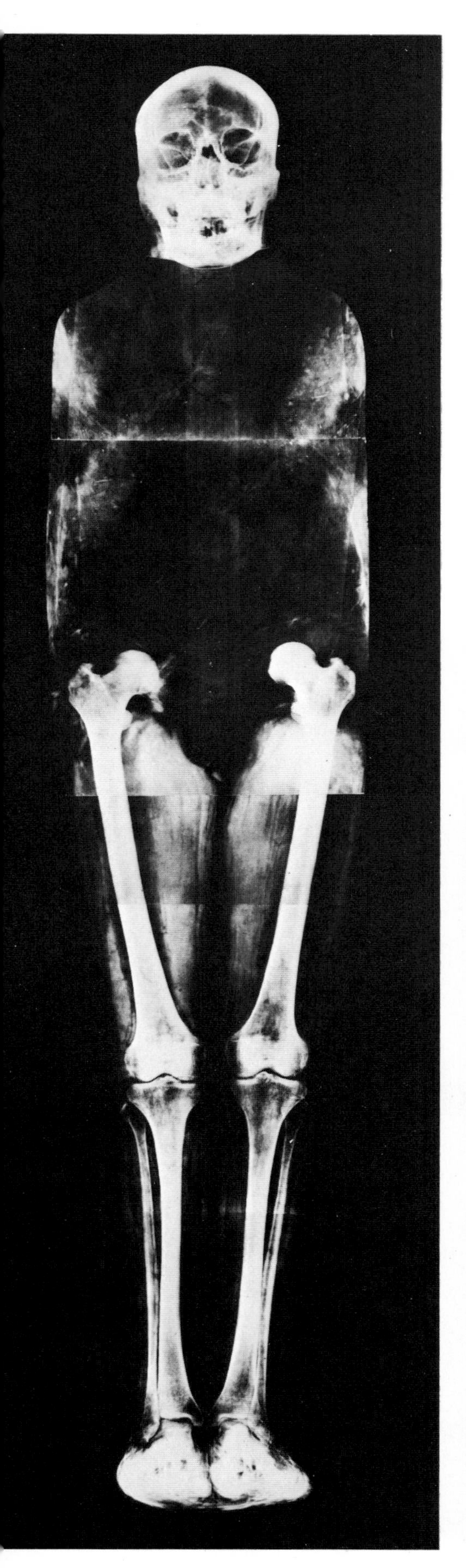

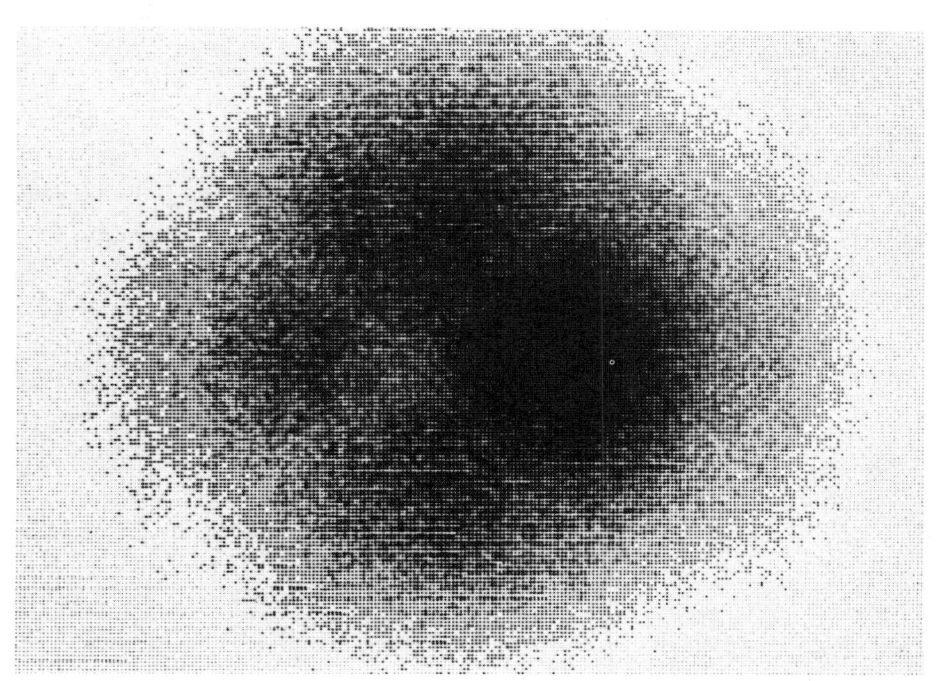

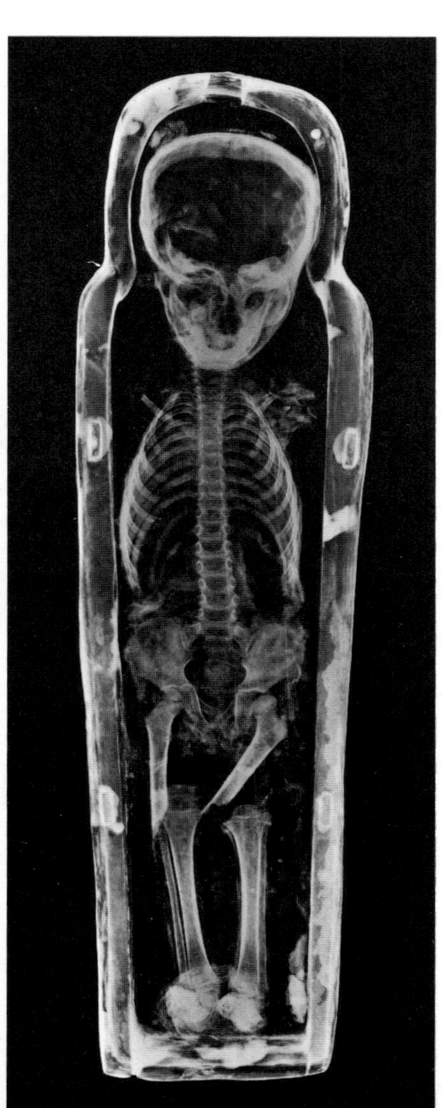

COSMIC PYRAMID

This is a photograph of the Great Pyramid of Chephren in Egypt. The picture was made with cosmic rays in an attempt to discover if the pyramid contained any hidden chambers.

Hundreds of thousands of invisible cosmic rays pass quietly through our bodies every day. They are mysterious particles that constantly shower down on us from outer space. They are so energetic and penetrating that they can easily pass through solid rock and bore deep within the earth.

With this in mind, a team of scientists headed by Dr. Luis Alvarez—a Nobel laureate from the University of California at Berkeley—placed a cosmic ray detector in a room at the base of the pyramid. If there were any secret rooms, they would have shown up as significantly darker areas in the computer-generated photograph.

Unfortunately no rooms were found . . . but it was an ingenious experiment.

The resulting photograph is a kind of x-ray image taken with cosmic rays. What you see here is what you would see if you were lying on your back in the center of the pyramid's base, looking straight up through it.

PEDIAMON

This baby received a less than noble burial. His arms were amputated and his legs were broken to fit into an undersized coffin.

SEEING WITH SOUND

Sound, like light or heat or x rays, radiates all around us in the form of vibrating waves. Sensitive sound-imaging cameras are now beginning to show us the world as it might look if our ears could see.

FETUS IN WOMB

Today, a mother's first picture of her baby is often made with sound before the child is born. A tiny developing fetus can now be safely seen and monitored during its growth in the womb. Complications during development can be quickly spotted. X rays would be harmful to the child, but sound waves apparently are not.

This ultrasound image is a cross-section view of the womb. The child's head is at the bottom right; its arm in the upper-left-hand corner.

The colors have been added by a computer imaging system to enhance our view.

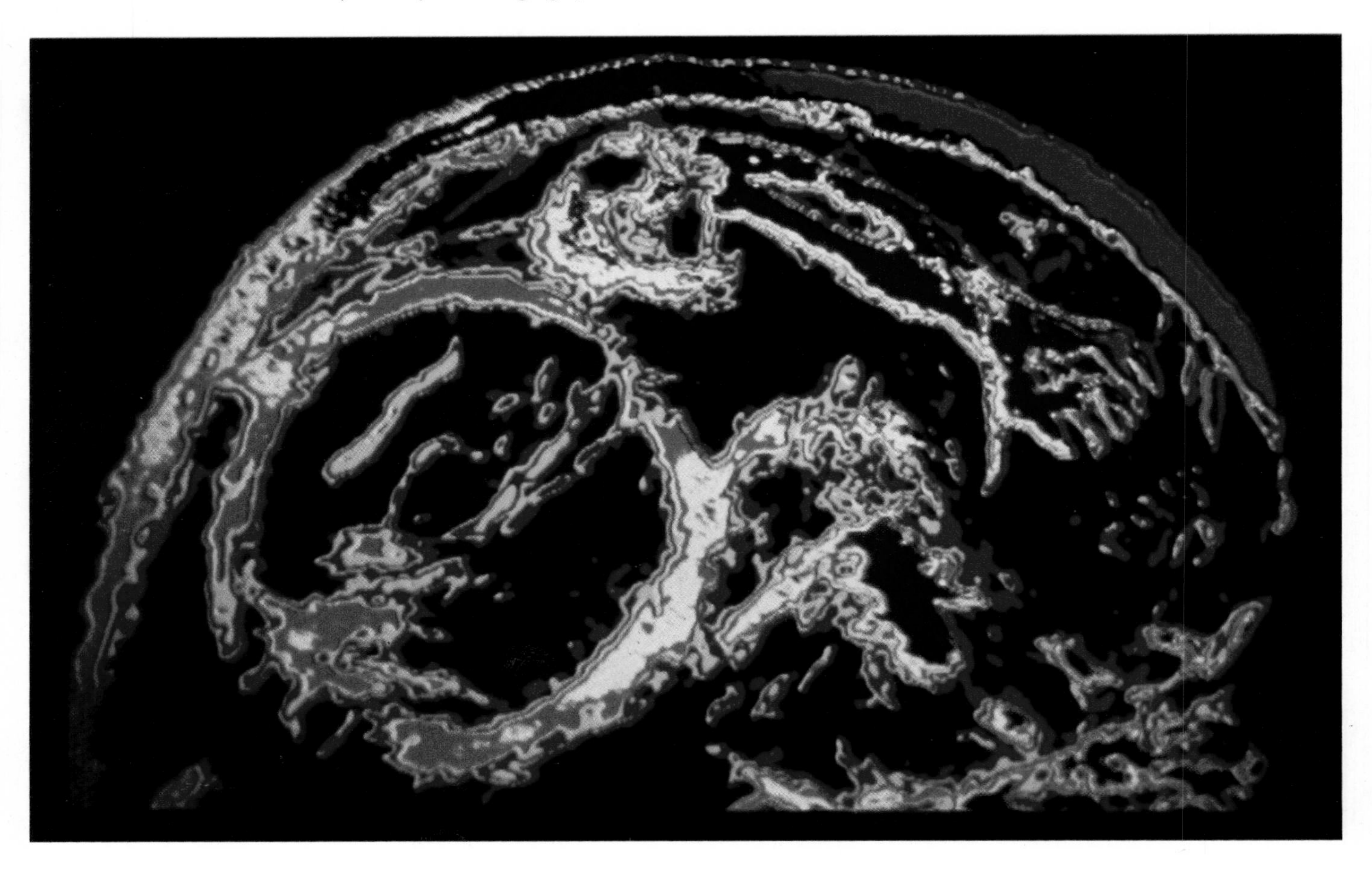

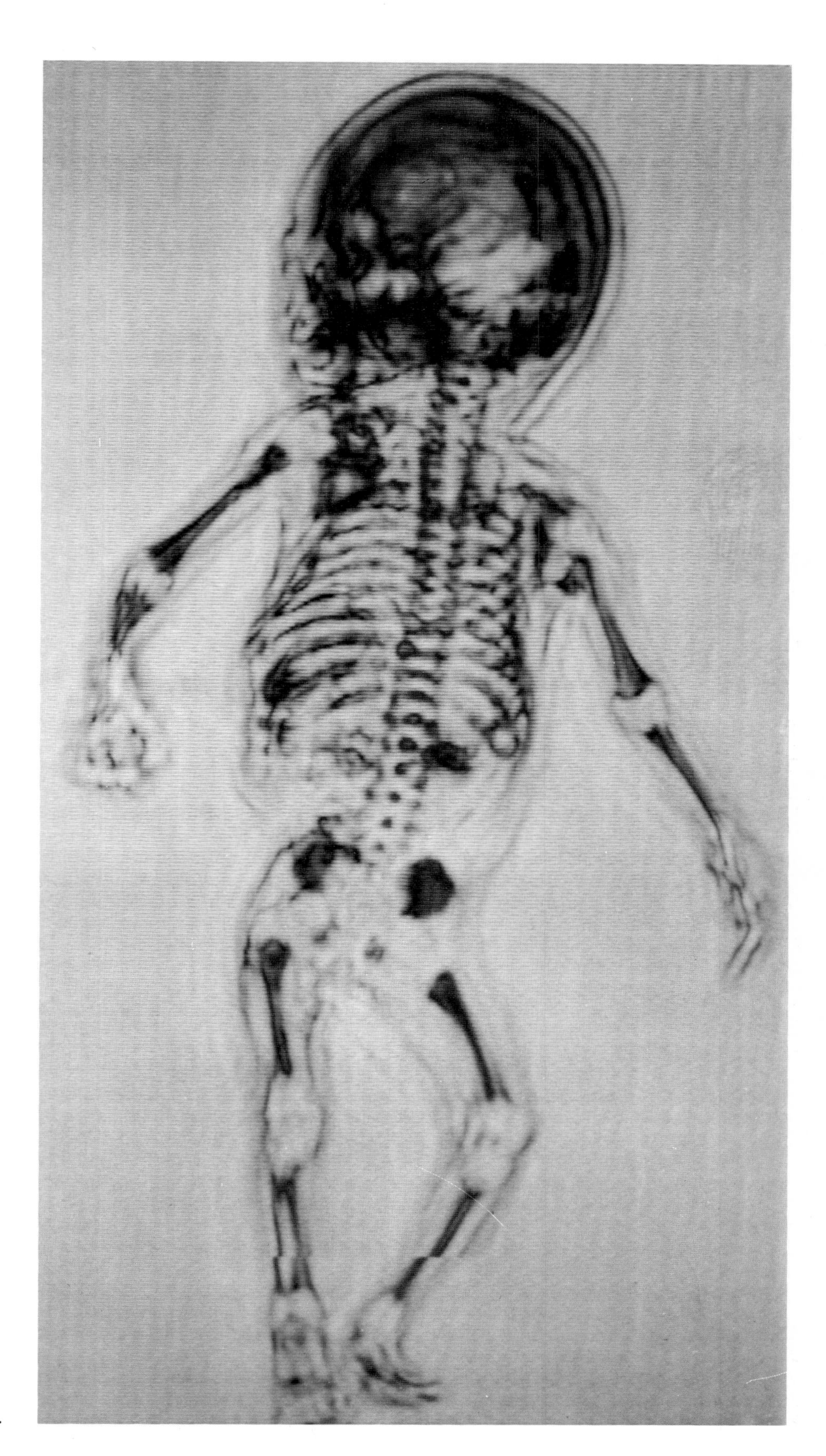

SONIC BABY

Unlike x rays, ultrasound images reveal soft tissue and muscle. This ultrasound image of a stillborn baby shows the early stages of skeletal development before cartilege has hardened into bone.

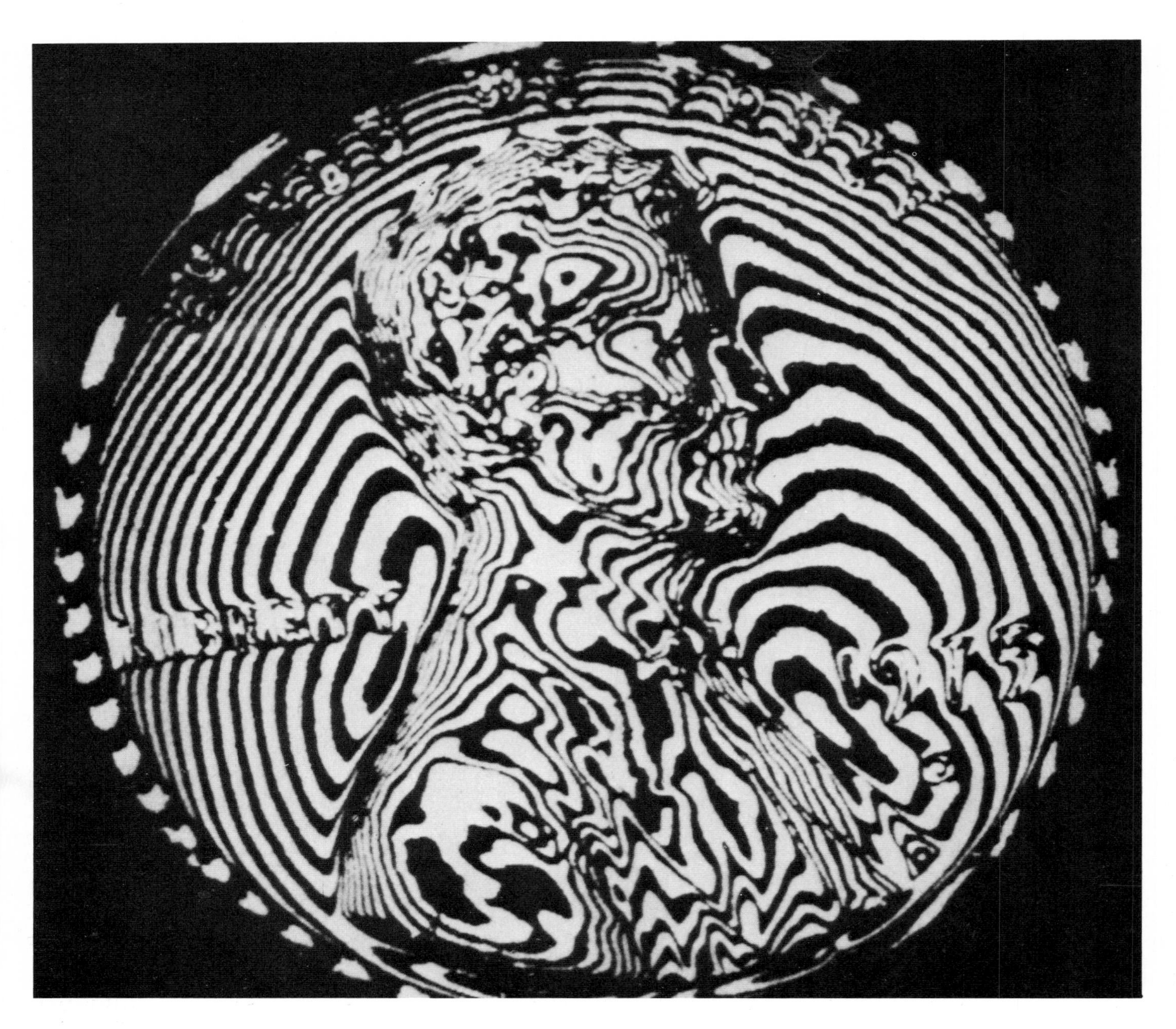

SOUND PENNY

When sound waves are bounced off a penny by an ultrasonic camera, a strange new dimension of this familiar object is suddenly revealed. The rippling pattern is a sonic reflection of the penny's metallic properties.

ULTRAVIOLET

Our world can also be seen in ultraviolet light—the invisible wavelengths of energy beyond the color violet.

The sun's ultraviolet rays can give us both tans and sunburns. Ultraviolet can also be used to reveal otherwise hidden structure.

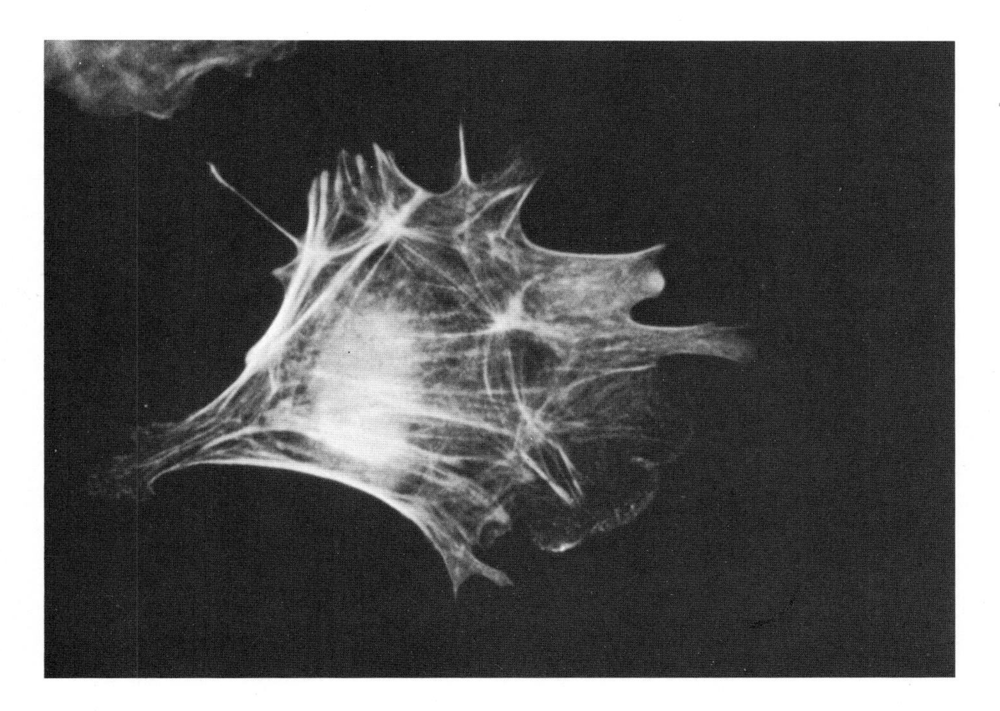

FLUORESCENT CELLS

Even cells have to flex their muscles to move. Tiny protein fibers known as actin filaments are relaxed when the cell is stationary. When the cell decides to travel, the fibers form themselves into a dynamically moving network that stretches and propels the cell.

These protein fibers were until recently invisible and unknown. They cannot be seen with normal light. Only when the cells are treated with a fluorescent dye and then viewed with ultraviolet light does the hidden microstructure become apparent.

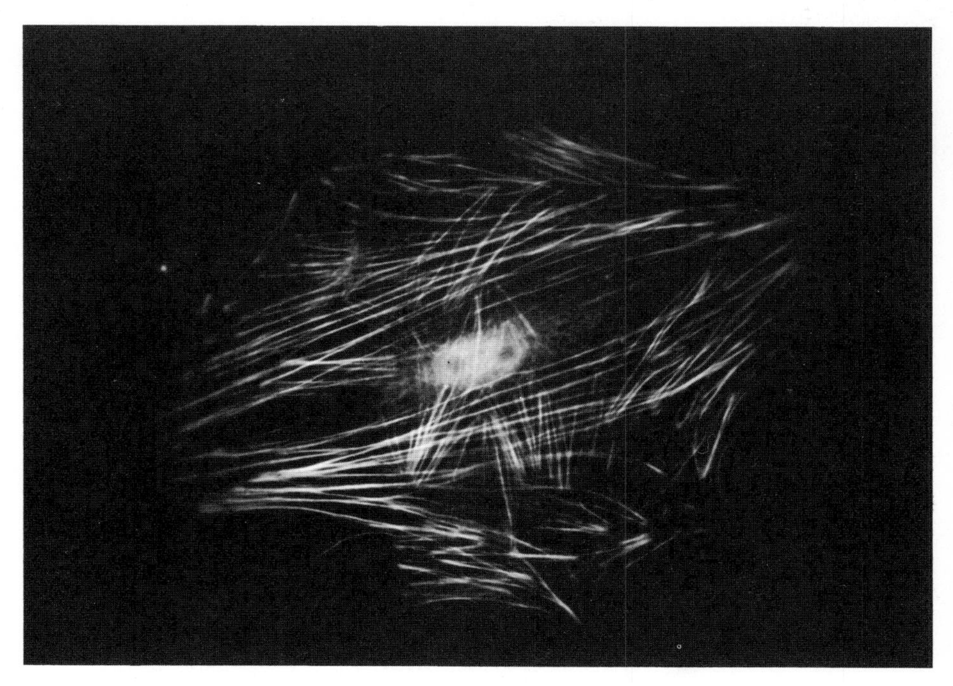

ELECTROPHOTOGRAPHY

A striking means of photography discovered at the turn of the century shows apparent fields of energy emanating from nearly everything. It is known as Kirlian photography, or electrophotography. Semyon Kirlian, a Russian scientist, did pioneering work in this field.

To make a Kirlian photograph, an object is placed over a sheet of unexposed film, which receives a burst of electricity from a metal plate beneath it. When the film is developed, the Kirlian corona appears.

Controversial and only partially understood, electrophotography is now undergoing serious examination as a possible diagnostic tool.

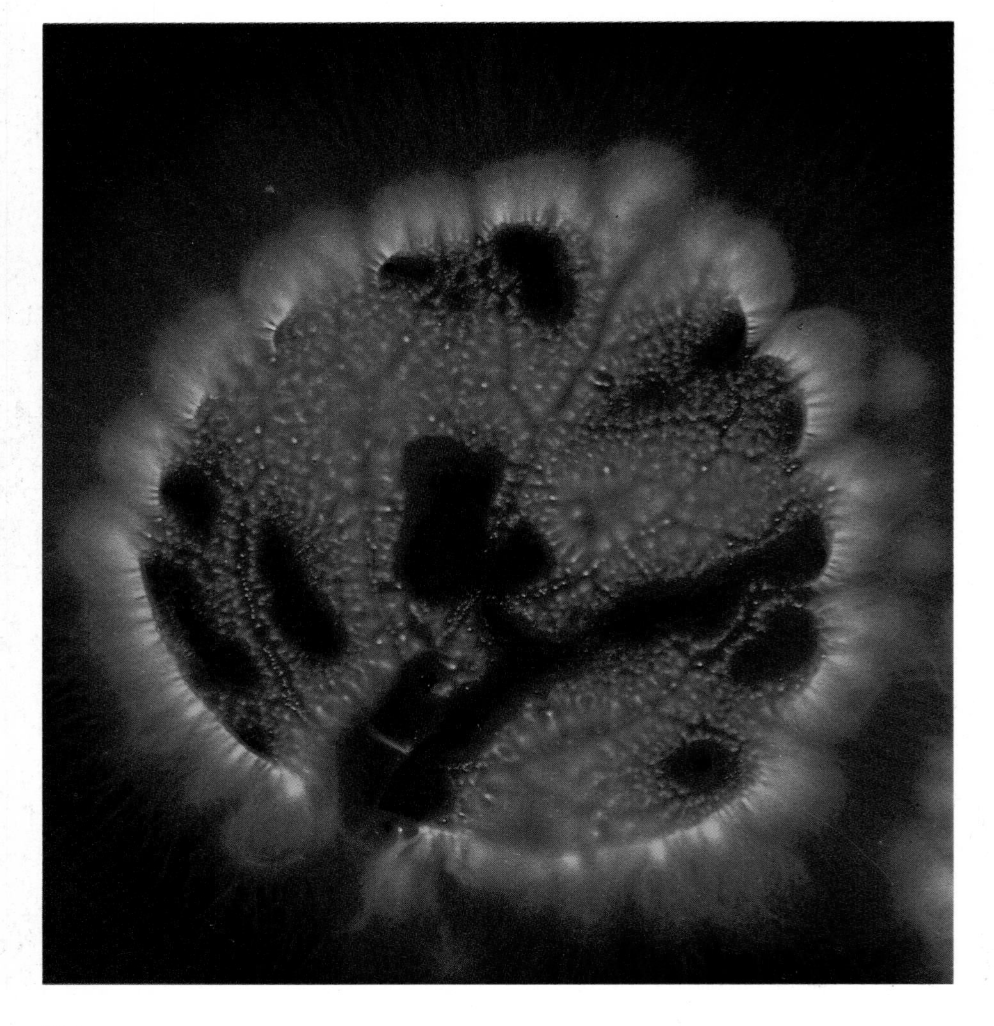

AIR ▷

A beautiful fantasy landscape results when air is photographed using a technique of electrophotography called energy imaging photography. It shows the form that electrical discharges take in the air under certain conditions.

PLANT POWER

A Kirlian photograph of a leaf shows the type of corona that is emanated when the plant is healthy.

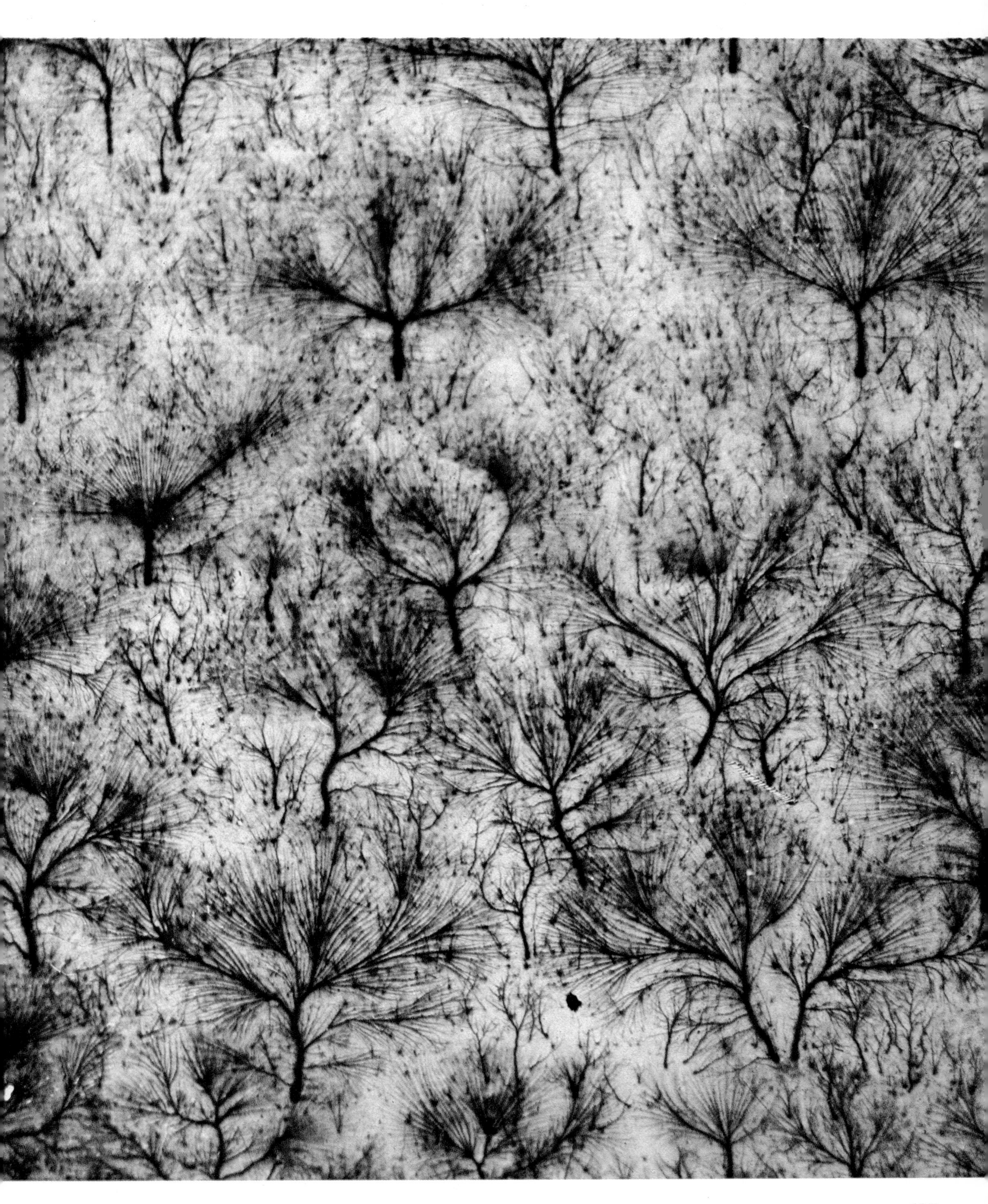

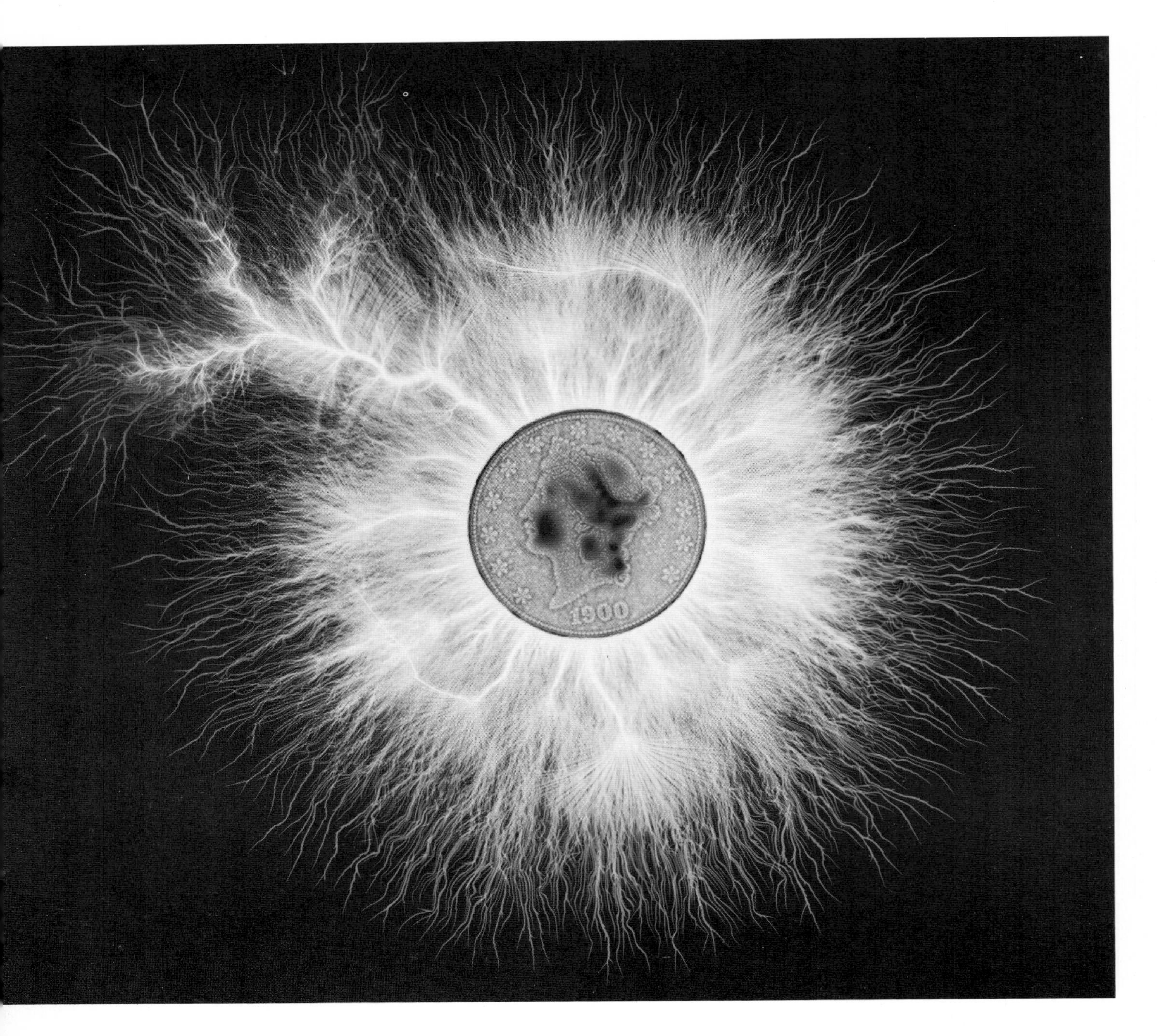

FLASHING MONEY
This electrophotograph of a $20 gold piece might also be called high-voltage currency.

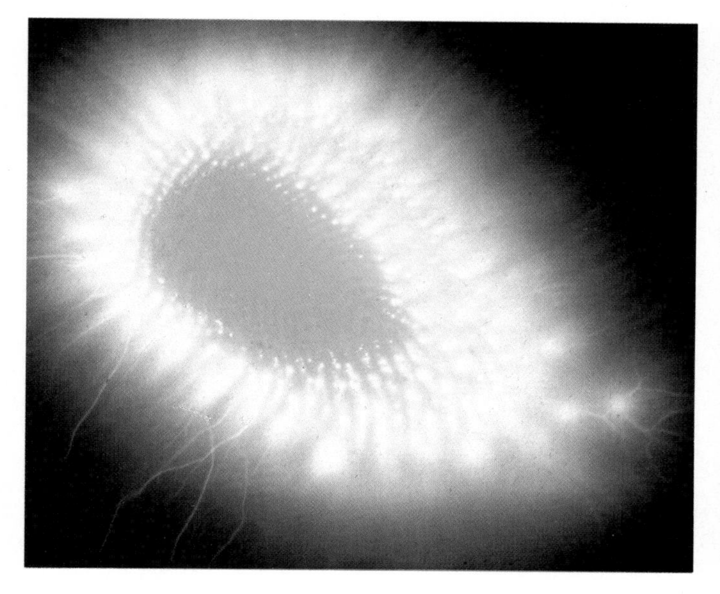

Love

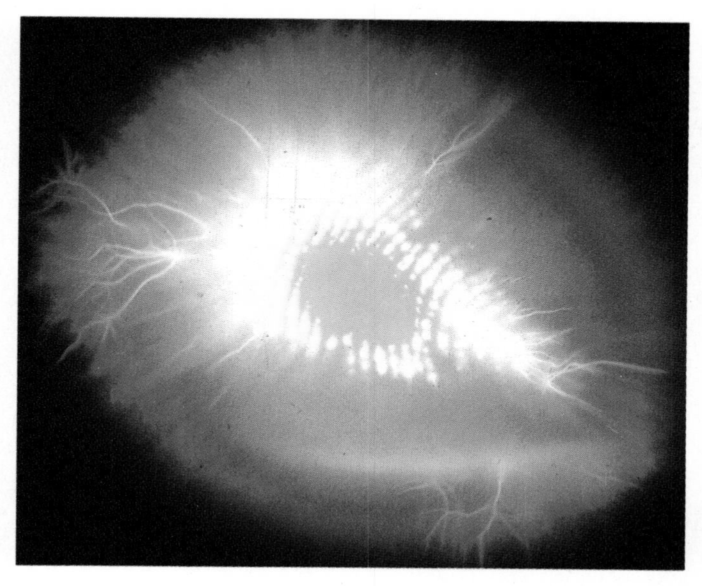

Anger

Vitality

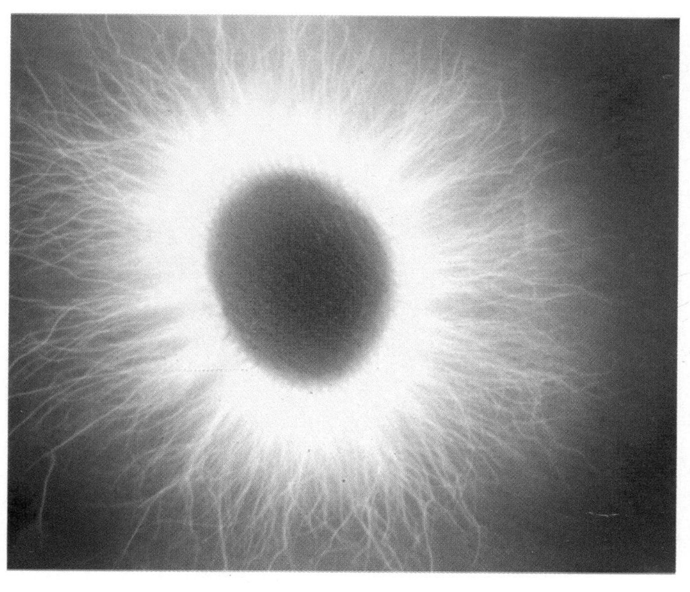

Dislike

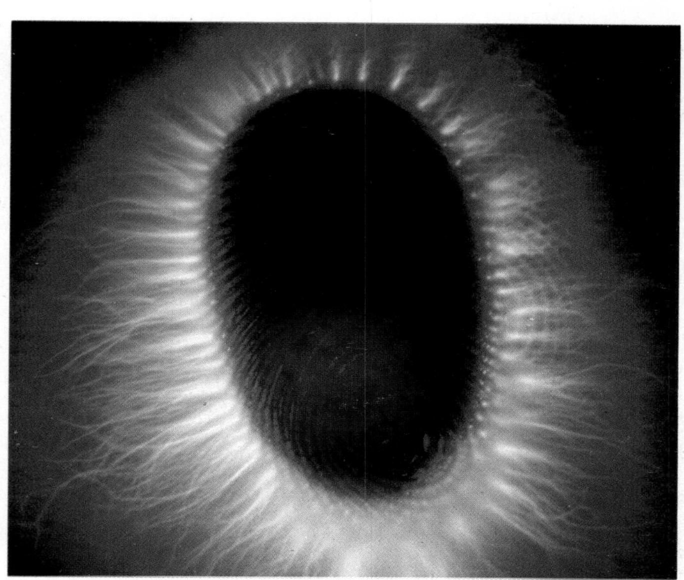

FINGERTIP EMOTIONS
Electrophotographs of human fingertips seem to reflect different emotional states.

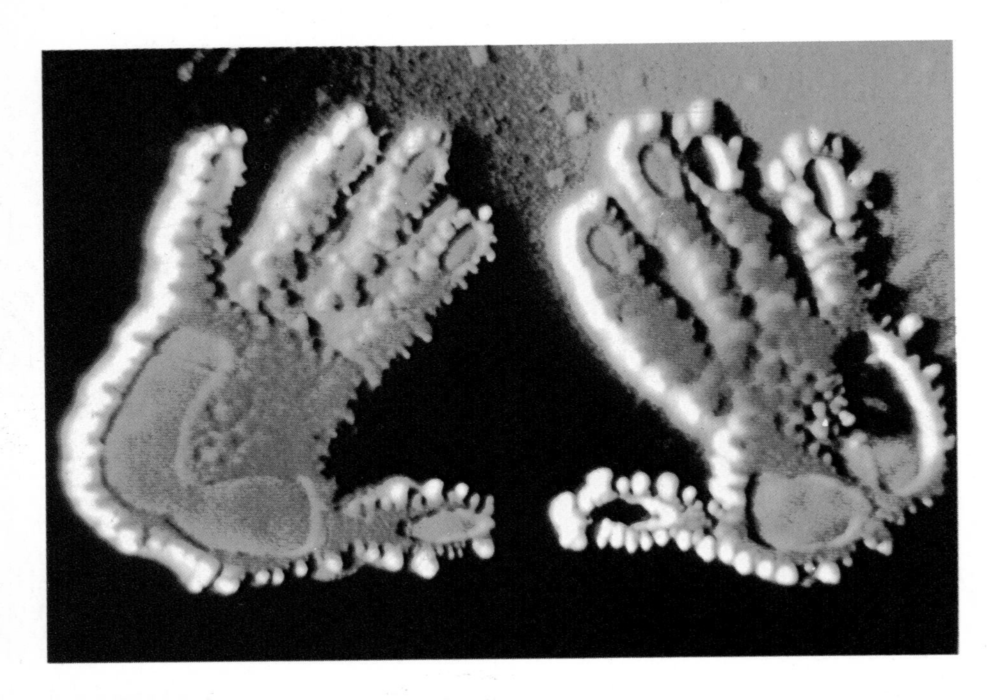

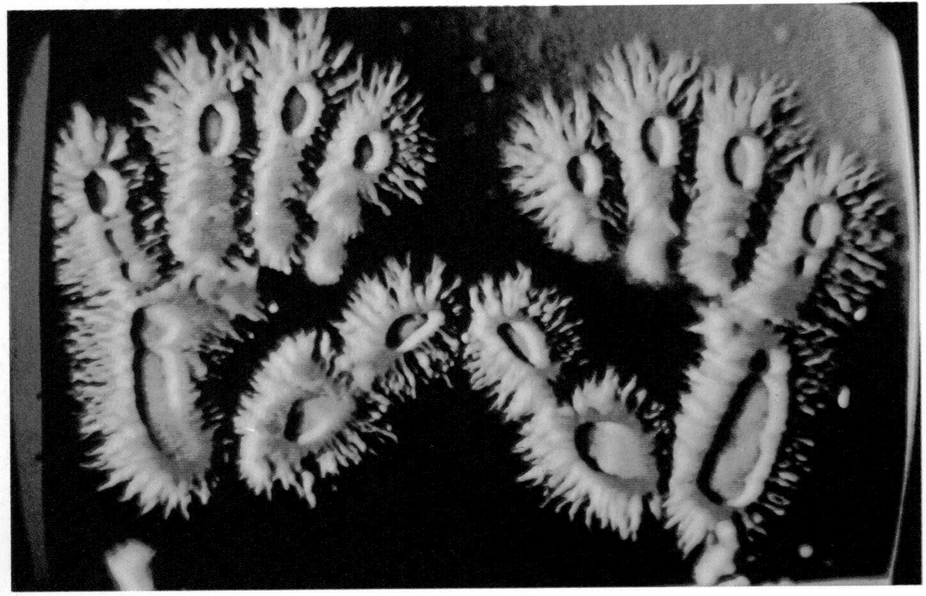

YOGI POWER
A yogi's hands before and then during a state of deep concentration.

COSMOS

Probing ever deeper into the enormity of the sky, the powerful eyes of telescopes are today extending our visual horizons toward the limits of space and time.
The telescope and the microscope are about the same age. Both were invented in the seventeenth century, and each expanded the known cosmos by extraordinary proportions.

Before the telescope, the universe consisted only of what the naked eye could see—the sun, the moon, several planets, and about two thousand stars. The telescope suddenly changed that. It revolutionized our image and understanding of the universe . . . and continues to do so.

Only sixty years ago, the existence of galaxies was a novel theory. With the building of larger and larger telescopes, thousands of galaxies were seen and photographed. Astronomers now estimate that the universe contains a hundred billion galaxies, each with at least a hundred billion stars.

Today we can see the heavens as never before. Telescopes sensitive to radio waves, x rays, heat, and ultraviolet light are unveiling awesome parts of the universe that were once completely invisible.

In the time since the telescope's invention, our methods of seeing into outer space have improved so enormously that we can now view countless distant objects that almost defy imagination.

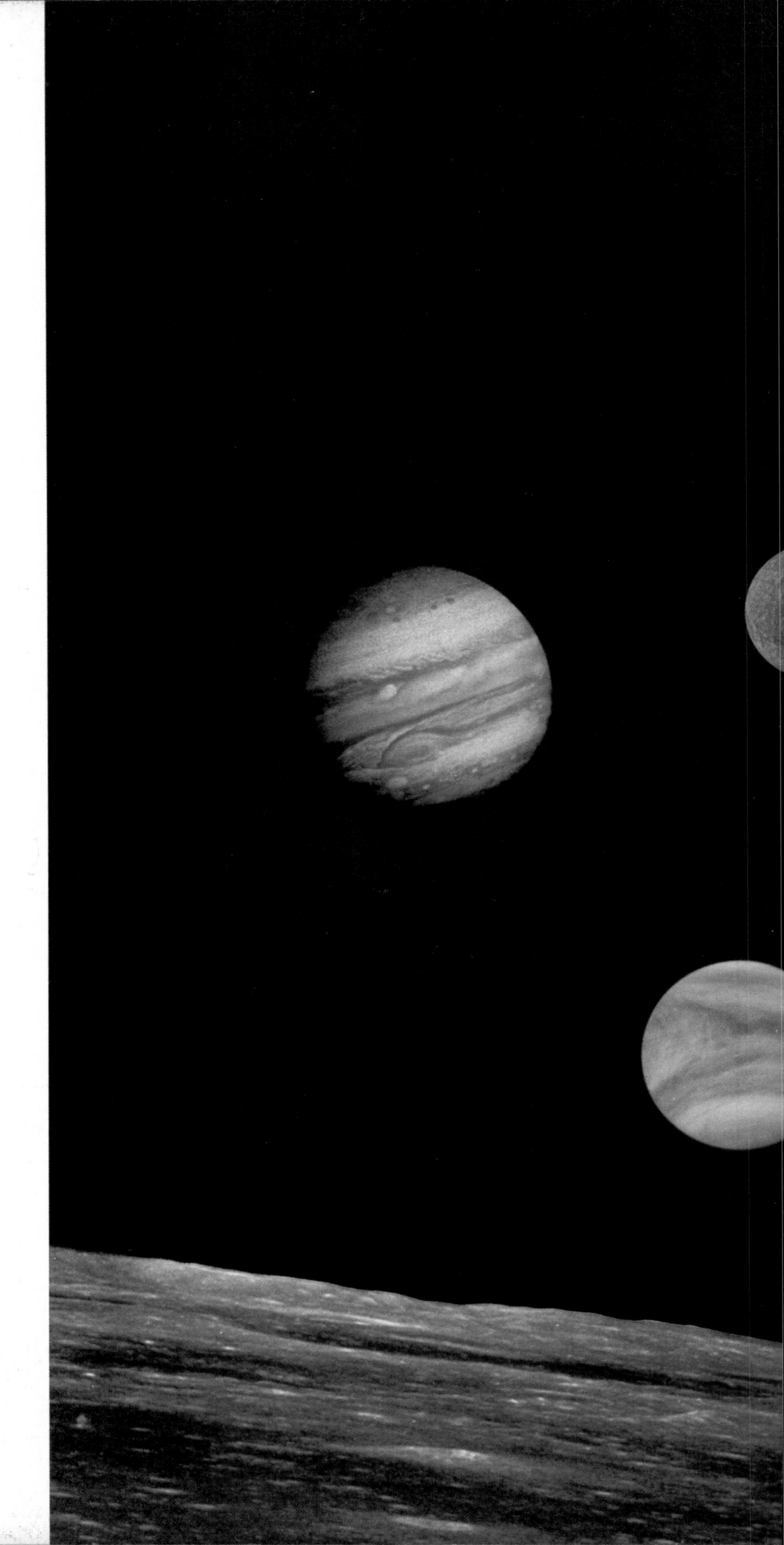

SPACESCAPE

The planets of our solar system seen from the surface of the moon. It is not an actual picture from space, but an imaginative photo-collage created by a NASA scientist.

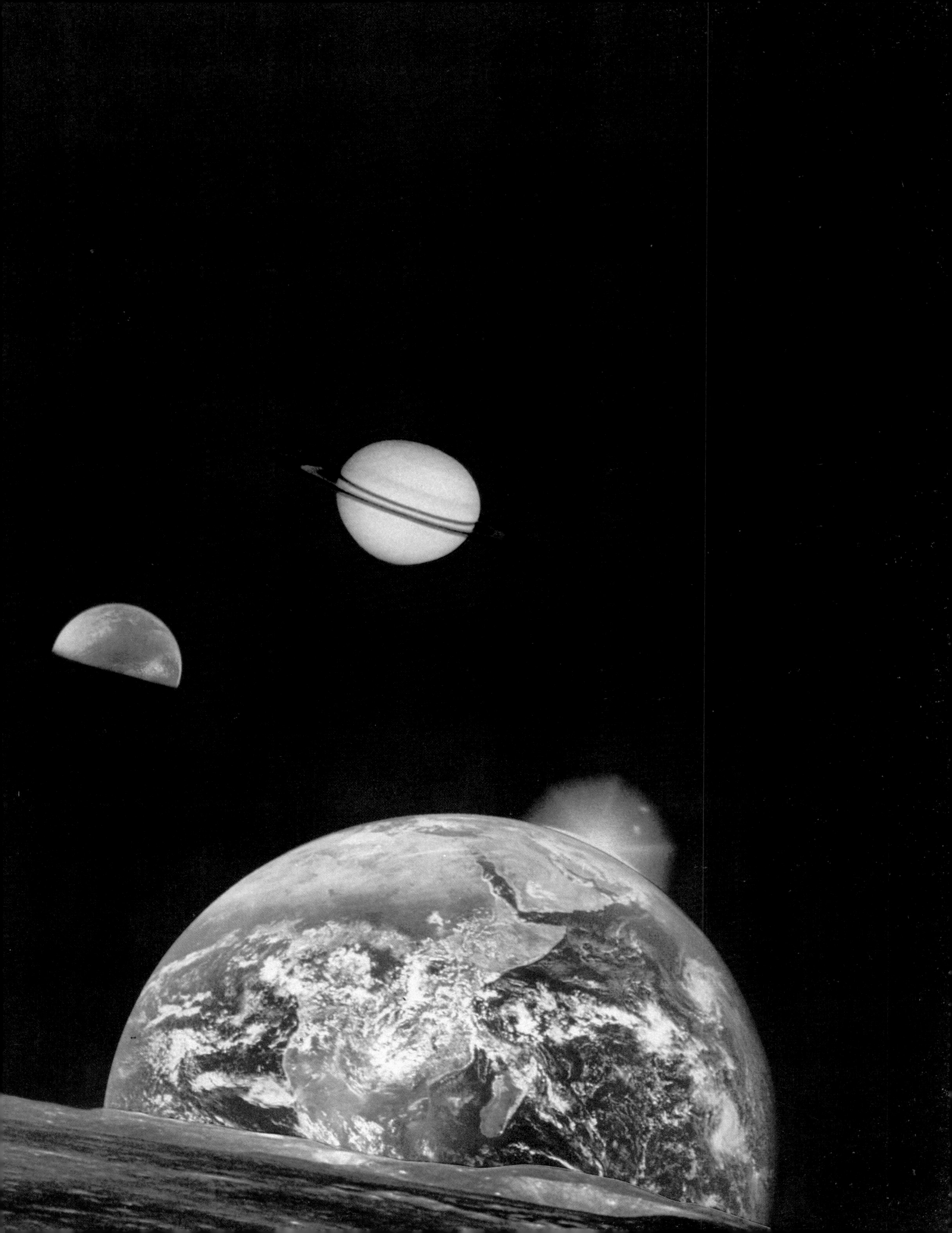

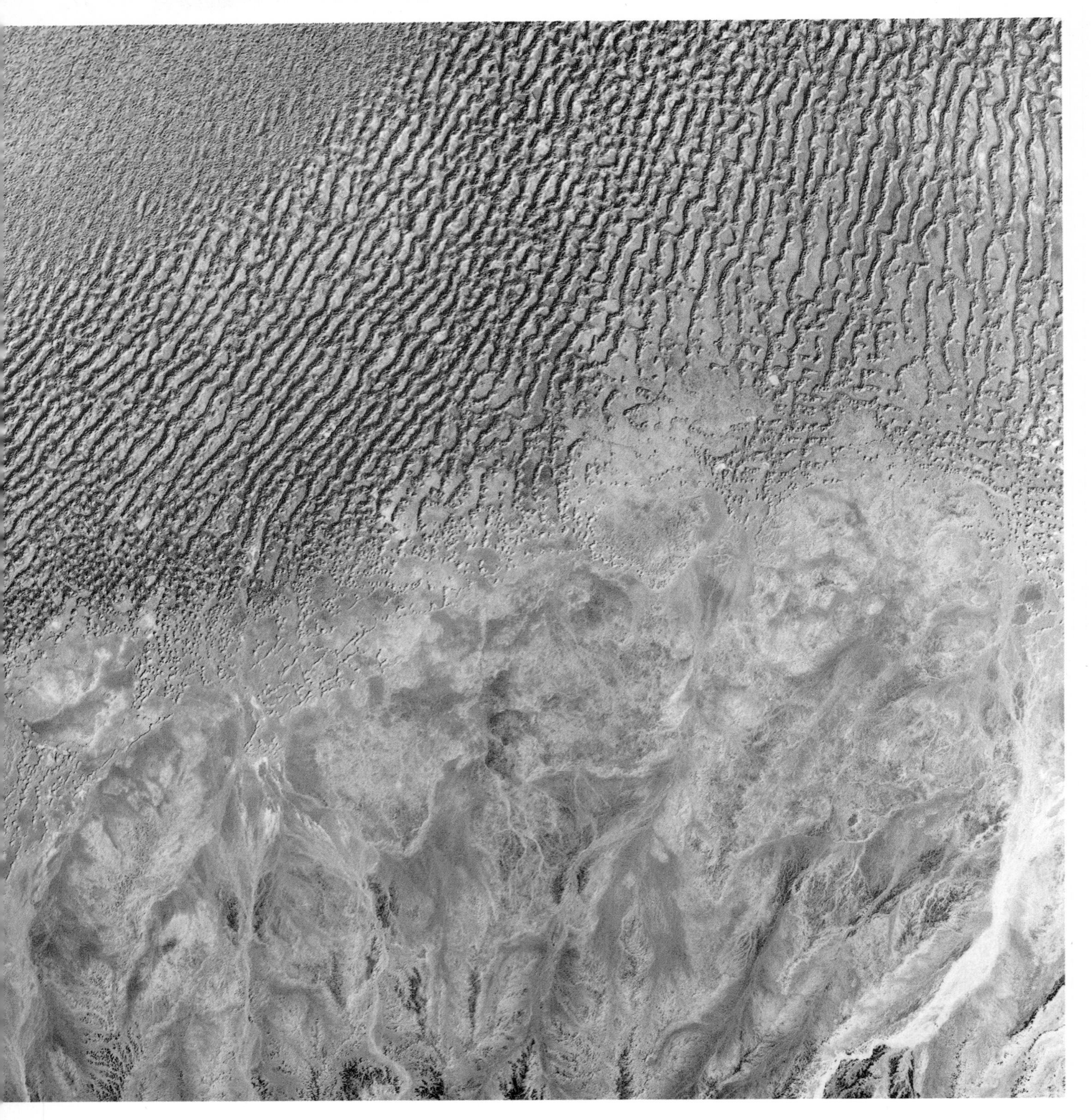

West Rub al Khali, Arabia

TERRA FIRMA

Snapshots of our planet, photographed from a satellite. Once the picture is taken it is converted into an electrical signal and broadcast back to earth. Computers then re-create and color the image. These glimpses of earth easily rival a beautiful abstract painting, but they are also a rich source of information about such things as agricultural potential and mineral resources.

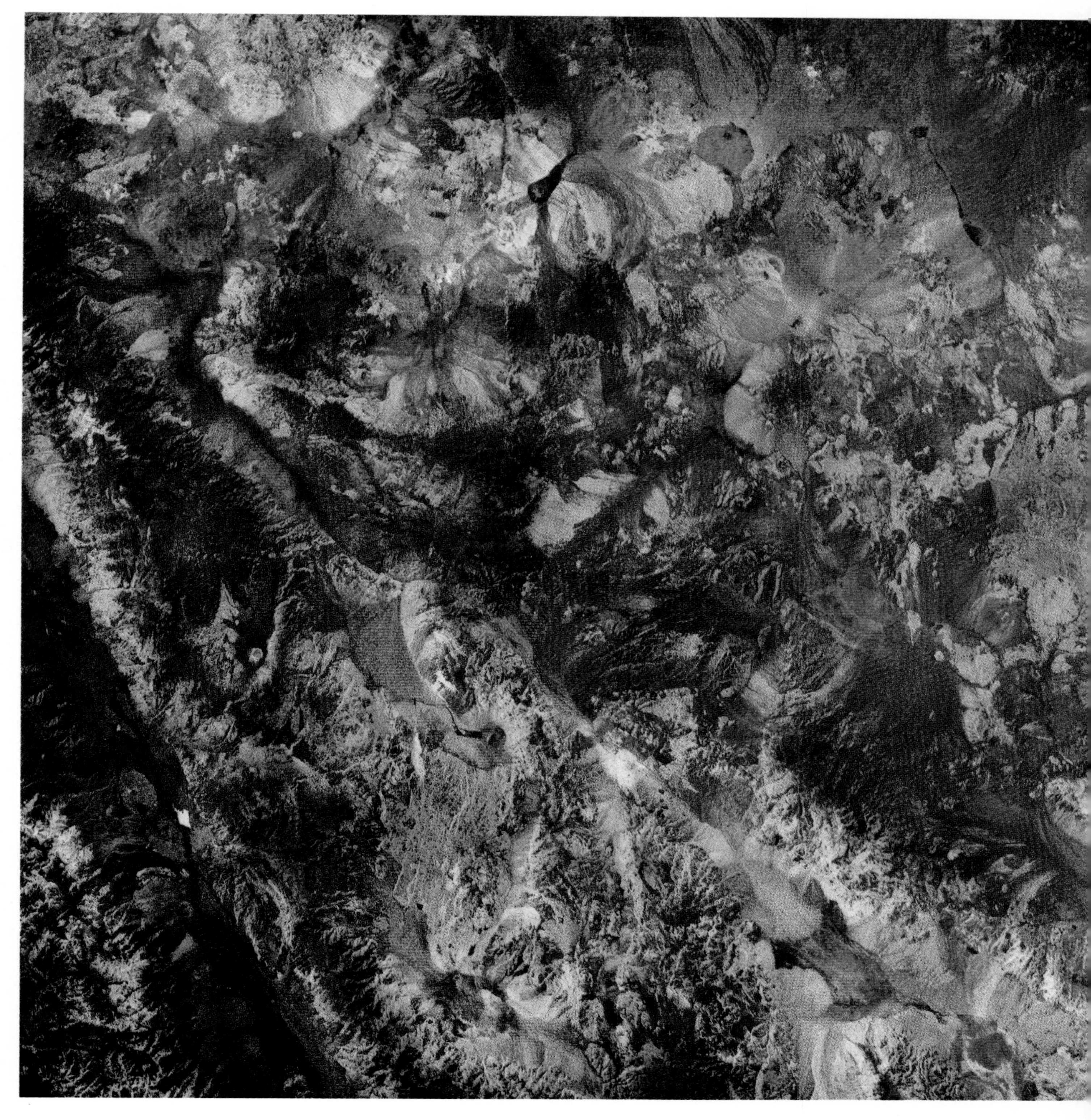

Lida, Nevada

SIX FACES OF THE SUN

Distance, heat, glare, and the meager power of our eyes prevent us from seeing the many aspects of the sun. Telescopes and cameras have recently provided a much more detailed view of this complex and beautiful star.

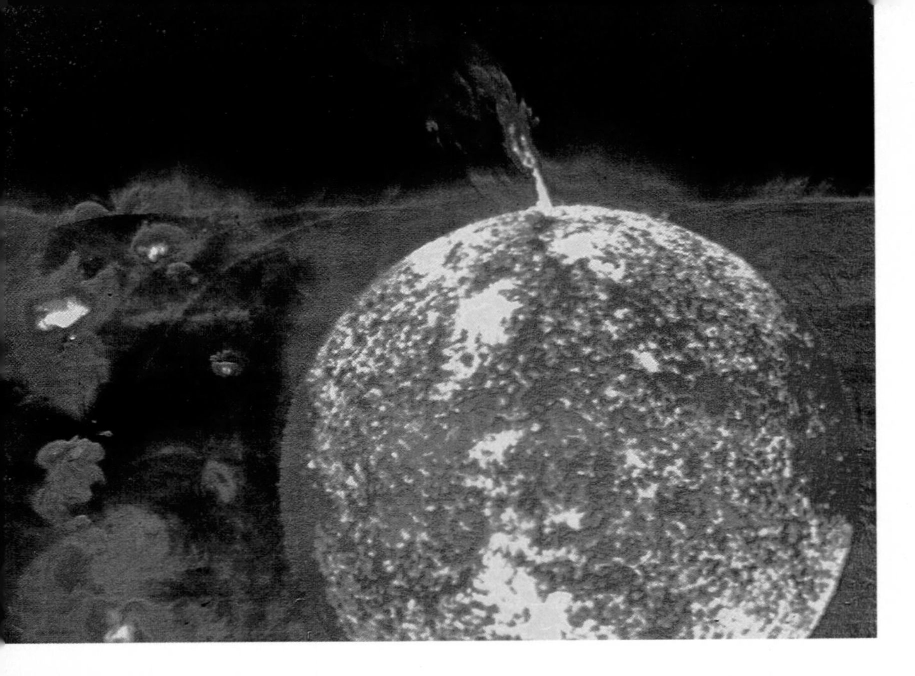

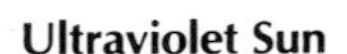

Ultraviolet Sun

When seen in ultraviolet light, the sun's roiling subsurface becomes visible. It is made up largely of helium, which boils at a temperature of about 25,000,000° F.

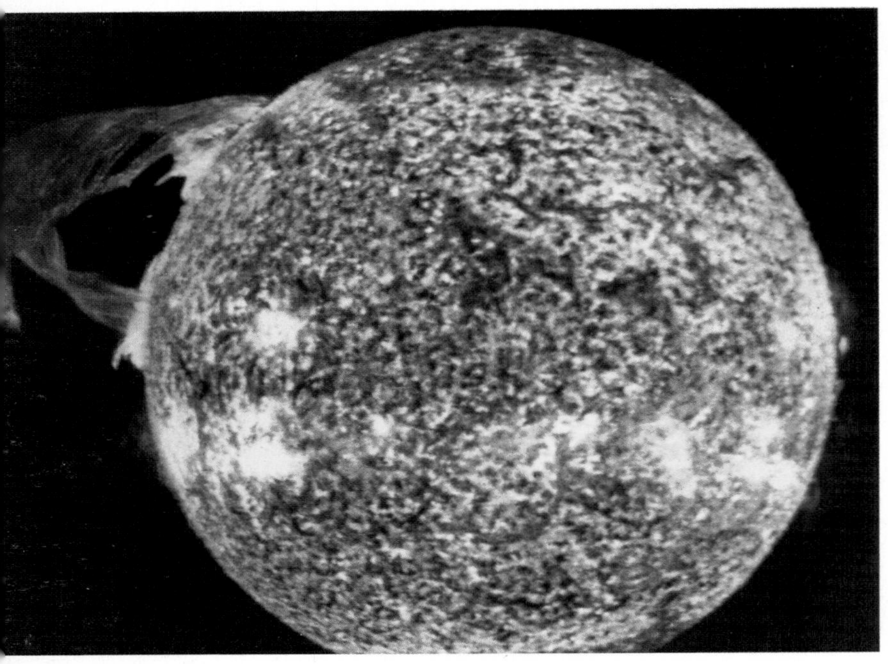

Flare-Up

Huge solar flares frequently erupt from the sun's surface. They are hundreds of thousands of miles long and move at nearly half a million miles an hour.

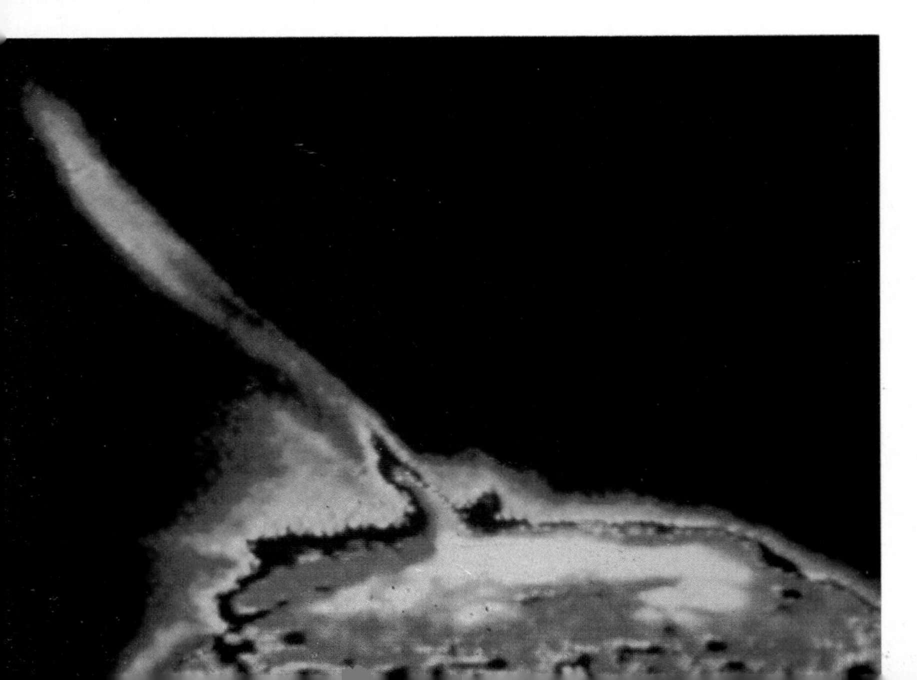

Solar Eruption

This image of solar violence was computer-enhanced and colored to show greater detail of the sun's dynamic surface.

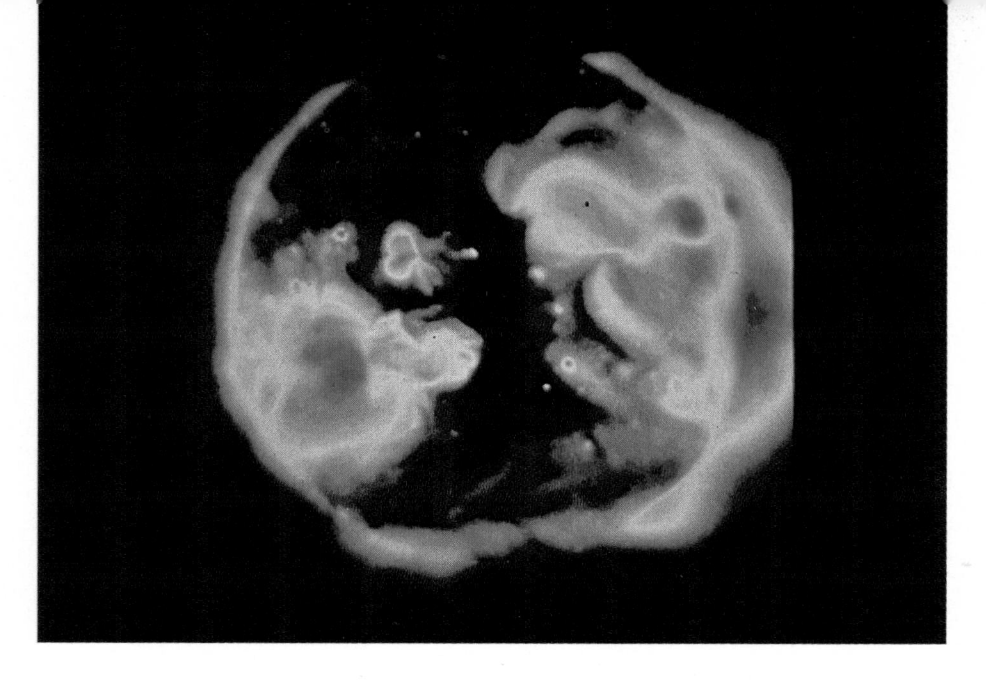

X-Ray Sun

The sun shines with lethal x rays as well as light. This picture was taken by an x-ray-sensitive telescope.

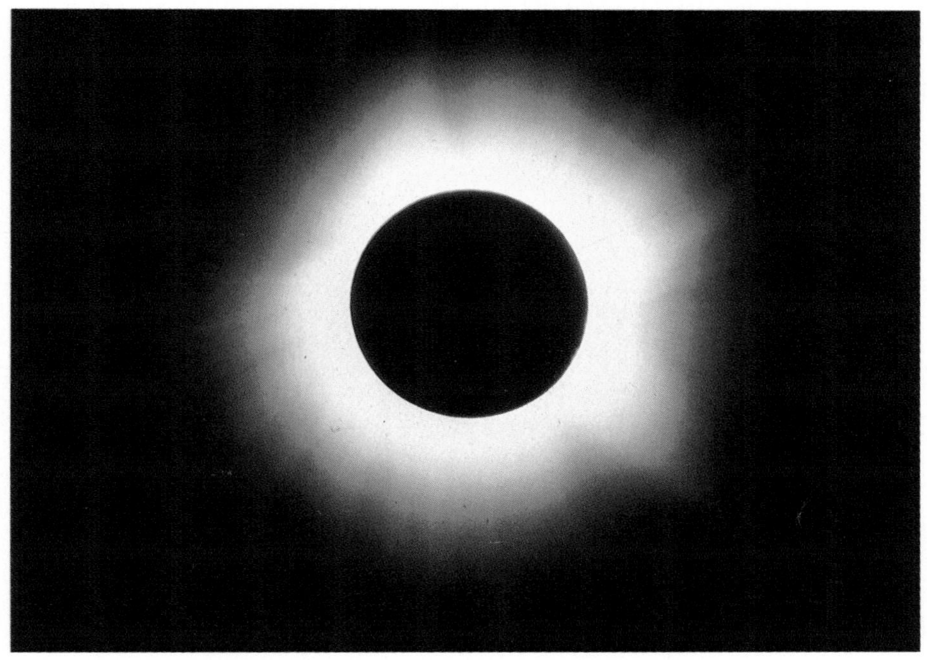

Solar Halo

During a total solar eclipse, the sun's shimmering corona can be seen from earth. It is usually invisible because of the sun's blinding glare.

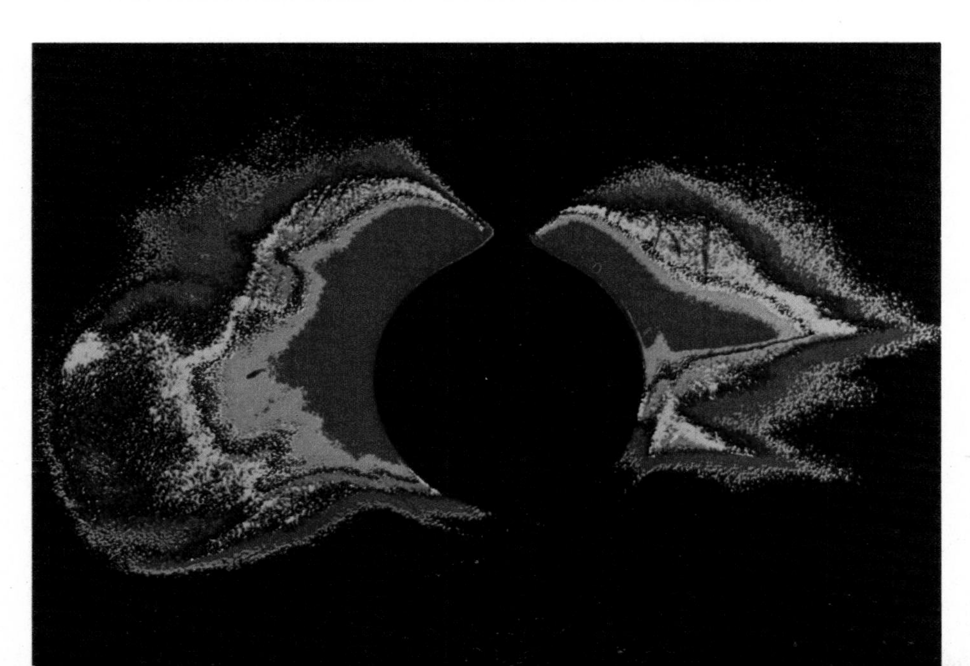

Invisible Sun

Vast streams of invisible gas, millions of miles long, constantly flow out from the sun's surface. This picture was taken with a sensitive solar telescope aboard *Skylab*.

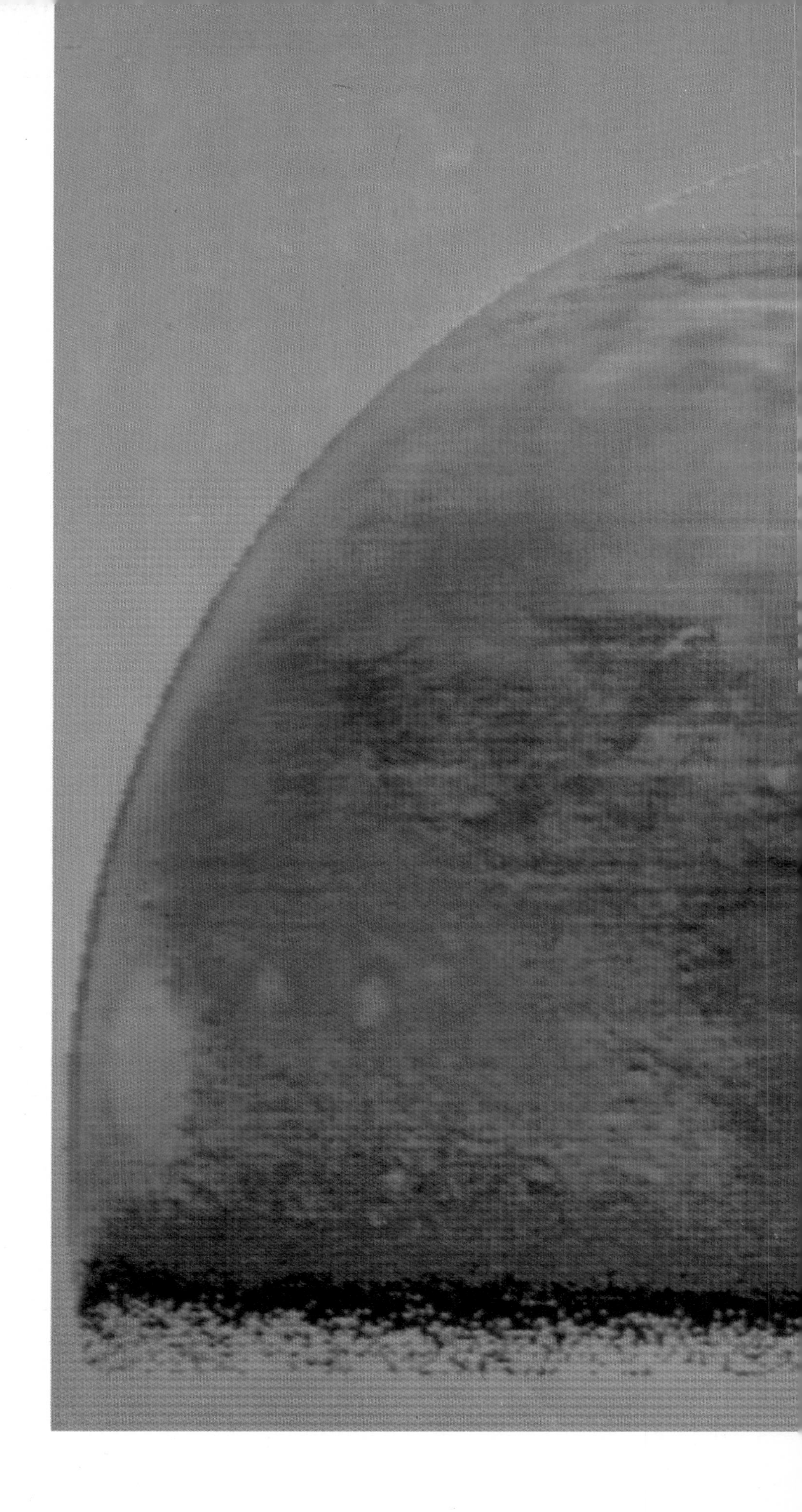

MARS

An eerie image of Mars, created by a computer from pictures broadcast by the *Viking* spacecraft.

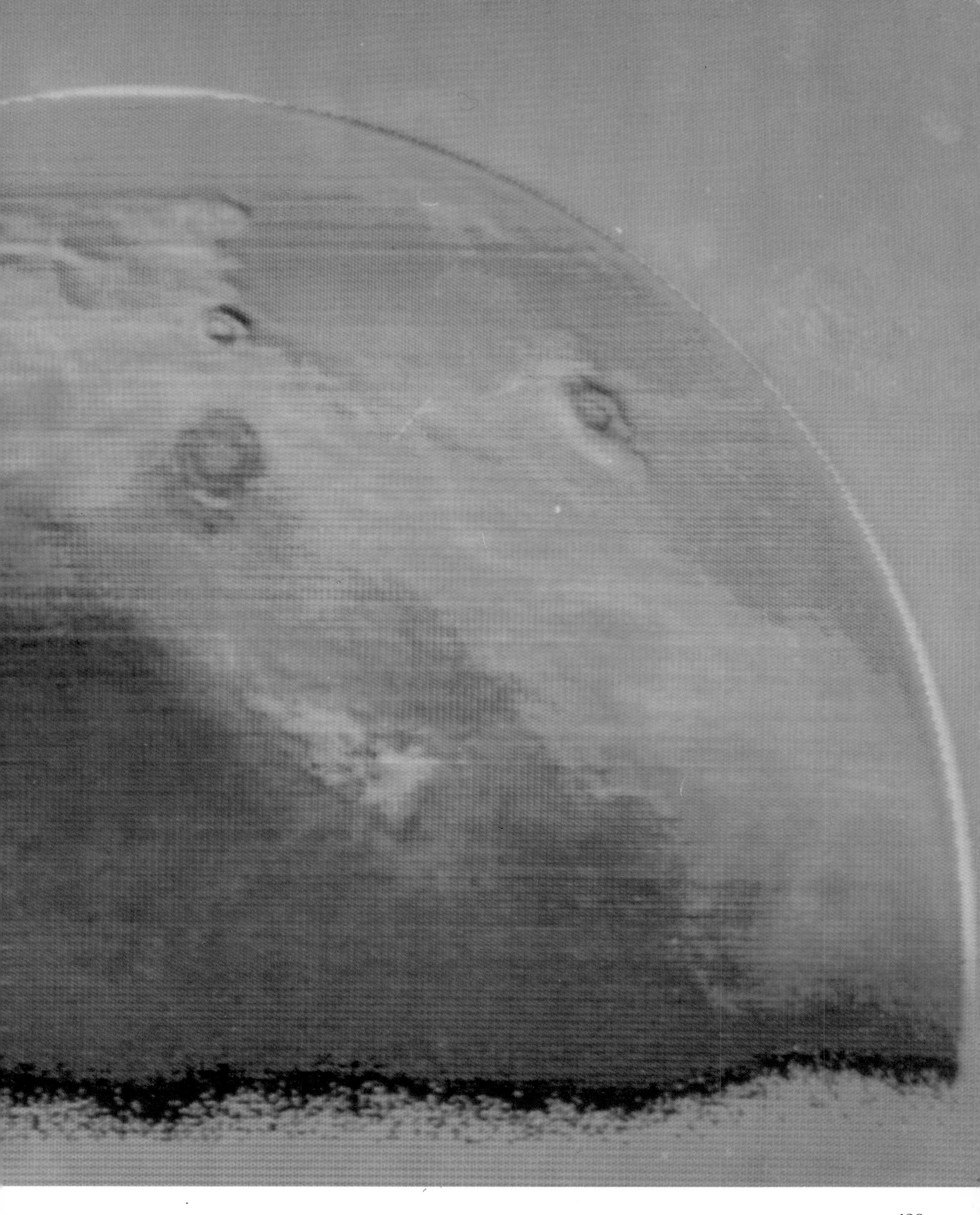

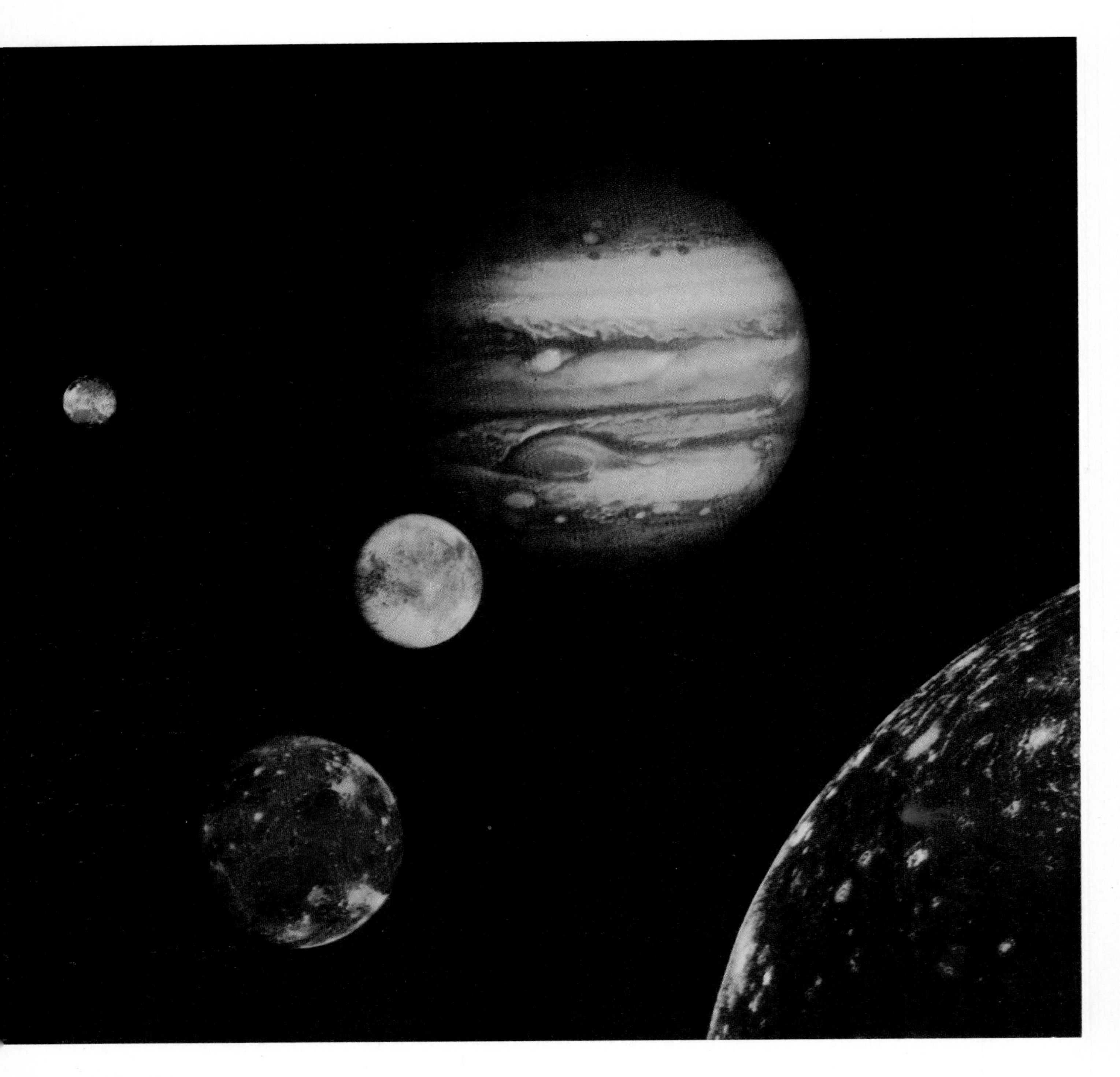

JUMPING JUPITER
The most massive planet of our solar system, Jupiter has thirteen moons. Four of them are featured in this composite photograph, created from pictures taken by the *Voyager* spacecraft. Jupiter itself is more than a thousand times larger than Earth. It orbits the sun every twelve years.

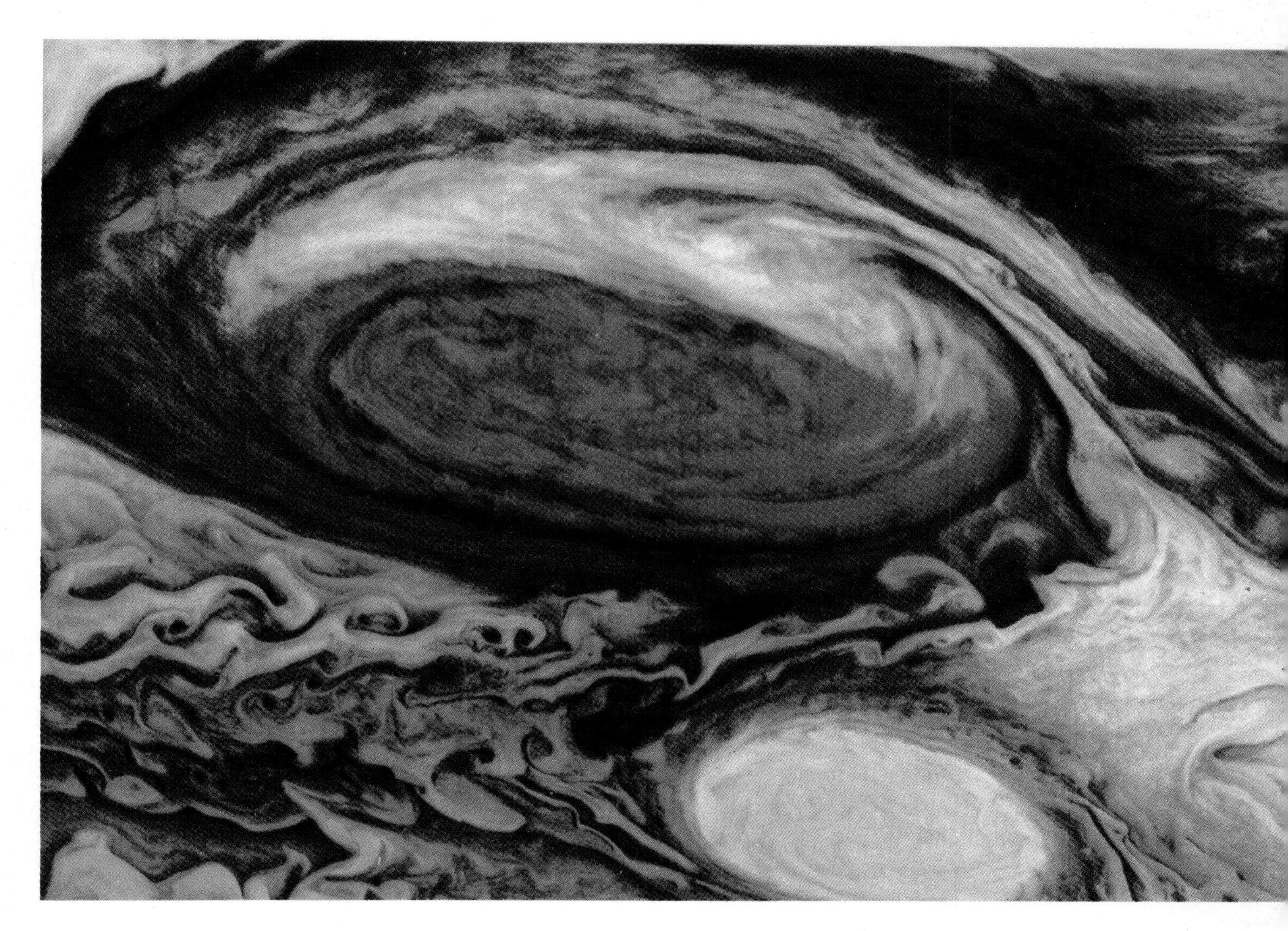

RED SPOT
This mysterious region on the face of Jupiter is 25,000 miles long. It rotates slowly around the planet, and is believed to be an immense and enduring Jovian storm.

HEAVENLY BODIES

Under ideal conditions, the naked eye can see but a few thousand stars. It is impossible to take an exact census, but astronomers estimate that there are at least a thousand billion billion stars twinkling in the sky.

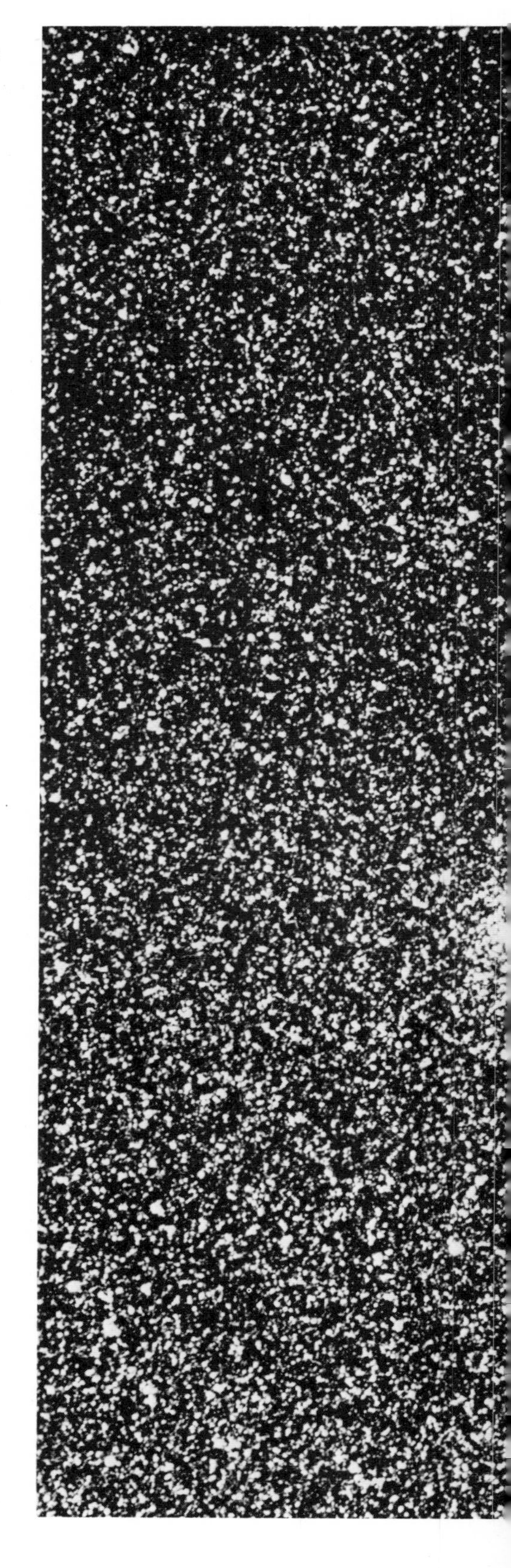

STARSCAPE
Countless stars often gather together into what astronomers call globular clusters. Exactly why such concentrations of stars are formed remains a beautiful mystery.

ETA CARINAE NEBULA (overleaf)
In the vast distances between stars lie enormous clouds of interstellar gas and dust. In these regions, when conditions are right, new stars are gradually formed.

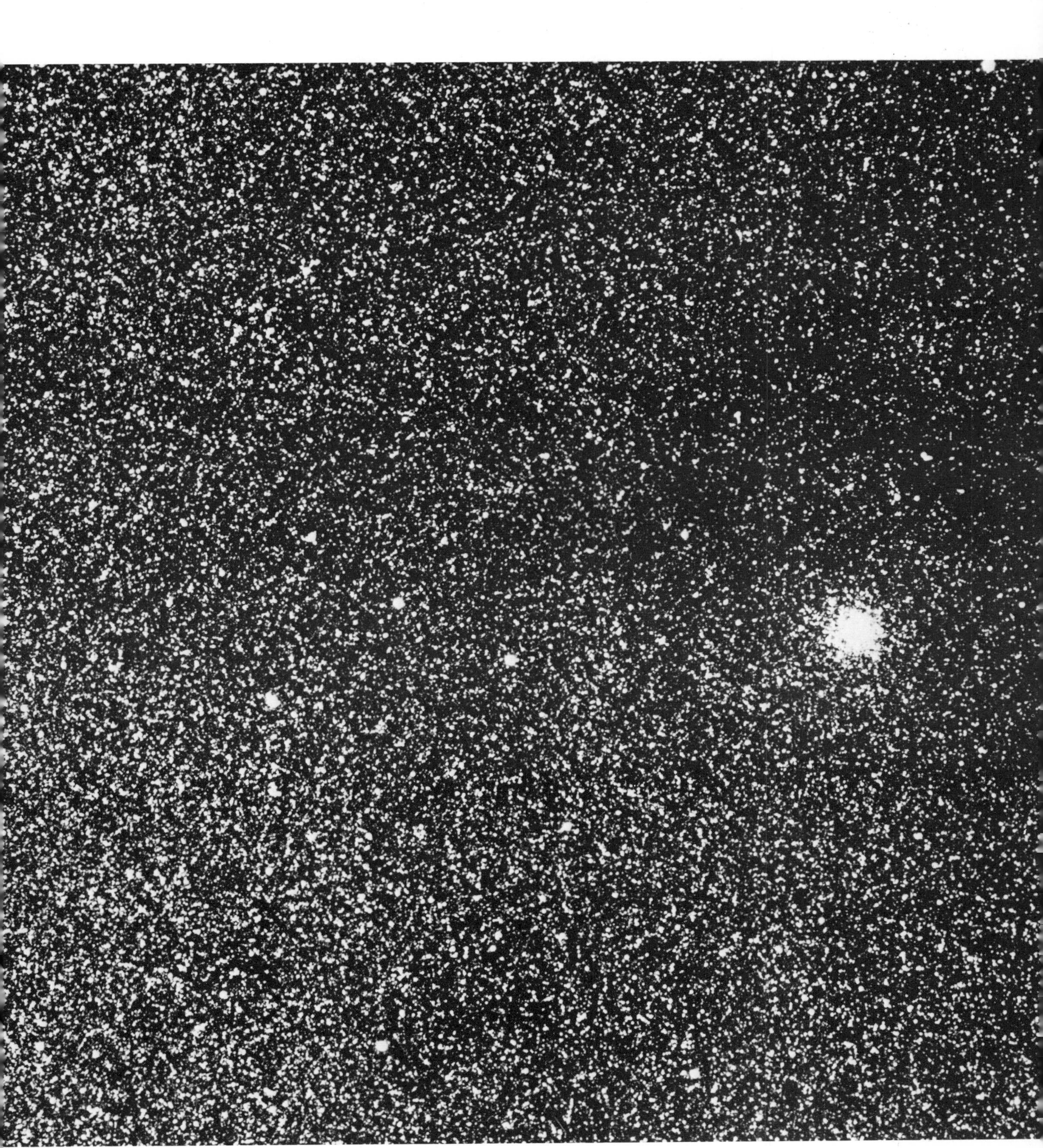

GALACTICA

We live on a small planet circling a medium-size star that revolves within a galaxy containing about a hundred billion stars. Our galaxy—the Milky Way—also slowly revolves. It is one of a hundred billion galaxies that make up the universe we know.

It was not until 1925 that galaxies became more than a theory. An American astronomer named Edwin Hubble pointed the world's largest telescope into the sky and photographed an "island universe" filled with countless stars. Before that, most astronomers thought that all of outer space was just a vague mass of stars.

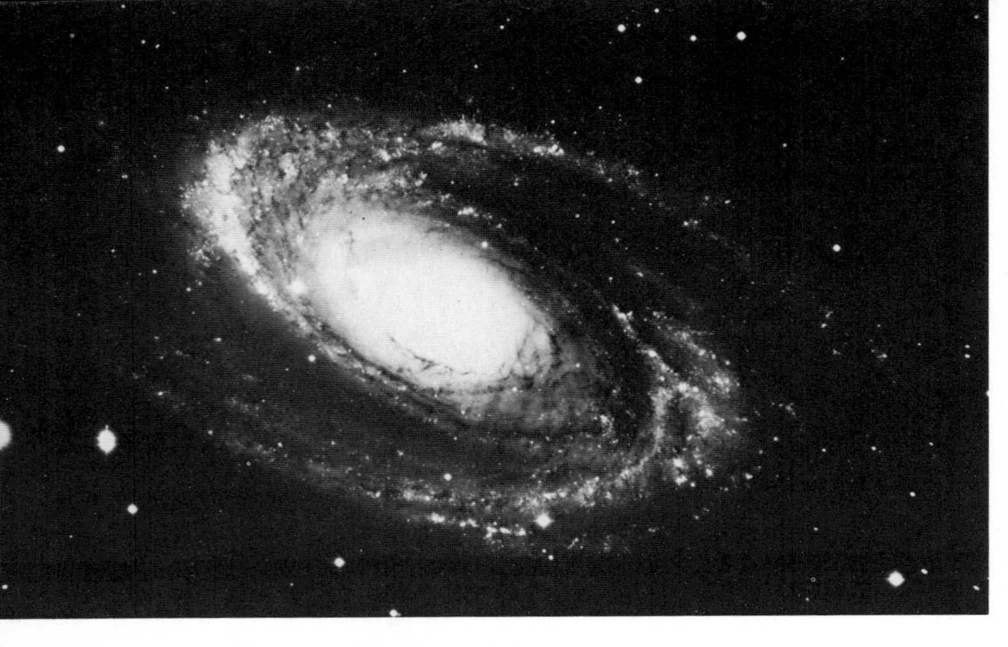

Spiral Galaxy in Ursa Major

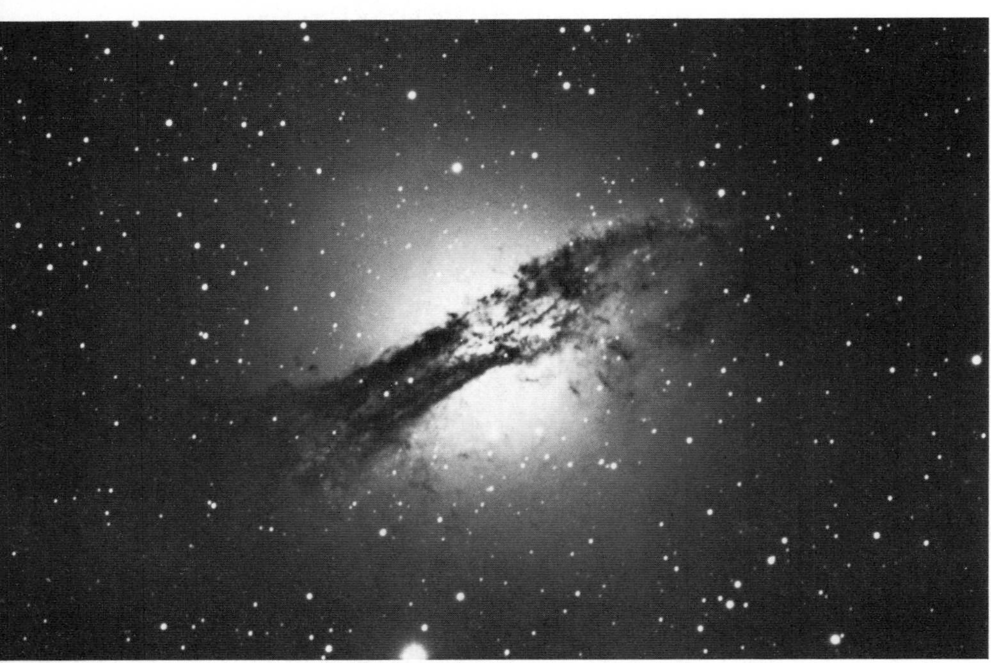

Peculiar Exploding Galaxy in Centaurus

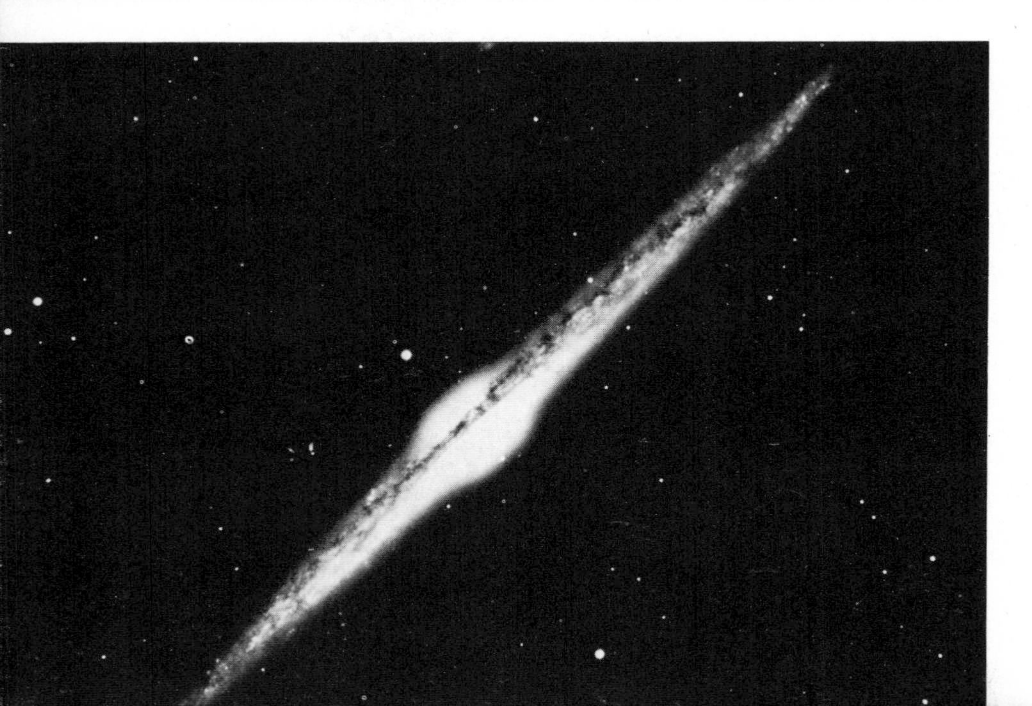

Spiral Galaxy in Coma Berenices

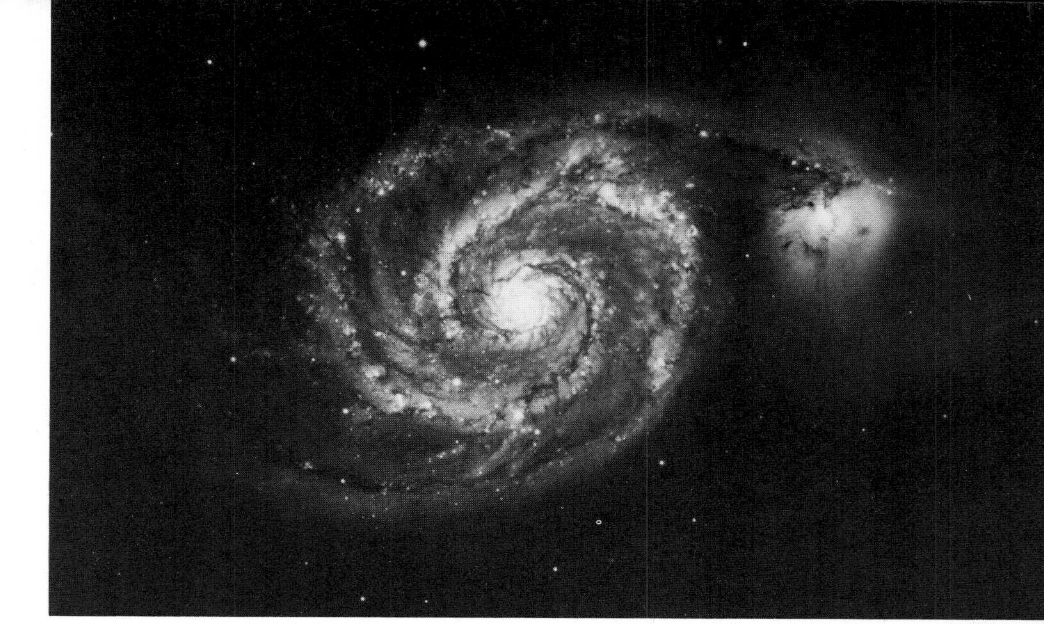

Whirlpool Galaxy in Canes Venatici

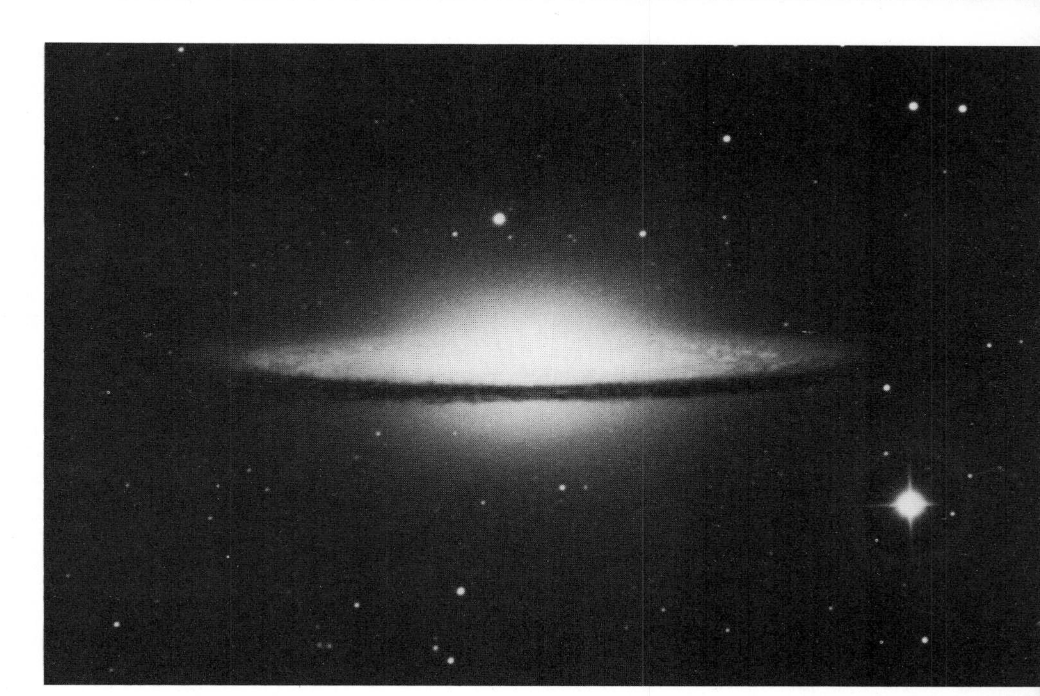

Spiral Galaxy in Virgo

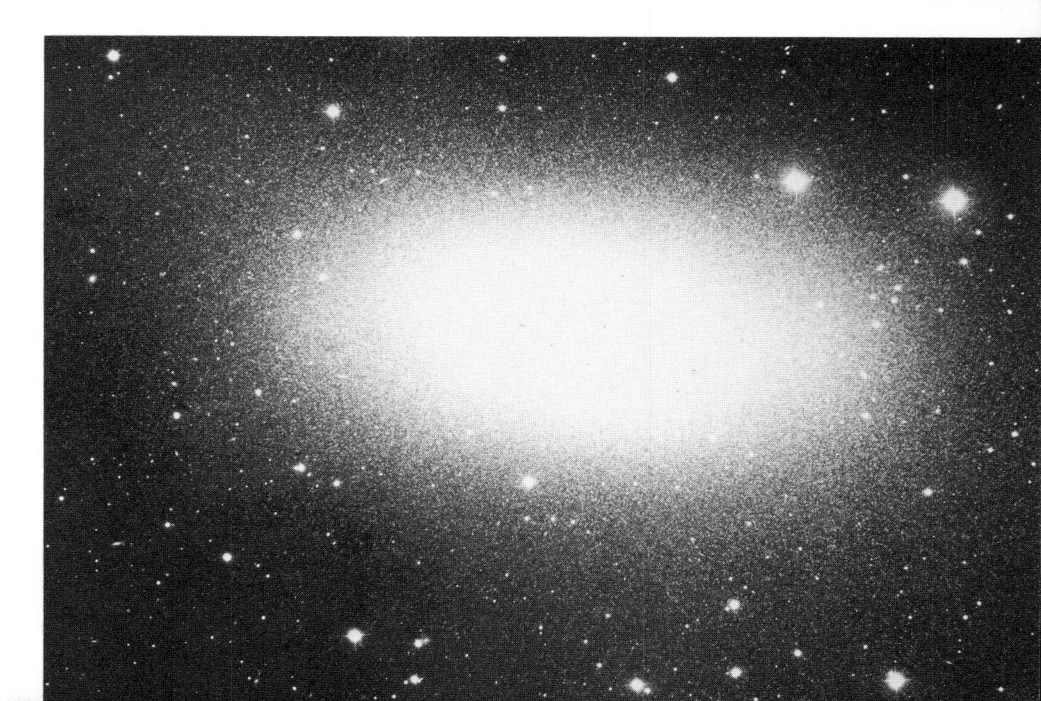

Elliptical Satellite Galaxy in Andromeda

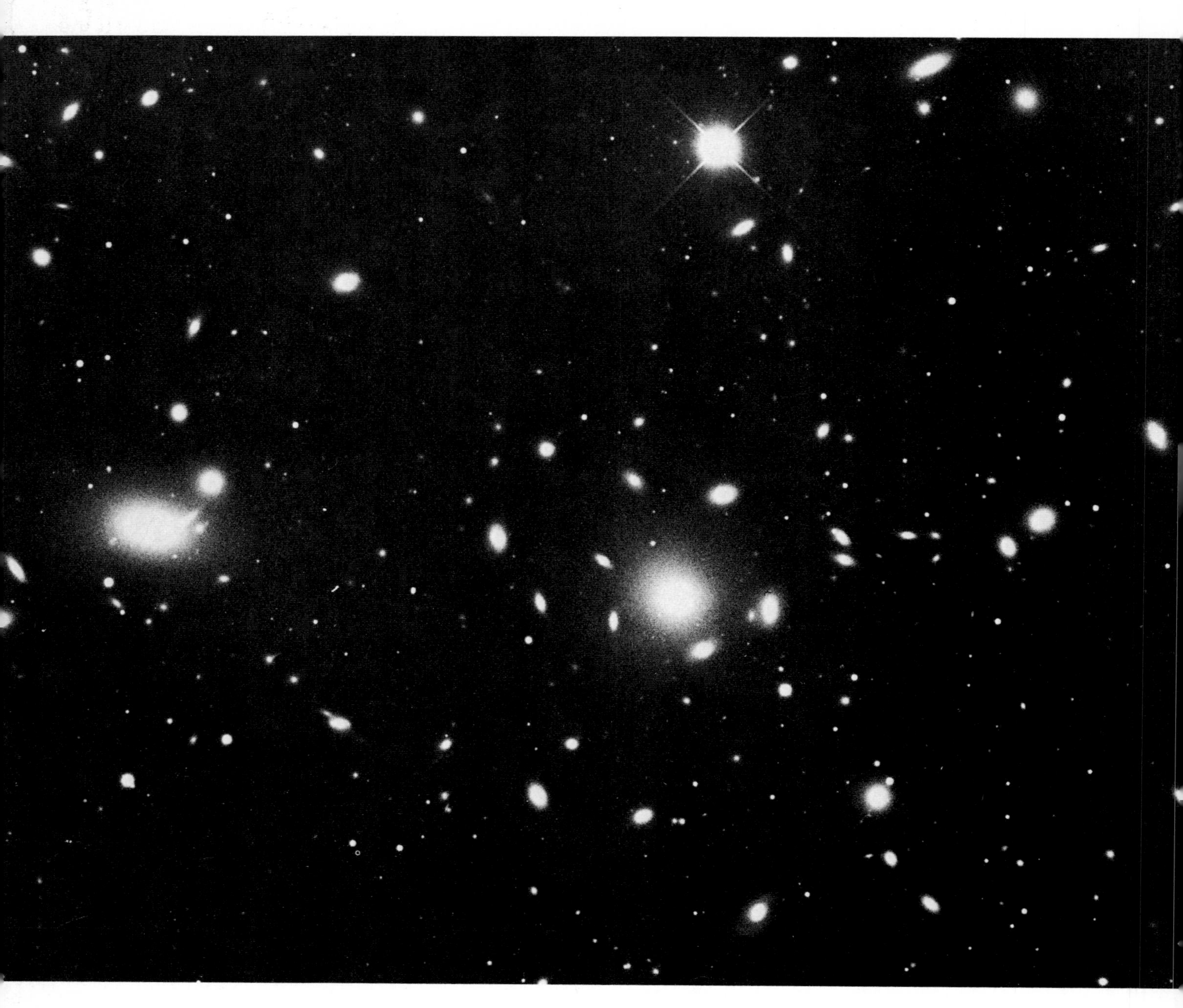

GALAXY CLUSTER

Galaxies, like stars, often group together into clusters. The dimensions of these cosmic groupings are awesome. A typical galaxy, for example, is about 600,000 trillion miles long.

ULTRAVISIONS

The powerful eyes of cameras are probing ever deeper into once-invisible worlds—revealing awesome images from the known limits of space and time.

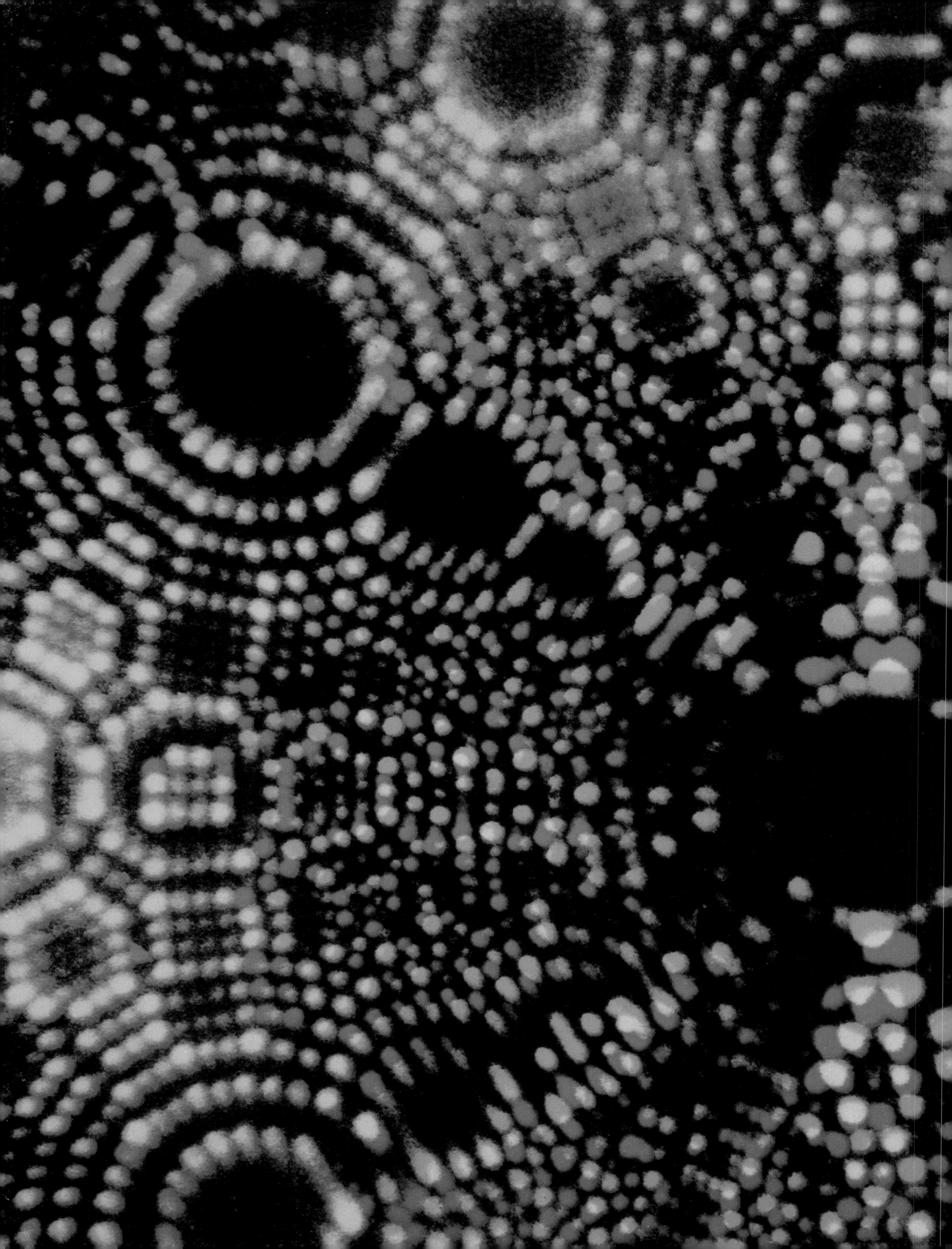

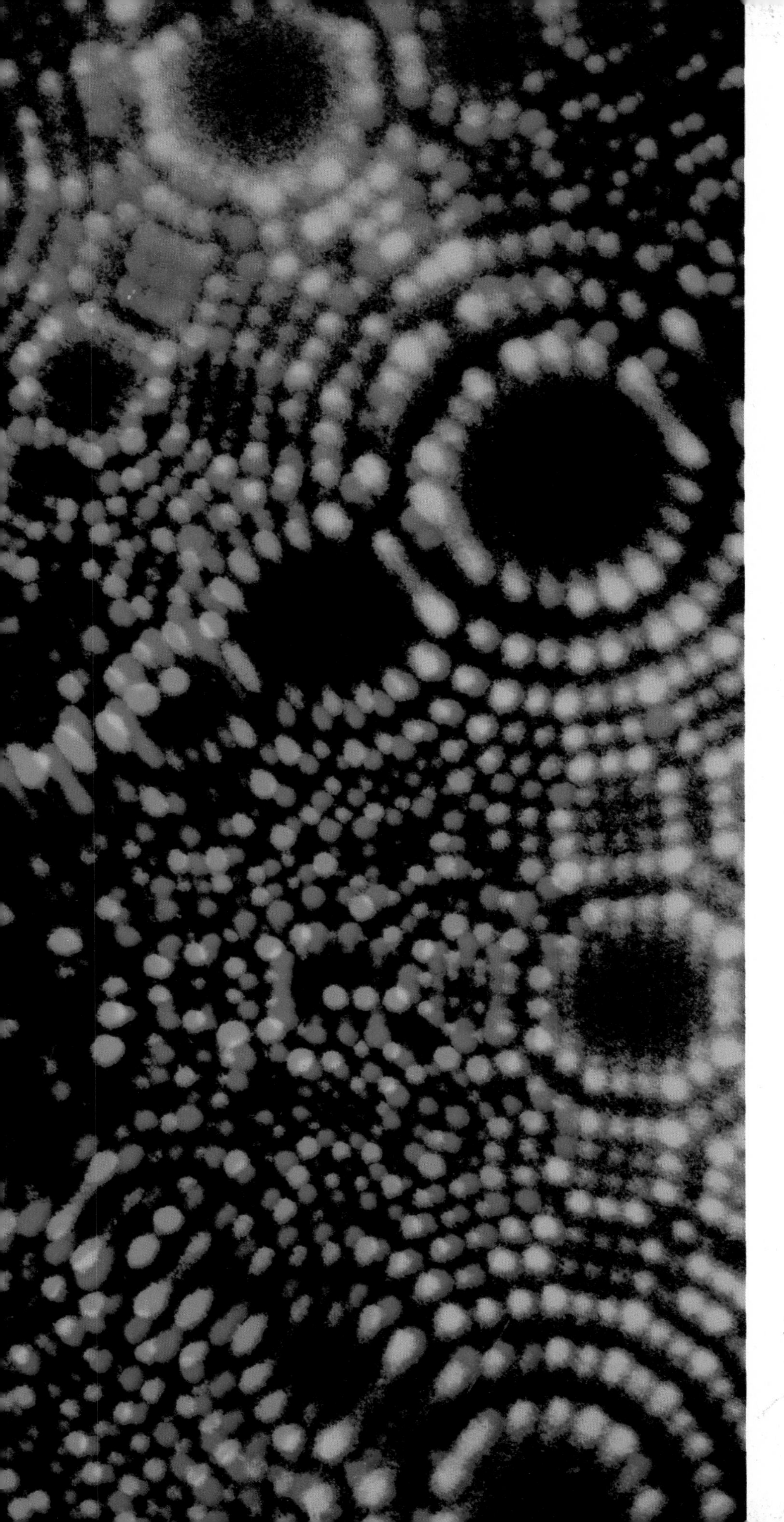

MOLECULE

When a piece of tungsten is magnified a half million times, we can see its molecular structure. This picture was made with an instrument called a field ion microscope.

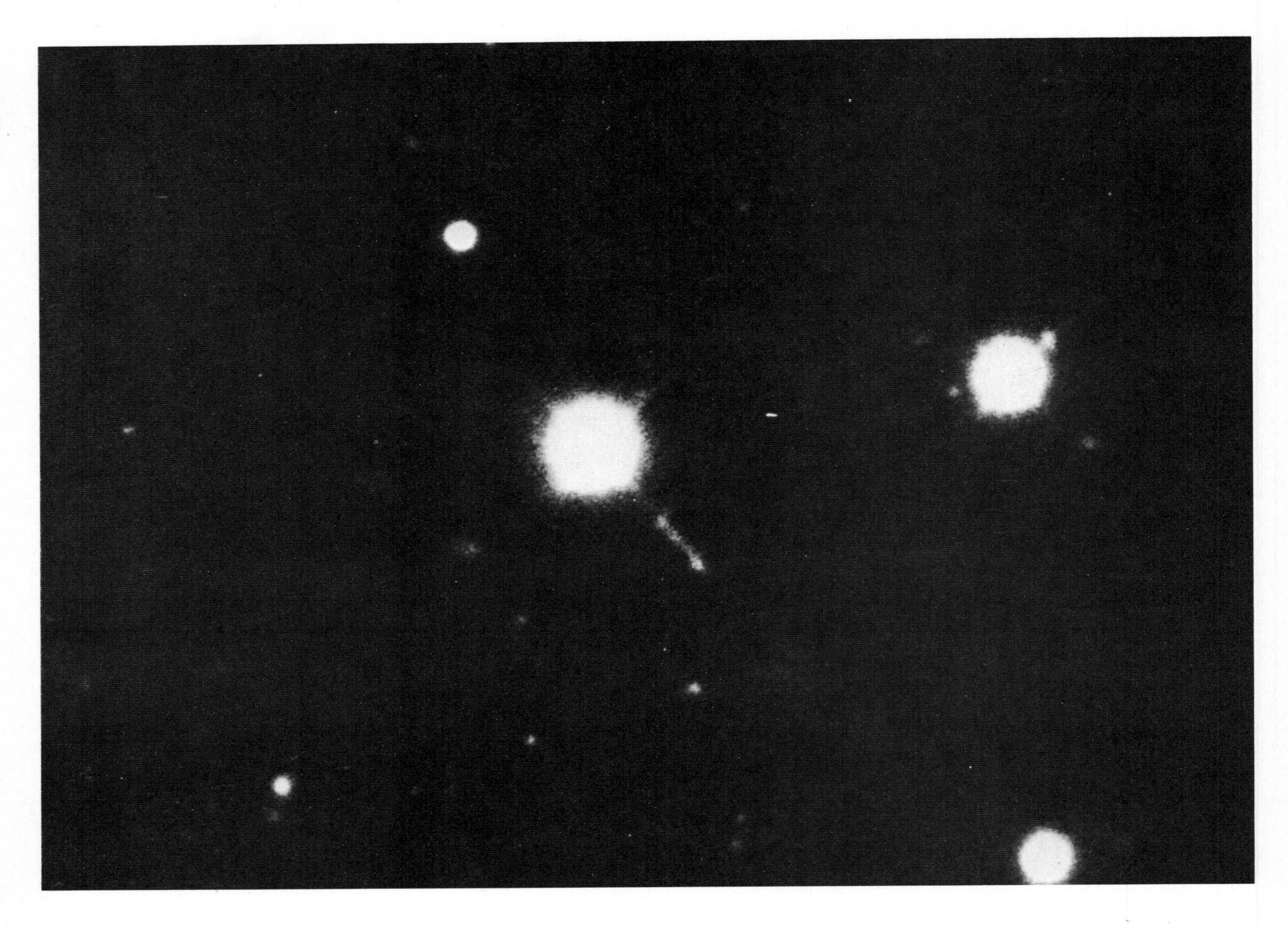

QUASAR

Quasar is short for quasi-stellar radio source. They are the brightest, most distant, and fastest moving objects ever seen.

Many lie at the edge of the known universe, and radiate as much energy as hundreds of galaxies. No one really knows what quasars are. This one is called Quasar 3C73.

SUBATOMIC PARTICLES

Only twenty-five years ago, atoms—made of protons, neutrons, and electrons—were regarded as the smallest basic objects. Today it seems that atoms are built of even tinier things.

This picture records the trails of minute subatomic particles released during the disintegration of an atom's nucleus.

It was taken in the hydrogen-filled bubble chamber of an atom smasher. Each type of particle has its own distinguishing signature of curving or spinning lines. By carefully studying these trails, scientists are learning more about the now-smallest and most elusive units of matter—the still unseen entities called quarks.

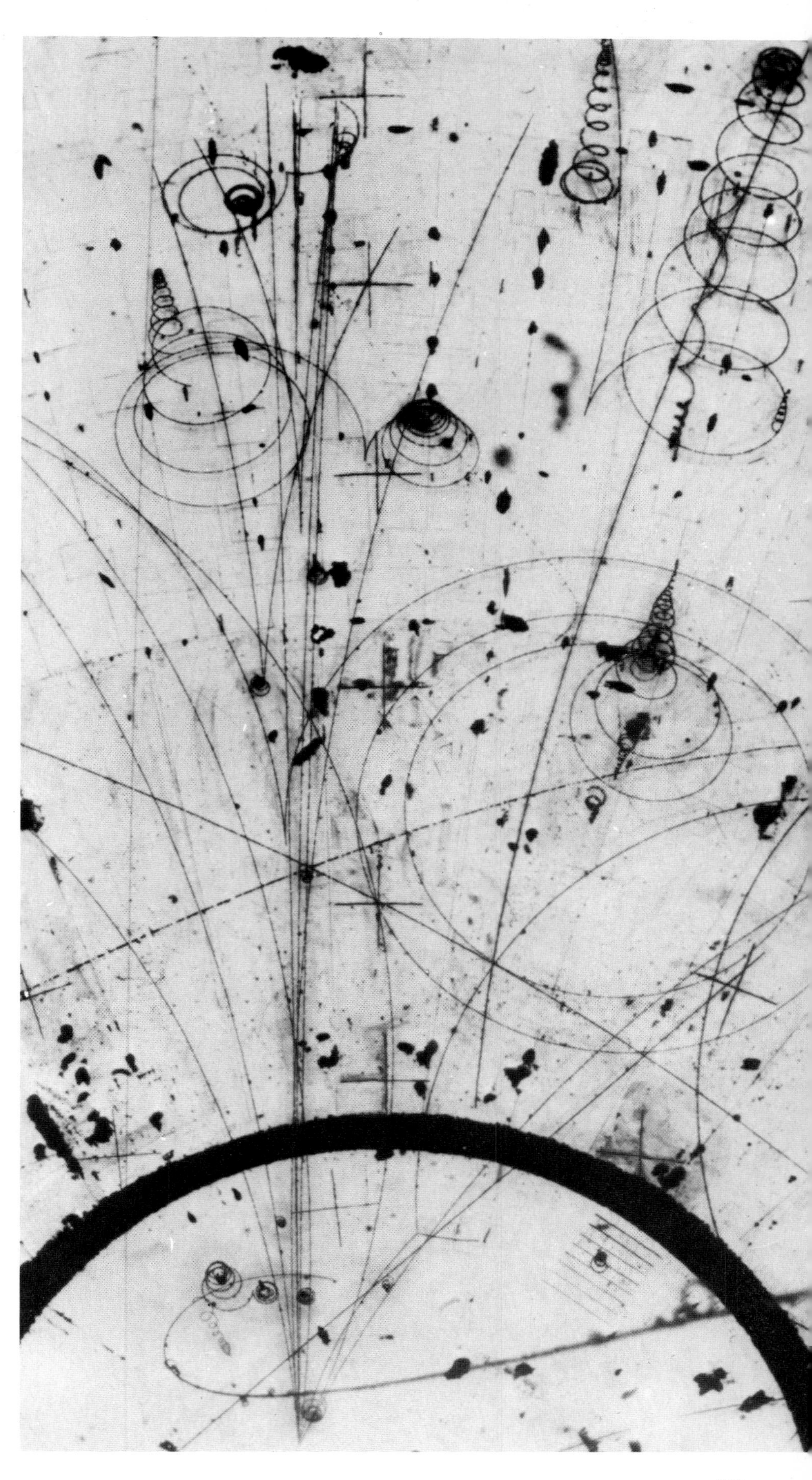

RED GIANT

This is the world's first image of the surface of a star other than the sun. Known as Betelgeuse, or Alpha Orionis, it lies 650 light years from earth and is 1200 times larger than our sun. The computer-colored contrasts on its surface are believed to be huge regions of hot and cold. Resolving this image through a telescope was like photographing a grain of sand from several miles away.

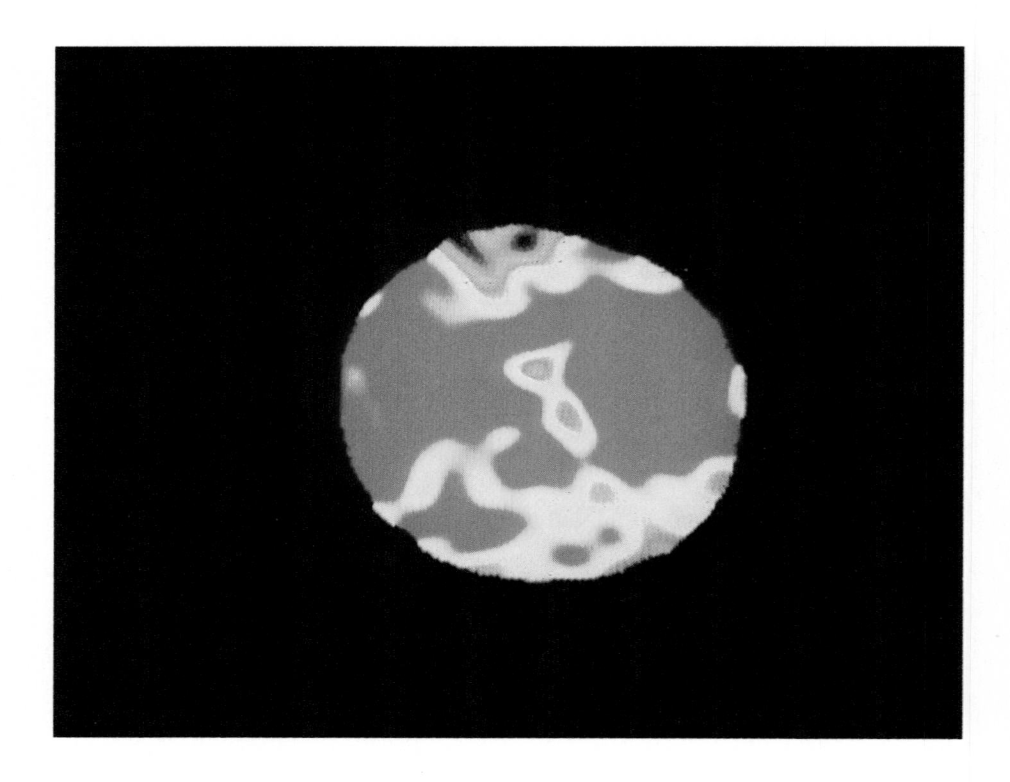

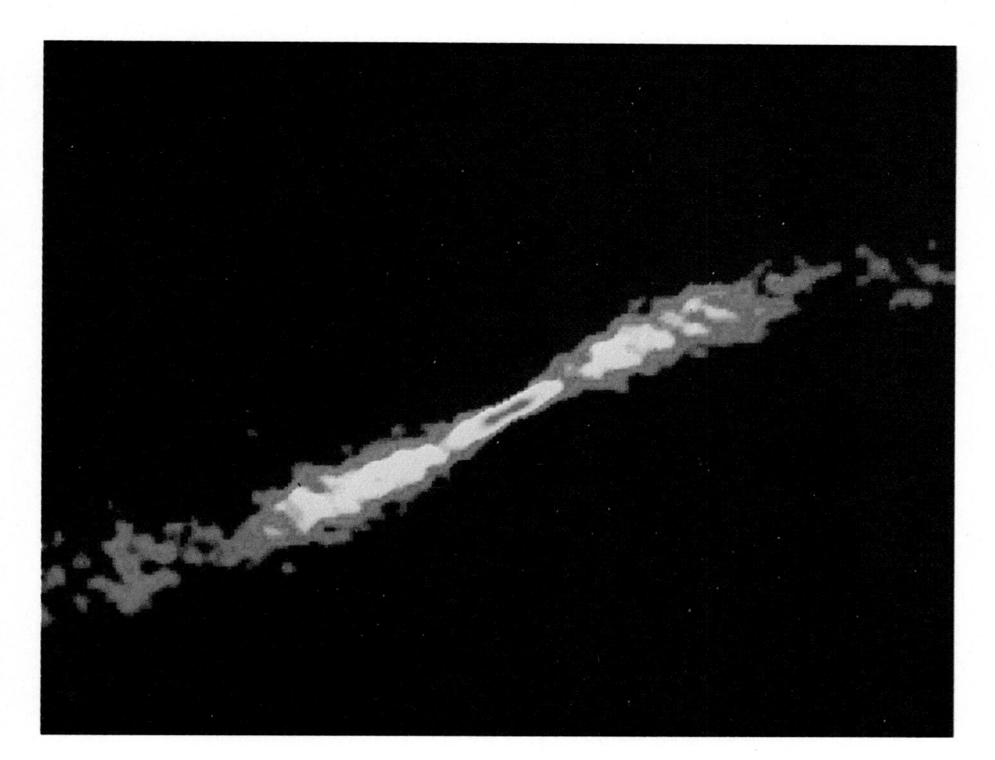

RADIO GALAXY

We can now listen to the universe, and make pictures of what we hear.

It is done with radio telescopes—huge dishes sensitive to the radio waves that constantly echo from outer space. The picture is of a galaxy called NGC326. Enormous streams of radio energy shoot out of the galaxy's red center. This phenomenon, and much of the galaxy, is invisible to telescopes sensitive to light.

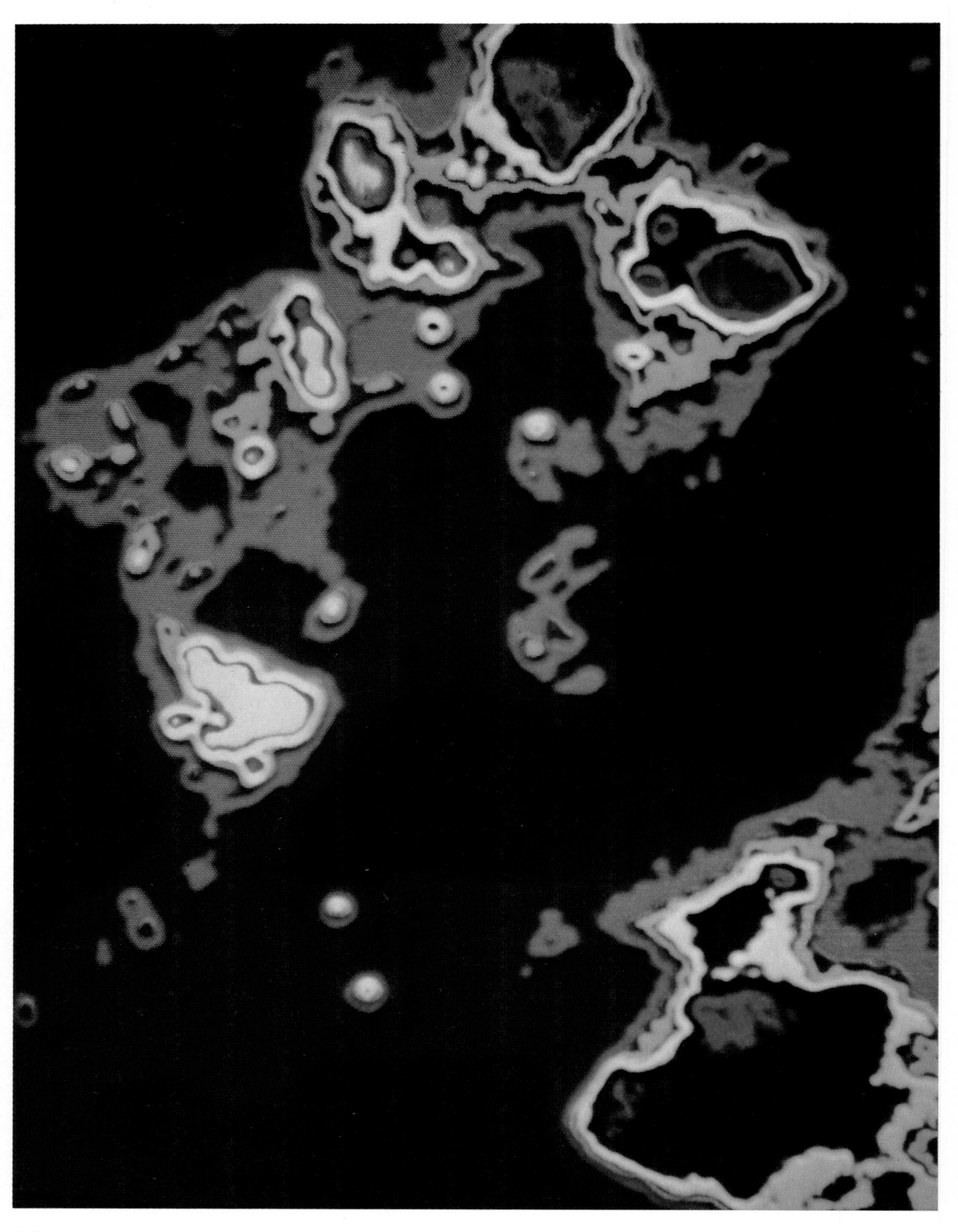

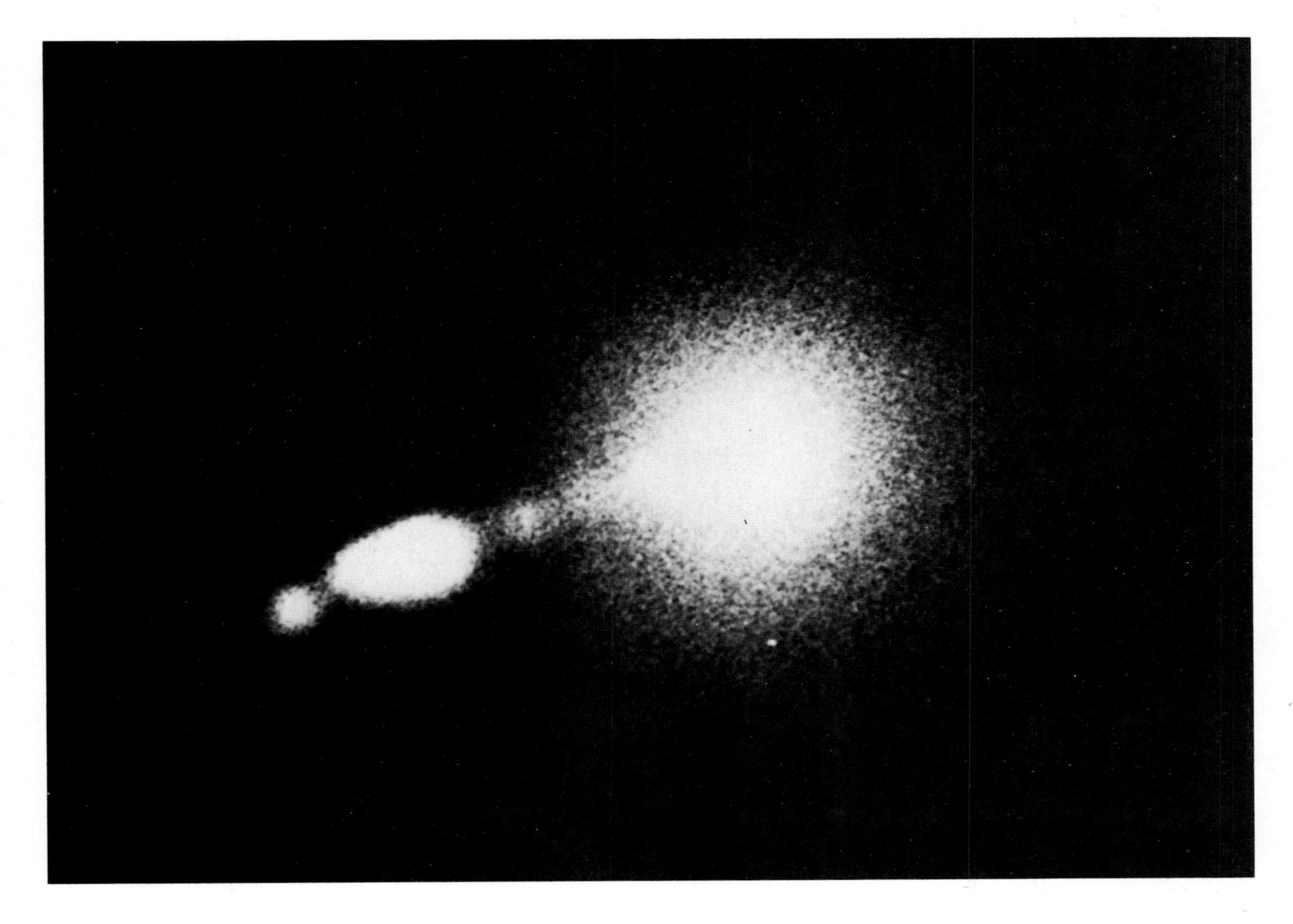

BLACK HOLE

This galaxy, known as M87, lies about sixty million light years from Earth. Some scientists suspect that it contains a black hole. It is the only way to account for the strange rotation of many of the galaxy's stars, as well as the huge stream of matter that pours from its center.

Black holes are theorized to be huge stars that have collapsed into nothingness. Their gravitation is so powerful that light cannot escape, and time ceases to exist. Black holes are completely invisible. Anything that is pulled inside can never emerge again. They are bizarre cosmic mysteries that may remain invisible forever.

◁ **ATOMS**

You are looking at atoms—atoms of gold. They are the smallest things ever photographed. The tiny specks are single atoms, each with a diameter of only a few billionths of an inch. The larger masses are clusters of several atoms.

This photograph was made with a special electron microscope. The atoms were magnified about ten million times —equivalent to enlarging a basketball to the size of Earth.

INVISIBLE WORLDS
In coming years our powers of vision will be stretched to newer boundaries. For today, we have only begun to see into the invisible world.

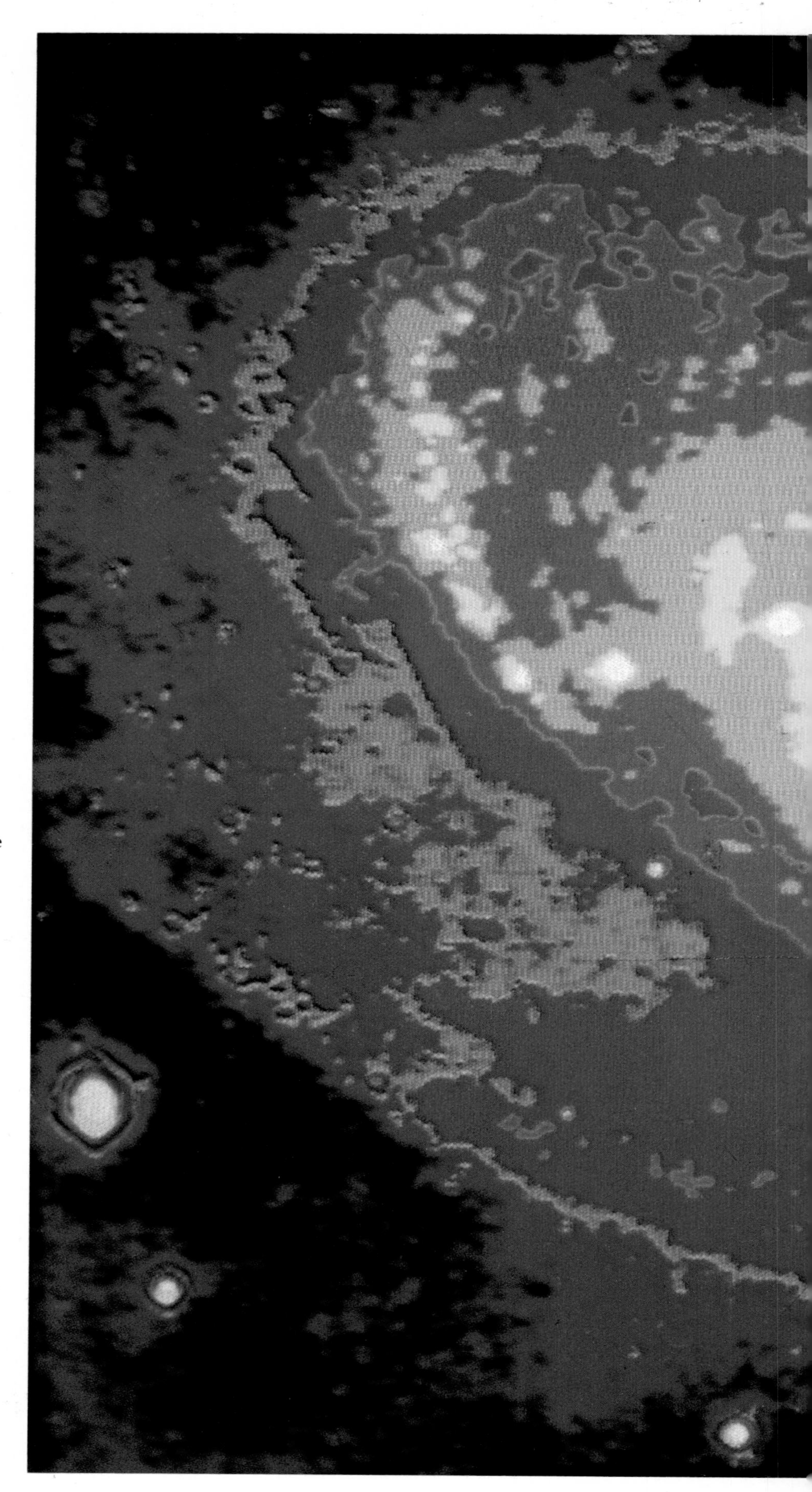

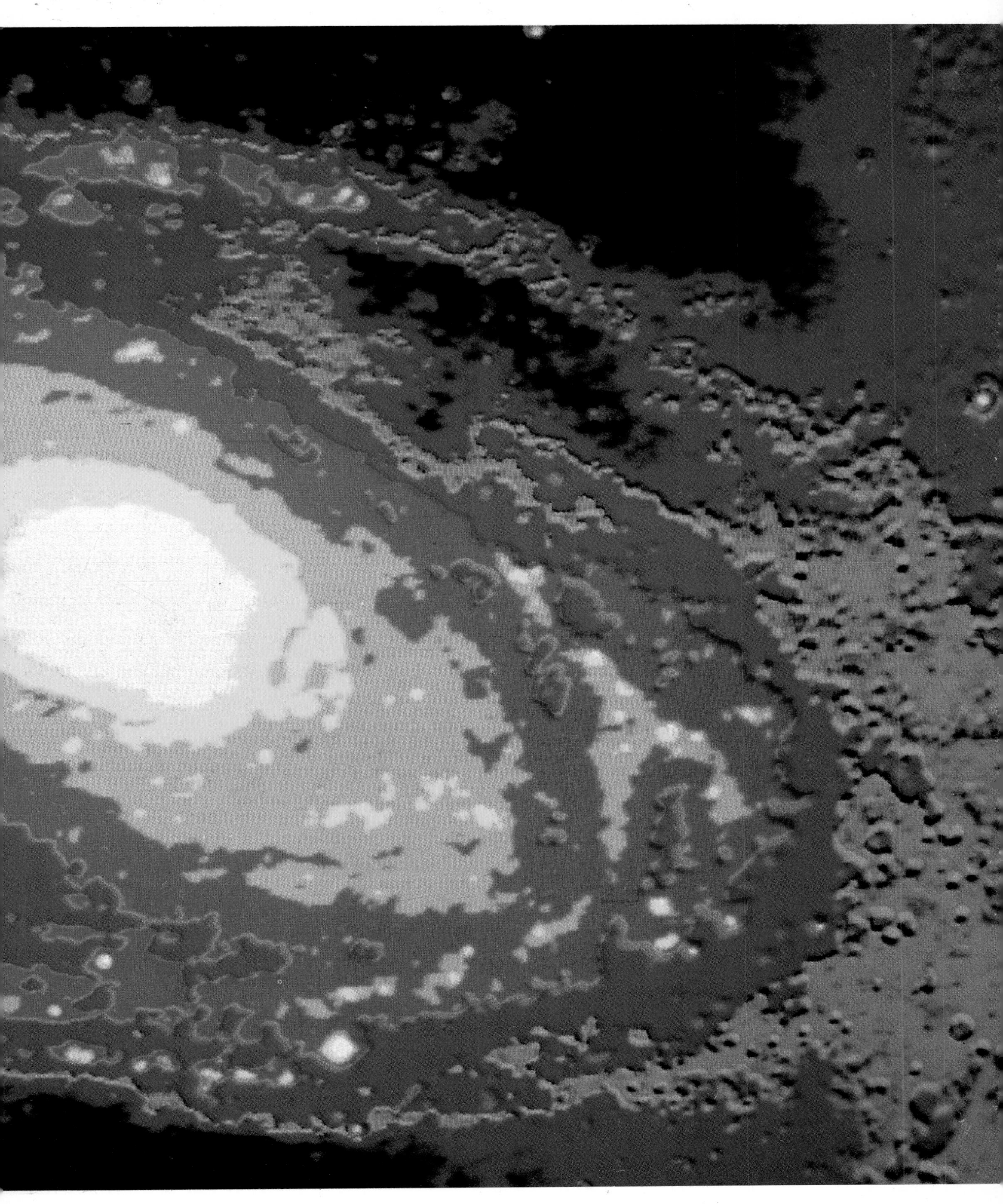

PICTURE CREDITS

The following photographs were supplied courtesy of Small World Competition, Nikon, Inc., Instrument Division, Garden City, New York: p. 30 (bottom), Art Hansen; p. 15, Joseph Goren; pp. 30 (top), 31 (top), 55 (top), David Gnizak; p. 18 (bottom), James M. Bell; p. 19 (top), John C. Walsh; p. 26, Dorothy Rutherford; p. 29, Robert C. Beebe; p. 33, George Brangan; p. 27, Stephen Skirius; p. 35, David Donofrio; p. 44 (top), Ralph L. Shook; p. 50, Andre Gorzynski; p. 59 (bottom), H. S. Baird; pp. 62–63, William A. Sokol; p. 66, DoSuk Duke Lee; p. 67, John V. Atkinson.

Other photographs are credited as follows: p. 2 (frontispiece), Photomicrograph by John Gustav Delly, Courtesy of Eastman Kodak Company; pp. 10, 12, 105 (bottom), 110, 111, 122, Howard Sochurek; p. 14, Dr. Donald Fawcett; pp. 18 (top), 19 (bottom), 99, Oxford Scientific Films; pp. 20 (top and bottom), 22 (top), Dr. Robert F. Smith, Cornell University; pp. 21, 23, 24 (bottom), 36, 37, 38, 39, 41, 43, 56 (top), Dr. David M. Phillips, Center for Biomedical Research, Rockefeller University; pp. 22 (bottom), 28, 31 (bottom), 34, 40, 44 (bottom), 45, 51 (top), 52, Jan Hinsch, Laboratory for Applied Microscopy, E. Leitz, Inc., Rockleigh, New Jersey; pp. 24 (top), 80, Dr. Garry T. Cole, Department of Botany, University of Texas, Austin; p. 25 (top), Dr. Lee D. Simon, Waksman Institute of Microbiology; p. 25 (bottom), Dr. Robley C. Williams, Virus Laboratory, University of California, Berkeley; pp. 32, 53 (bottom), 81 (top), Dr. A. J. Gwinnett, Department of Oral Biology, State University of New York at Stony Brook.

Pages 42, 54 (top right), 55 (bottom right), 69, 82, Dr. Jean-Paul Revel, California Institute of Technology; pp. 46–49, 51 (second from bottom), 60, 61, 53 (top), 58, 65, David Scharf; pp. 51 (second from top), 54 (top left, bottom left and right), 110–117, Courtesy of Eastman Kodak Company; pp. 51 (bottom), 55 (bottom left), 56 (bottom), 57, Dr. Roderick MacLeod, Center for Electron Microscopy, University of Illinois; p. 59 (top), Dr. William Jordan; p. 64 (top), Parker Pen Company; p. 68, Dr. Wolf H. Fahrenback, National Institute of Health; p. 64 (bottom), Dr. Guenther Albrecht-Beuhle, Cold Spring Harbor Laboratory.

Pages 70, 71, 74, 75, 76, 77, 79, Dr. D. A. Griffiths and V. Cowper, Pest Infestation Control Laboratory, M.A.F.F., Crown Copyright; pp. 72, 73, 81 (bottom), 104, Arcarology Laboratory, Ohio State University; p. 78, Dr. J. D. H. Andrews, Victoria University of Wellington, Dr. William Nutting, University of Massachusetts, and Louis Raboni; pp. 84–85, 86–87, George Eastman House; pp. 88, 89, 90, 91, 92 (top left), 93 (top right), 94 (bottom), 96, Dr. Harold E. Edgerton, Massachusetts Institute of Technology; p. 94 (top), Charles Miller, Massachusetts Institute of Technology; p. 93 (bottom), Michael Hadland, John Hadland, Ltd.; p. 95, David Gorham and Dr. Ian Hutchings, Cavendish Laboratory, University of Cambridge; pp. 98 (top), 154, AURA, Inc., Kitt Peak National Observatory; p. 98 (bottom), Carl Zeiss, Inc.; pp. 100–101, Dr. J. Kim Vandiver, Massachusetts Institute of Technology.

Page 102, Dr. Gary S. Settles; p. 103, Battelle Memorial Institute; p. 104, Dan McCoy, Rainbow; p. 105 (top), AGA Corporation; pp. 106–107, VANSCAN™ Thermogram, courtesy of Daedalus Enterprises, Inc.; pp. 108, Theodore Thomas and AGA Corporation; p. 109, Hawker-Siddeley Dynamics, Ltd.; p. 118, Joseph D. McKenzie, New England Baptist Hospital, Boston, Mass., and Robert E. Wise, M.D., Lahey Clinic Foundation, Burlington, Mass.; pp. 119, 158–159, Alex Pomasanoff; p. 120, Kodak Pathe/The Louvre; p. 121 (left and bottom), Field Museum of Natural History, Chicago; p. 121 (top right), Dr. Luis Alvarez, University of California, Berkeley; p. 124, Holosonics, Inc.; p. 123, Stanford Research Institute; p. 125, Dr. E. Lazarides, California Institute of Technology; p. 127, Kendall Johnson; p. 126, Dr. Thelma Moss; p. 130, I. F. Dumitrescu; p. 129, Dr. Alfred Hulstrunk; p. 128, G. Marshall, H. S. Dakin Laboratory, San Francisco.

Pages 132–133, 136, 137 (top and bottom), 138–139, 140, 141, NASA; pp. 134, 135, Earth Satellite Corporation; p. 137 (middle), Kitt Peak National Observatory; pp. 142–143, 148, 152, Kitt Peak National Observatory and Cerro Tololo Observatory; p. 144–145, Cerro Tololo Observatory; pp. 146, 147, Palomar Observatory, California Institute of Technology; p. 153, Fermi Lab Photo; p. 155, Dr. Edward Fomalont, National Radio Observatory; p. 156, courtesy of A. V. Crewe, The Enrico Fermi Institute, University of Chicago; p. 157, Dr. Halton Arp, Palomar Observatory, California Institute of Technology.